Live Well, Live Long

KEEP UP TO DATE

Visit the Live Well, Live Long website

www.livewelllivelong.com

The Live Well, Live Long website provides:

- new medical information to help up-date the information provided in this book.
- new information resources, including websites and publications.
- information about how this book can be purchased.

The Live Long, Live Well Preventative Health Clinic

The preventative health practice of Dr Paul Goyen in Sydney. Visit the above website for contact details and further information.

Live Well, Live Long

A lifetime of healthy living

DR PAUL GOYEN

ALLEN&UNWIN

For my family, Robyn, Leigh and Anna
and
for all those who have suffered from the premature loss of loved ones.

First published in 2003

Allen & Unwin
83 Alexander Street
Crows Nest NSW 2065
Australia
Phone: (61 2) 8425 0100
Fax: (61 2) 9906 2218
Email: info@allenandunwin.com
Web: www.allenandunwin.com

National Library of Australia
Cataloguing-in-Publication entry:

Goyen, Paul, 1955- .
Live well, live long : a lifetime of healthy living.

Bibliography.
Includes index.
ISBN 1 86508 927 3.

1. Medicine, Preventive - Popular works. 2. Self-care, Health. I. Title.

613

Set in 11/13 pt AGaramond by Bookhouse, Sydney
Printed by Shannon Books, Melbourne

10 9 8 7 6 5 4 3 2 1

Contents

PART 4 Obesity and physical inactivity

PART 5 Preventing heart attacks and strokes

PART 6 CANCER PREVENTION

Appendices

Foreword

In *Live Well, Live Long* Dr Paul Goyen achieves his laudable aim of providing knowledge to enable the general reader to attain a longer and happier life protected from physical and mental disability.

After acknowledging the difficulty of changing entrenched harmful behaviour patterns such as sedentary lifestyle and unbalanced diet, Dr Goyen provides a practical roadmap to initiate positive behaviour and preventative approaches. Clear summaries and practical approaches abound, with key points highlighted and web references listed.

A comprehensive range of topics, relevant for each age group, is covered, including cancer and heart disease prevention, depression, hearing loss and osteoporosis. There is a useful focus on Australian resources and context.

While this book could happily be a well-thumbed reference, its easy style enables it to be a pleasurable cover to cover read for the general reader, providing help and insights from childhood to old age. Doctors and other health professionals will also find the book useful in discussions with patients, even when future advances modify some of the specific recommendations.

The value of a responsive, engaged GP is emphasised. Indeed, most people would be fortunate to have someone like Dr Goyen as their GP. Dr Goyen also stresses the importance of the informed individual as partner.

Dr Goyen notes that one of life's mysteries is that routine car maintenance is considered essential but routine body maintenance is not. *Live Well, Live Long* does an excellent job in redressing this paradox.

Geoffrey Tofler, Professor of Preventative Cardiology, Sydney University
Senior Staff Specialist, Royal North Shore Hospital

Acknowledgements

A preventative book of this kind covers by necessity many varied health topics. It is not possible for a general practitioner to be an expert in all fields. For this reason, numerous specialist practitioners were approached to comment on the information contained in this book. I would like to sincerely thank the following practitioners who have provided information and support that has been invaluable to me in this project: Dr Robert Coles, Professor Ron Rapee, Dr Greg Crossland, Dr Susan Cornish, Dr Philomena Renner.

I would especially like to thank Dr Rosemary Stanton for her evaluation of an early version of this book and for her help and encouragement in getting the book published; Professor David Sullivan for giving freely of his time to help with my numerous enquiries; and my friends, both in the medical profession and outside, for their guidance regarding the content of this book as it slowly evolved over several years.

Numerous medical organisations and government bodies have permitted the use of material from their publications. For this I am also sincerely grateful. I would especially like to thank the Australian Institute of Health and Welfare, which provided most of the statistical information used, and the Royal Australian College of General Practitioners for its general assistance and its permission to use College material.

The lengthy process of transforming my initial rudimentary efforts into the well-crafted publication you now hold was a formidable task. Rebecca Kaiser and all those associated with the book at Allen & Unwin deserve special praise for their patience and hard work while helping me along this long and at times very winding road.

My final thanks go to all those practitioners who give unselfishly of their time to publish articles that help keep Australia's general practitioners up to date on best current medical practice.

Introduction

Most of the major illnesses facing people in Western societies can be prevented, postponed or significantly reduced through good preventative health strategies. The aim of this book is to provide the knowledge necessary to prevent illness so you can live a longer life that is happy and less subject to suffering from physical and mental disability.

This knowledge is presented in two forms. Firstly, the book identifies and describes the preventable illnesses most likely to affect you. It outlines their deleterious effects and discusses the behaviours you need to adopt to minimise your risk of being affected. Secondly, and perhaps most importantly, the book describes how to go about accomplishing the changes you need to make to live this healthier life. Premanently modifying entrenched behaviours, such as dietary habits, is a very difficult task that should not be underestimated. A considerable part of this book examines the general principles involved in accomplishing such changes and should be read thoroughly before you attempt to change your lifestyle.

As well as advice regarding lifestyle changes, the first section of this book identifies the preventable illnesses that affect each age group, from the very young to the very old. It then sets out a timetable for your 'prevention program'. The subsequent sections look at different illness groups with regard to their prevention and there is also a large section on numerous health topics related to nutrition. To be comprehensive, it has been necessary to cover many different illnesses and the length of this book reflects this fact. Thankfully, it is unlikely that you will be affected by them all and, for most people, a few long-term changes will make a huge difference to your health!

While mental illness is not the major cause of death and disability in Western societies, it is mentioned first because it has a history of being neglected by governments, the medical profession and the general population, and because it causes massive amounts of disability in relatively young people. This section also includes segments on relationship problems and alcohol abuse, two of the major causes of unhappiness in Western society. It is a section that everyone should read.

The information contained in this book will help you devise your personal preventative health program with your general practitioner. Your GP can provide any additional information you require and give the continuing guidance and support that is necessary if you are to successfully improve your health. Additional information can also be gained from the numerous websites and publications mentioned throughout this book. This information has been produced by experts in their fields and contains a wealth of helpful information. All this information will hopefully ensure that you live well and live long.

In order to make this book both friendly and informative, I have purposely written in the manner of a friendly GP giving information and advice to a patient. Throughout the book, you are directly advised to adopt certain practices to improve your health. The advice offered is the sort of advice you would receive from a mainstream medical practice, although it needs to be stressed that medicine is not an exact science and some health professionals will have views that differ from those given. Also, we do not live in a perfect world, so differing life circumstances mean it is unlikely that you will be in a position to adopt all the recommendations made in this book, even if you wanted to. They are offered as a 'best health' guide; the final choice is up to you.

This book deals with how you can improve your own health. The other cornerstone of preventative medicine is public health. This includes areas such as the provision of medical facilities, ensuring our food and water are safe to consume, sewage and waste disposal, and initiating and managing healthcare programs that target major health problems or groups at risk of illness. While public health is very important, it is mainly the concern of government and health authorities and is thus mentioned only occasionally.

Good health!

Disclaimer

The information and recommendations contained in this book are, by necessity, general in nature. They are designed to act as a guide only and should not be used as your sole source of information or advice regarding your preventative health. You will have your own health problems that will affect the preventative health options you adopt. Also, advances in medical knowledge will mean that some informaton in this book will need updating. For these reasons, it is essential that you seek regular advice from your general practitioner when developing, implementing or modifying your personal preventative health program.

Conflict of interest statement

Other than for being an associate member of the Royal Australian College of General Practitioners, the author is not associated in any way with any of the organisations mentioned in this publication. No benefit of any kind has been received by the author, his medical practice or any related party for the information included and the comments made in the book. Some of the publications recommended in the 'further information' sections have been written by health professionals who have contributed to this book. Their inclusion was based solely on merit. No payment has been made by the author for any of the book's endorsements. The author does have a minor interest in the wine industry, being a part owner in a small vineyard producing grapes for table wines.

Dr Paul Goyen

Part 1

Preventing illness—the basics

Identifying preventable adult illnesses

The duration of your life and the degree of physical disability you may have to endure are very important factors in determining your achievements and your level of happiness. Fortunately Australians have access to a high standard of public health and one of the world's best health systems and it is thus not surprising that most of us enjoy a long and healthy life. We have one of the longest life expectancies in the Western world at 75.9 years for males and 81.5 years for females.

Having said this, many still die prematurely or suffer unnecessary disability due to diseases that can mostly be prevented by living a healthy lifestyle. In 2000, 27 per cent of males and 16 per cent of females died before the age of 65. The aim of this book is to provide the essential information you need to avoid these preventable diseases and to assist you in incorporating all this advice into your lifestyle.

While this book provides much information that can be used by the individual, it was written with the partnership between general practitioner (GP) and patient in mind, as many aspects of illness prevention require the assistance of a supportive GP. Together, you should be able to identify and co-ordinate the preventative measures you need to adopt to minimise your medical problems. Through regular visits to your GP, your management plan can be monitored and modified as necessary to address any changing circumstances. All this is very difficult to achieve on your own.

Burden of disease

Table 1 shows the 16 leading causes of death and disability (or burden of disease) in Australia, most of which are significantly preventable. The figures used in this book to grade the death and disability caused by each illness are derived from information gathered and interpreted by the Australian Institute of Health and Welfare (AIHW). When assessing the importance of an illness, the AIHW does not just look at its incidence. It also measures carefully the extent to which the illness causes premature death and the length and degree of disability the illness causes. Diseases that on average occur earlier in life, and thus cause earlier deaths or lengthier periods of disability, are given a higher rating. Both the disability and death caused by the particular illness are given a value in terms of years of healthy life lost and, when added together, give an overall 'burden of disease' rating for the illness (measured in disability adjusted life years or DALYs) (see appendix 1). This allows comparison of the harm caused by all illnesses, whether they cause predominantly death or disability.

Illness and lifestyle choices

Burden of disease values have also been calculated for lifestyle options and it is estimated that adopting poor lifestyle health options is responsible for 44 per cent of all male burden

Table 1 The leading causes of burden of disease in Australia (1996)

Cause	*Percentage of total burden of disease*
Coronary artery disease (heart attacks)	12.4
Stroke	5.4
Depression (including bipolar disorders)	4.4
Chronic obstructive lung disease	3.7
Lung cancer	3.6
Dementia	3.5
Anxiety disorders	3.0
Diabetes	3.0
Colorectal cancer	2.7
Asthma	2.6
Alcohol dependence/harmful use*	2.2
Suicide and self-inflicted injuries	2.2
Road traffic accidents	2.2
Breast cancer	2.2
Osteoarthritis	2.2
Adult-onset hearing loss	1.9

* The figure for alcohol combines the harmful effects (4.9%), which mainly occur in younger people, with the beneficial cardiovascular effects (2.7%) which occur mostly in older people.

Source: Adapted from Australian Institute of Health and Welfare: Mathers, 1999.

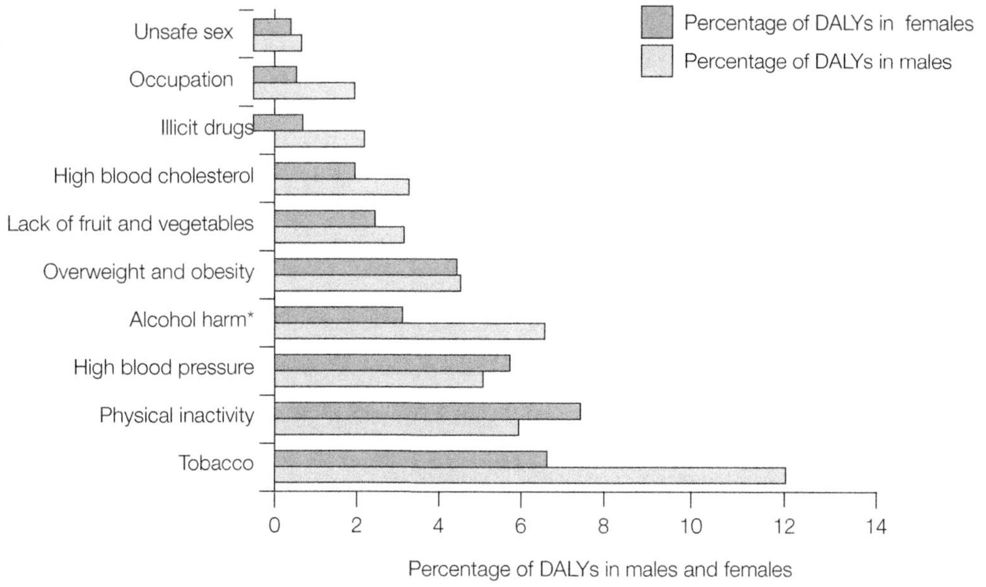

* Figures for alcohol harm do not include the potential health benefits from reduced cardiovascular disease that alcohol can give older people if taken in moderation (i.e. two drinks or less per day). This amounts to about 2.4 per cent in males and 3.2 per cent in females. It needs to be emphasised that the harmful effects of alcohol affect a predominantly young age group; mainly the 15 to 35 year olds (especially males).
Source: Adapted from Australian Institute of Health and Welfare: Mathers, 1999.

Figure 1 Proportion of total burden of disease (DALYs) attributable to lifestyle risk factors (1996)

of disease and 32 per cent of all female burden of disease. This is a huge amount. Figure 1 provides a breakdown of which poor lifestyle options are most responsible for disease burden in both males and females.

By avoiding these poor lifestyle options you can significantly reduce both premature death and the length of time that you are likely to suffer from disability. Most disability occurs in the final 12 years of life and it is estimated that living a healthy life can reduce this period by almost half. Sounds good!

Illness variation with age and sex

The illnesses causing the most burden of disease vary markedly between different age groups, a fact that is well demonstrated in Table 2. You should look carefully at these figures as they show the diseases that are going to cause you harm, and most of them are significantly preventable. These are issues of life and death that concern you now.

Table 2 Leading causes of burden of disease in Australians according to age (1996)

Males		Females	
Cause	*% of total disease burden in each age group*	*Cause*	*% of total disease burden in each age group*
15 to 35 year age group		**15 to 35 year age group**	
Road traffic accidents	10.8	Depression	19.1
Suicide and self-injury	10.8	Anxiety disorders	11.9
Depression	9.9	Alcohol	5.2
Alcohol	8.0	Asthma	5.0
Anxiety disorders	7.3	Eating disorders	4.8
Heroin/poly-drug use	6.1	Road traffic accidents	3.9
36 to 54 year age group		**36 to 54 year age group**	
Coronary artery disease	11.1	Breast cancer	9.4
Depression	6.2	Anxiety disorders	8.8
Suicide and self-injury	5.8	Depression	8.7
Alcohol	4.2	Osteoarthritis	5.0
Chronic obstructive lung disease	3.8	Diabetes	4.9
Anxiety	3.7	Chronic obstructive lung disease	3.1
55 to 74 year age group		**55 to 74 year age group**	
Coronary artery disease	19.2	Coronary artery disease	12.8
Lung cancer	8.4	Breast cancer	6.9
Stroke	6.1	Stroke	6.1
Chronic obstructive lung disease	5.8	Osteoarthritis	5.5
Colorectal cancer	4.7	Lung cancer	5.2
Adult-onset hearing loss	4.4	Alzheimer's disease, dementias	5.1
75 years and over age group		**75 years and over age group**	
Coronary artery disease	23.1	Coronary artery disease	23.0
Stroke	10.3	Stroke	12.8
Alzheimer's disease, dementias	7.3	Alzheimer's disease, dementias	10.6
Chronic obstructive lung disease	5.8	Age-related vision disorders	4.2
Prostate cancer	5.6	Chronic obstructive lung disease	3.2
Lung cancer	4.9	Colorectal cancer	2.8

Source: Adapted from Australian Institute of Health and Welfare: Mathers, 1999.

While many of the illnesses mentioned in Table 2 might not surprise most readers, several points are worth noting. Firstly, mental illnesses (including alcohol abuse) account for a huge proportion of the burden of disease in younger age groups. Secondly, breast cancer is a very important illness because of its high incidence and the fact that it occurs earlier than most other cancers. Finally, although melanoma is not mentioned in any age group, it is important because it is still fairly common, especially in men, is potentially fatal, and almost always preventable.

It is important to note that in the majority of cases preventing these illnesses requires action before you reach the age they are likely to affect you. You therefore need to concentrate not only on illnesses in the age group that you are in at present, but also on the illnesses that will affect you in the future. For example, prevention of cancer and vascular disease are lifelong projects. You will not provide your best chance of avoiding them by acting at age 60, although starting at a later age is much better than never starting at all and can still give significant benefit.

As would be expected, the burden of disease increases with age. However, a considerable proportion of diseases still occur between 15 and 55 years. Males have more illness than females in all age groups other than those 75 years of age and older.

The least you need to do

Health monitoring program

Women are usually good at having their health regularly monitored. Men unfortunately are not. The fact that routine car maintenance is considered essential but routine body maintenance is not is another one of life's mysteries.

You should have routine check-ups at least every second year up until the age of 40 and then yearly. Routine screening will need to be organised at these visits as appropriate and may include any or all of the following: blood pressure and urine checks, Pap smears for cervical cancer, mammograms for breast cancer, faecal occult blood tests for colon cancer, eye pressure checks to exclude chronic glaucoma, and blood tests for cholesterol and diabetes. Immunisations also need to be kept up-to-date.

Table 3 indicates a lifetime timetable for acting on preventative health issues. It is the foundation upon which your medical prevention program should lie. Some of these topics, such as depression, cancer prevention or stress, may seem unusual for discussion at a routine medical. However, they are the problems most likely to cause you harm and they are all significantly preventable with good preventative advice and treatment. Please study the tables well and refer to them before each GP check-up.

Maintain healthy lifestyle options

The principal components of a healthy lifestyle appear on the next page. As well as keeping to them yourself, you need to encourage your family to do the same, especially your children.

- Maintain a healthy weight (a BMI of between 20 and 25).
- Incorporate as much physical activity into your daily routine as possible and exercise for 30 minutes a day for at least four days a week. (Do not suddenly start exercising at this level if you have not been routinely doing so.)
- Maintain a healthy diet. (See page 9.)

Table 3 Illness prevention program

Age Group	*0–9*	*10–14*	*15–19*	*20–24*	*25–29*	*30–34*	*35–39*	*40–44*	*45–49*	*50–54*	*55–59*	*60–64*	*65–69*	*70–74*	*75–79*	*80+*
• General check-ups[1]																
– Blood pressure			•	•	•	•	•	•	•	•	•	•	•	•	•	•
– Weight	•	•	•	•	•	•	•	•	•	•	•	•	•	•	•	•
– Exercise	•	•	•	•	•	•	•	•	•	•	•	•	•	•	•	•
– Smoking		•	•	•	•	•	•	•	•	•	•	•	•	•	•	•
– Alcohol and illicit drugs			•	•	•	•	•	•	•	•	•	•	•	•	•	•
– Stress levels			•	•	•	•	•	•	•	•	•	•	•	•	•	•
– Skin cancer check			•	•	•	•	•	•	•	•	•	•	•	•	•	•
– Anxiety and depression (and suicide)	•	•	•	•	•	•	•	•	•	•	•	•	•	•	•	•
– Sexually transmitted diseases and contraception			•	•	•	•	•	•	•							
– Dementia												•	•	•	•	•
– Parental concerns							(as appropriate)									
– Immunisations (see schedule on p. 368)	•	•	•	•	•	•	•	•	•	•	•	•	•	•	•	•
– General cancer prevention				•			•									
• Genetic counselling				•					•							
• Pre-pregnancy (both partners)				•				(earlier or later if appropriate)								
• Vascular disease prevention discussion[2]				•					•							
• Cholesterol[3]—low vascular disease risk[4] (assess every 5 years)									•	•	•	•	•	•		
• Cholesterol[3]—high vascular disease risk[4] (assess yearly)				•	•	•	•	•	•	•	•	•	•	•		
• Diabetes[5]—low risk (assess every 3 years)													•	•	•	•
• Diabetes[5]—medium risk (assess every 3 years)										•	•	•	•	•	•	•
• Diabetes[5]—high risk (assess yearly)								•	•	•	•	•	•	•	•	•
• Stroke prevention (high vascular disease risk groups—check for stroke symptoms[6])										•	•	•	•	•	•	
• Osteoporosis prevention	(at menopause or before for females)								•	•	•	•	•	•	•	
• Colorectal cancer (assess every 2 years with FOB test)										•	•	•	•	•		
• Fall prevention in the elderly (yearly)													•	•	•	•
• Chronic glaucoma[7]													•	•	•	
• Females—Breast cancer (assess every 2 years with mammogram)[8]										•	•	•	•	•		
• Females—Cervical cancer (Pap smear every 2 years)				•	•	•	•	•	•	•	•	•	•	•		

Notes:
1. At least every second year until 40 then every year. All check-ups need to include an assessment of weight, exercise levels, a full skin examination and urine testing and the issues of depression and alcohol.
2. Vascular disease risk factors should be assessed at 20 years of age in people with a strong family history of vascular disease (i.e. coronary artery disease in a first-degree relative under the age of 60). Otherwise assessment should first be done at 45 years of age.
3. Checking the cholesterol level of well people who are over the age of 70 and have a low risk of heart disease is of questionable benefit.
4. Criteria for high vascular disease risk appears in section on cardiovascular disease.
5. Criteria for various diabetes risk levels appear in boxed section in section on diabetes.
6. Symptoms of stoke can include dizzy turns or funny turns, weakness or numbness in the arms or legs, speech disturbance or blurred/double vision.
7. Test for chronic glaucoma from age 40 years if at high risk. (Those at high risk include people with a first-degree relative with chronic glaucoma or who have already been found to have a raised pressure in either eye.)
8. Women with an increased risk of breast cancer may need to start screening mammography earlier. (See section on breast cancer.)

Source: Adapted from National Preventive and Community Medicine Committee, 'Guidelines for preventive activities in general practice', *Australian Family Physician*, 2002, 31 (5): SI XIV–SIXV, The Royal Australian College of General Practitioners.

- Do not smoke.
- Minimise harm from alcohol. (The optimum level is one to two standard drinks per day.)
- Minimise harm from illicit drugs.
- Ensure your work and home environments are as safe as possible.
- Minimise harm from sun exposure.
- Recognise, treat, and where possible, help prevent mental illnesses.
- Participate in disease screening programs.
- Regularly monitor your health (check-ups with your GP).
- Ensure you look after your important relationships.

Healthy Diet

- Maintain total dietary fat intake at about 25 to 30 per cent of total energy intake.
- Ensure dietary fat intake is mostly unsaturated fat, especially monounsaturated and omega-3 polyunsaturated fatty acids.
- Minimise saturated fat intake.
- Ensure that energy intake is in the normal range for your energy expenditure level.
- Ensure you eat at least five (preferably seven) serves of vegetables and fruit per day.
- Maintain an optimum level of alcohol consumption for good health; one or two standard drinks per day with at least two alcohol free days each week. This does not mean that you cannot have an occasional night out (as long as you don't put yourself at risk and it doesn't occur too often).
- Eat plenty of wholegrain breads and cereals to increase dietary fibre.
- Use minimal amounts of spreads.
- Maintain an adequate calcium intake.

Preventative health questions you need to address

1. Do you have a family GP you see regularly for check-ups? When is your next check-up due?
2. Are your vaccinations up-to-date?
3. Does your GP inspect your body for skin cancers at your regular check-ups?

4. Does your GP check your urine at your regular check-ups?
5. Do you know your BMI (body mass index) and waist measurement? If they are excessive, have you sought advice regarding reducing them?
6. Do you eat well? (See boxed section on page 9.)
7. Do you partake in adequate physical activity?
8. If you are over 45, have you had your cholesterol checked? If it was not normal, have you taken measures to reduce it?
9. What is your blood pressure? Has it been tested within the last two years?
10. If you are over 55 or at increased risk of diabetes, have you been checked for diabetes within the last three years?
11. Are you aware of the symptoms of depression? If you know someone with depression, have you discussed the problem with them or a medical practitioner?
12. Are you at risk from your alcohol consumption? Do you pass the AUDIT alcohol test? (See Part 2 in the 'Alcohol use and abuse' section.) Do you have at least two alcohol-free days each week?
13. If you smoke (or take illegal drugs), have you looked into stopping? If you smoke and are over 35 years of age, have you had your lung function checked?
14. Do you spend time each day thinking about issues relating to improving relationships with family and friends? How do you fare in the Relationships Australia relationship test? (See Part 2 'Functioning in our society' section.)
15. Do you have a family history that may increase your risk of any disease, especially cancer, heart disease or diabetes? If so, have you discussed this with your GP?
16. If over 50, do you have a check for blood in your bowel motions (faecal occult blood test) at least every second year?
17. If you are female and have been sexually active at any time, do you have Pap smears every second year?
18. If you are female and over 50, do you have mammograms every two years?
19. If you are female and approaching menopause or have gone through menopause, have you discussed osteoporosis with your GP?
20. If you are planning a family, have you planned medically?
21. Do you suffer from any urinary incontinence at all? If so, have you sought help from your GP?
22. Have you investigated your work and hobbies to determine any specific health risks they may pose?
23. If elderly, have you been assessed for risk of falls?
24. Do you take precautions to protect your hearing when exposed to high noise levels?
25. Do you spend time planning your future activities?

Choosing your family doctor

Hopefully you will already have a good long-standing relationship with a GP. If not, you should get to know one and make sure you are comfortable with his/her attitudes and manner so that you can build a trusting relationship. In the future you may need to rely on medical judgments made in an emergency situation and it is important to have confidence in your doctor at such a stressful time. This can only be achieved by visiting a practice where continuity of care is available.

Your GP needs to be easily accessible, located close to home and preferably amenable to doing house calls. It is often good to get to know two doctors in a practice as your doctor will get sick and will sometimes have holidays too.

Further information

Cochrane Institute
This is the best source of medical advice based on good quality evidence. It has a consumer-oriented site and a site with more detailed information. Both can be accessed free of charge. Websites: www.cochraneconsumer.com or www.cochranelibrary.com

Government-sponsored health education resources
The website for these resources links to many health-related sites. All connected sites have been assessed as providing accurate medical information that you can rely upon (unlike many websites). Website: www.healthinsite.gov.au

NSW Health
NSW Health gives a very wide-ranging list of reliable sources of medical information that have been accredited by the NSW Department of Health. Websites: www.health.nsw.gov.au (general) or www.health.nsw.gov.au/hospitalinfo/hotlinks.html (for other endorsed information resources)

Multicultural information
This is provided on a wide variety of health matters in many different languages in a downloadable form from www.mhcs.health.nsw.gov.au

Commonwealth Department of Health and Aged Care
Website: www.health.gov.au

National Health and Medical Research Council
A good source of information about government-recommended standards regarding investigation and treatment of medical conditions. Website: www.nhmrc.gov.au

Australian Institute of Health and Welfare (AIHW)
A great source of up-to-date statistics about all health issues in Australia. Website: www.aihw.gov.au

Identifying preventable childhood illness

> 'Fifty years from now it will not matter what kind of car you drove, what kind of house you lived in, how much you had in your bank account, nor what your clothes looked like. But the world may be a better place because you were important in the life of a child.'
>
> Anonymous

The causes of childhood illness are fundamentally different from those responsible for adult illness. However, like adult illness, many are preventable. The burden of disease caused by childhood illnesses is shown in Table 4.

There are a few noticeable differences between illness in boys and girls. Importantly, boys experience about 57 per cent of the burden of disease from all childhood illness and girls only 43 per cent. Significant contributors to this difference are accidental injury, with boys experiencing 64 per cent of all accidental injury burden of disease, and attention deficit disorder, with boys experiencing 72 per cent of the burden of disease from this condition.

Several of the major childhood illnesses, including neonatal causes, accidental injury and sudden infant death syndrome, can be significantly prevented. It is also worthwhile noting that the reason infectious disease contributes only 5.6 per cent to total disease burden is that Australian children are immunised against most serious infections. Without immunisation, this situation would be very different. Despite this, over 5000 children suffer vaccine preventable illnesses in Australia each year, the most common being whooping-cough, measles and rubella.

Table 4 Burden of disease caused by childhood illness

Important illnesses in children 0 to 14 years of age	*% of total burden of disease in boys*	*% of total burden of disease in girls*
Asthma	17.9	18.6
Mental health disorders including attention deficit hyperactivity disorder, autism and depression	17.3	14.1
Neonatal causes including low birth weight, birth trauma, neonatal infections	13.8	14.9
Congenital abnormalities	12.6	13.2
Accidents	11.9	8.6
Infectious disease	5.8	7.2
SIDS (Sudden Infant Death Syndrome)	3.2	3.3
Cancer	2.3	2.3

Source: Adapted from Australian Institute of Health and Welfare: Mathers, 1999.

The rest of this chapter deals with other preventable childhood illnesses, with special emphasis on parent and mental health issues (something all parents need to address). Reducing the incidence of asthma and accidental injury are covered in separate sections of this book.

Mental disorders The influence of parental behaviour on children can not be underestimated. Good parenting techniques and refraining from substance abuse, especially alcohol, are major factors in producing healthy, well-adjusted children and can significantly reduce the incidence of mental illness in childhood. For example, parental conflict has been shown to impact negatively on childhood mental illness, causing fear, anger and stress, whereas an encouraging parenting style using rewards and reinforcement has the opposite effect. Divorce and separation interestingly have a negative emotional and mental impact in the short term but in the long term children are not detrimentally affected. The topic of parenting is dealt with in more detail in the sections on anxiety and relationships.

Neonatal causes The main causes of neonatal illness are low birthweight and birth trauma, including breathing problems at birth (asphyxia). Babies with a low birthweight (less than 2500 g) are more likely to suffer illness at the time of birth, such as infections and neurological complications, and are more likely to develop diseases, including high blood pressure and diabetes, in later life. The incidence of low birthweight can be significantly reduced by refraining from smoking and alcohol and eating a healthy diet while pregnant, and by ensuring you receive good obstetric care. Similarly, good obstetric care is of paramount importance if birth trauma and asphyxia are to be prevented. Ensuring you have an experienced and caring practitioner delivering your child in a well-resourced hospital is the best start you can give your baby. In childbirth, problems are not always predictable and can occur quickly. Home is not the place to be. Medical preparation for producing a healthy baby and mother needs to start prior to conception and this topic is covered in the section on preparation for pregnancy.

Congenital abnormalities The causes of most congenital abnormalities are unknown; however, about 5 per cent are due to maternal illness, including diabetes and infections such as rubella, and drugs (teratogenic drugs) that cause foetal abnormalities. Environmental substances, such as mercury, and nutrient deficiencies, especially folate, are also causes. The incidence of some congenital malformations can be reduced through neonatal diagnosis of the conditions and subsequent termination of the pregnancy, for example in Down syndrome. Reducing congenital abnormalities is covered in the section on preparation for pregnancy.

Sudden infant death syndrome (SIDS) Most cases of SIDS occur in the first six months of life. The incidence of SIDS can be drastically reduced (by up to 70 per cent) by ensuring children are not placed on their stomachs to sleep and are positioned so they can not roll over onto their stomachs. (They should be placed at the foot of the cot.) Not smoking during pregnancy and not smoking near babies is also a very important way to reduce the risk of SIDS. Sleeping with an infant on a sofa or a chair can increase the SIDS risk and should be avoided. There is still debate as to whether sleeping with your baby in your bed increases the risk of SIDS. Certainly, it should not be combined with smoking in bed. Breastfeeding may reduce the incidence of SIDS. Through the adoption of the above recommendations, the incidence of SIDS reduced by 62 per cent from 1990 to 2000 and it is still falling.

Obesity and physical inactivity Dietary excess and physical inactivity are major problems for Australian children. Their consequences mainly occur, however, in adult life and thus they are reflected in adult rather than childhood burden of disease. Dietary deficiencies are uncommon in Australian children. The only exception is anaemia due to iron deficiency, which is responsible for just under 2 per cent of the total burden of disease. A list of foods rich in iron appears in Appendix 5.

Finally, it is important to make sure that children, especially young children, are regularly checked for medical problems. Many childhood medical problems that can lead to significant disability are correctable if found early, including congenital hip dislocation, squints and hearing/speech abnormalities. This process starts in the hospital with baby checks and should be continued on a regular basis. Visits for routine immunisations are a good opportunity to have your baby checked and to mention any concerns you have. Presented in the boxed section following is a timetable for addressing childhood and adolescent preventative health issues.

Childhood and adolescent preventative health timetable

Early parenting issues

- Early parenthood is a difficult period and it is common for parents to have difficulty coping. If you are worried that you are not coping, see your GP before the problem becomes too serious. (Depression is a major problem at this time.) Any family member or friend who is concerned about the well-being or safety of a child or mother should seek help as soon as possible.
- Contraception needs to be discussed at the first post-natal visit with your GP.

Babies

- The first post-hospital GP check is important for detecting congenital problems, including hip problems, heart murmurs, and undescended testes in boys. It is also a good time to check that blood tests taken in hospital for phenylketonuria, cystic fibrosis and hypothyroidism were normal and to check whether a vitamin K injection was given in hospital. (Occasionally vitamin K is given orally.)
- SIDS is an important concern in the first two years of life and particularly in the first six months.
- Breastfeeding is best.

0 to 5 year olds

- Growth should be checked every three to six months in the first two years of life by measuring height, weight and head circumference. From 3 to 5 years of age, yearly growth checks should include height, weight and BMI.
- Developmental progress, including speech, hearing, sight and mobility, should be actively monitored by parents. Abnormalities should be discussed with GPs. A table detailing developmental milestones appears in Appendix 4.
- Squints (turned eyes) should be searched for by parents and GPs from a very early age as successful treatment relies on early detection.
- Accident/injury prevention. (See Part 8, 'Accidents and injuries' section.)
- Dental care should include an annual visit to the dentist from 3 years of age. Children who do not have fluoride in their water supply should have regular fluoride supplements.
- Sun protection is an important health issue from birth. Your pre-school or school should have good sun protection policies, such as the no-hat-no-play rule, and promote education about sun protection. (See Part 6, 'Skin cancer prevention' section.)
- Optimum nutrition and physical activity levels need to be encouraged.
- Immunisations. (See immunisation schedule on page 368.)

6 to 14 year olds

- Accident/injury prevention. (See Part 8, 'Accidents and injuries' section.)
- Assessment of growth progress through assessing height, weight and BMI should be done if there is concern about progress.
- Educational progress should be assessed at least yearly.
- Sun protection should continue.
- Awareness of mental health problems, especially anxiety and depression, needs to be a priority in this age group. (See Part 2.)
- Immunisations should continue.

Adolescents

Parents, GPs and other adults, including teachers and friends, need to be both observant and inquisitive so that any adolescent health problems can be found and addressed early. Parents and schools need to be active in providing information to all adolescents about the following health issues and discussing appropriate preventative strategies. Don't assume it won't happen to your child.

- Depression/suicide.
- Obesity and physical inactivity.
- Smoking.
- Risk-taking behaviours, including alcohol and other drug abuse.
- Social problems at home, including the risk of abuse.
- Teenage pregnancy.

A child's approach to illness prevention

> 'Children have never been very good at listening to their elders, but they have never failed to imitate them.'
>
> James Baldwin (1924–87)

As you read through the chapters of this book, it should become obvious that many serious adult health problems have their foundations in inadequate child upbringing. Poor behaviours learned at home by children and carried into their adult lives can lead to a very impressive list of health problems including:

- obesity
- physical inactivity
- poor dietary choices.

These three problems can lead to high blood cholesterol, diabetes, coronary artery disease and many cancers.

Other health problems that can occur in later life include:

- depression and anxiety
- drug and alcohol abuse
- skin cancers due to inadequate sun protection
- poor attitudes to illness prevention (i.e. not having regular check-ups).

The behavioural patterns that are the underlying cause for the above diseases are usually well entrenched by adulthood and are difficult to treat. A large part of this book is about overcoming these inappropriate behaviours and the change that can be achieved by most people. However, it is much easier not to have the problems in the first place. This is why the current epidemic of obesity and lack of physical activity in children is such a disaster! Parents are responsible for providing a caring and nurturing environment for their children. They should:

- Provide a good example for children to follow in all aspects of life. This can be achieved by demonstrating the following attributes.
  - Planning for the future and maintaining a sense of purpose in the home.
  - Developing trusting and loving family relationships.
  - Maintaining an optimistic outlook when dealing with family problems.
  - Maintaining a flexible outlook towards problem-solving and trying to maintain control of the situation when solving problems.
  - Showing how to learn from mistakes.
  - Anticipating and planning ahead for stressful situations.
  - Taking care of yourself and appreciating yourself. (This includes keeping yourself healthy by exercising and eating well.)
  - Demonstrating responsible attitudes to alcohol use.

- Encourage children to become self-reliant. This can be done by encouraging the development of good problem-solving and social skills and increasing 'success experiences' by encouraging hobbies/interests.
- Encourage children to participate in family decision making, such as meal choices.
- Ensure that their children's school has in place teaching strategies to improve coping skills and self-esteem. An example is the FRIENDS program (pages 66–7), which aims at preventing childhood anxiety.

This will at times seem like an insurmountable hurdle. However, the effort involved will provide parents with their greatest lifetime reward—well-adjusted and happy children who love and respect you.

HOW DO YOU ACHIEVE THIS?

Parenting is not a skill you are born with and your main education in this field is most likely to have come from watching your parents have a go at it. This may or may not be a good thing.

As bringing up your children is likely to be the most important thing you do, it is worthwhile becoming educated about how to do it well. This requires two things.

First, you need to allocate enough time to educate yourself properly. It is vital that both parents participate, as raising children is a shared responsibility and it is important parents are consistent in their approach to their children.

Second, you need to access good sources of information about child rearing. Information about many health issues is contained in this book. More detailed information about specific topics and additional topics not covered can be sourced from other texts. The Kids Health Bookshop at The Children's Hospital at Westmead (in Sydney) is a wonderful source of information about rearing children and childhood illness. The books it sells have been read and approved by staff at the hospital. (See boxed information below.)

Finally, you need to access help when you are in trouble. Start with your general practitioner, your child's teacher or your school counsellor.

Further information for parents

The Children's Hospital, Westmead

This hospital is one of the two main paediatric teaching hospitals in Sydney. Its website www.chw.edu.au/parents is a great source of information on children's health topics. It provides fact sheets about many child health issues that are free and downloadable and lists books on most child health topics all of which have been assessed by members of the medical staff at the hospital. These books are available for purchase from the Kids Health Bookshop at Westmead (02 9845 3585) or they can be purchased via the 'e-shop' on the website. All profits go into supporting the work of the hospital.

Some suggested books on parenting

All these books and many more appear in the 'self-esteem, behaviour and family life section' of the books section on the hospital's website.

- *Every Parent: A positive approach to children's behaviour* by Matthew R. Sanders, PhD.
- *Who'd Be a Parent* by Dr John Irvine.
- *Raising Kids—A parent's survival guide* by Charles Watson, Dr Susan Clarke and Linda Walton.
- *Reviving Ophelia* by Mary Pipher.
- *Teen Esteem* by Dr P. Palmer and M. Froehner.
- *Bully Busting* by Evelyn M. Field.
- *Raising Boys* by Steve Biddulph.
- *Helping Your Anxious Child—A step by step guide for parents* by R. Rapee, S. Spence, V. Cobham and A. Wignall.

Population groups with special health needs

Some population groups in Australia have special health needs or have an increased risk of developing particular illnesses. This chapter attempts to highlight these problem areas so that individuals in the groups concerned can anticipate and prevent their occurrence. However, the solutions for solving many of these issues lie in the domain of public (government) health policy and a detailed discussion of such matters is beyond the scope of this book. It is important that readers are aware that such issues exist and are supportive of government funding initiatives to help overcome them.

Health in Indigenous people

The health of Indigenous Australians is one of the major health problems facing Australia today. Across all age groups, Indigenous Australians are significantly worse off in almost all illness categories. Death rates are much higher than those of average Australians. For example, in 1996 the death rate of Indigenous Australians in the 35 to 54 year age group was six times that of the Australian average.

Illnesses that are of particular concern include cardiovascular disease, hypertension, respiratory diseases, depression and suicide, cancers, diabetes, eye disease including traucoma, kidney disease, especially kidney failure, and maternal and infant/child health problems (babies of Indigenous mothers are twice as likely to die at birth). Social and emotional well-being needs to be addressed, with critical issues including youth suicide, substance abuse, education, family violence and family network disruption (e.g. the stolen generation).

The main health risk factors for aboriginal people are:

- *Low birth weight.* Babies with a low birth weight are more vulnerable to illnesses in childhood and to some adult illnesses such as kidney disease. This common problem in Indigenous Australians is due to a multitude of factors including socioeconomic disadvantage, maternal smoking and other risk-taking behaviours.
- *Obesity.* Indigenous people have a higher incidence of obesity than the general population.
- *Poor nutrition.* Restricted access to healthy foods and traditional foods, lack of knowledge about nutrition, and financial constraints all contribute to poor nutrition. A change in the traditional Indigenous high fibre, high protein, low fat diet to one based on fat and refined carbohydrates is a particular problem.
- *Alcohol and other drug use.* Fewer Indigenous people actually consume alcohol than the general population but those who do are much more likely to consume at hazardous levels. About 20 per cent of Indigenous people consume at levels that will cause long-term harm and 49 per cent consume at levels that cause short-term harm. Cigarette smoking is about twice as common in Indigenous people. The use of inhalants (petrol, glue and aerosols) is a particular problem in some communities.
- *Living conditions.* Many Indigenous people do not live in housing that provides adequate shelter, safe drinking water or adequate sewerage. Overcrowding encourages the spread of numerous infectious diseases such as respiratory infections, rheumatic fever and tuberculosis. While living conditions are a particular problem in rural communities, urban Indigenous people also have relatively poor housing standards with inadequate bedroom numbers.
- *Lack of access to suitably trained health workers.* Many remote communities have no access to free GP services and specialist care is almost always a great distance away. Thus, Indigenous people tend to under utilise primary health care services with the consequence that they develop illnesses that mean they over utilise hospital services. A cervical cancer rate that is 14 times the incidence experienced by white Australian women is a good example of the consequences of this situation.

Most of these problems are public health issues and many appropriate responses are already being implemented. They include:

- The provision of adequately trained health workers who are well resourced and supported. Crucial in this training is education regarding cultural issues that impact on developing trusting relationships with Indigenous people and their acceptance of medical advice.

- The education of local people in the provision of health services to their own communities. This is of paramount importance as they are in a much better position to promote and improve the acceptance of mainstream medical advice and treatment. They also do not experience the communication problems that non-Indigenous health workers experience. Most successful interventions are accomplished when there is Indigenous community control of health programs.
- Continuing evaluation of the adequacy of health worker training and medical resources.
- The provision and maintenance of adequate housing, water resources and sewerage systems.

It is important that all Australians are aware of the seriousness of the health problems facing Indigenous people and that they support and encourage adequate funding for government initiatives to help reverse this situation.

Health in overseas-born people

About 25 per cent of people living in Australia were born overseas, with over half coming from non-English speaking countries. Overall, people who immigrate to Australia have better health when they arrive than the average Australian. This is mostly because they are carefully screened medically before arrival. Illness and disability levels, however, do increase with length of residence in Australia. (Cardiovascular disease is one illness that follows this pattern.) Overseas-born people have lower rates of suicide, motor vehicle accidents and especially skin cancers throughout their lives.

There are some illnesses that occur more commonly in certain ethnic groups or in people from certain countries. Most of these differences are due to different levels of exposure to disease risk factors such as smoking, rather than any differences in genetic make up. Thus, many individuals at increased risk can be identified by assessing their risk factors for particular diseases. Illness levels in overseas-born Australians that vary from average levels include the following:

- Males and females from the United Kingdom and Ireland have an increased risk of lung cancer, as have males from other European countries.
- Women from the UK and Ireland have higher rates of breast cancer.
- Rates of cervical cancer are higher in women born in Asia and from European countries other than the UK and Ireland.
- The incidence of diabetes is higher in people from Asia, the Pacific Islands and Europe (excluding the UK and Ireland). Education regarding the management of diabetes is needed as these groups often have poor control of their disease.

- Some genetic diseases are more prevalent in specific ethnic groups. These are discussed in the section on preparation for pregnancy.

  Public health issues related to overseas-born people include:

- Ensuring that information about public health issues and individual diseases is available in both English and other languages.
- Ensuring that health professionals are aware of cultural issues that may impact on the provision of health care.
- Ensuring that there are adequate numbers of health care workers able to speak languages other than English and that hospitals and other health services have translators available.
- Ensuring that specific health problems affecting overseas-born people, such as the treatment of diabetes, are addressed in health promotion campaigns.

Health in rural and remote communities

Looking at illness in rural and remote communities is complicated by the fact that a relatively higher proportion of Indigenous people live in these areas and their significantly higher mortality/disability rate distorts the figures. For this reason, this discussion will deal with illness in non-Indigenous Australians in these areas.

For people over the age of 65 years, death rates are actually slightly lower for those living in remote areas. For people under the age of 65 years, death rates in rural and remote communities are about 10–20 per cent higher than in metropolitan areas. The main contributing factors in both men and women are higher rates of death from cardiovascular disease, respiratory disease and injury. Motor vehicle accidents are considerably more common in rural communities due to a variety of factors such as longer distances travelled, poorer roads and increased alcohol consumption in young people. A significant issue for people living in rural and remote communities is the high incidence of male suicide (see pages 76–7). This is dealt with in the section on suicide. Relative isolation also means that many rural people find obtaining appropriate treatment for their medical problems more difficult. This is a particularly true with mental illnesses. In children, injuries are the main problem, especially those involving farm equipment and drowning. (See the section on childhood injuries and the farmsafe websites at the end of this chapter.)

Several risk factors for poor health are more common in rural communities and help explain this increased mortality rate in people under 65 years. These factors include higher levels of smoking, obesity and physical inactivity. Hazardous alcohol consumption in young adults (20 to 29 age group) is twice as common in rural/remote areas compared to their metropolitan counterparts (Australian Institute of Health and Welfare 2002). Reduced availability of medical services and restricted access to healthy food in very remote areas are also important issues. Lower incomes and higher food prices also restrict healthy food choices.

Other than for public health issues, such as the availability of health professionals, the issues identified above are all discussed in detail in this book. And on a positive note, rural people are less likely to report unhappiness and rural women have lower stress levels (Australian Institute of Health and Welfare 2002).

Health in socioeconomically disadvantaged groups

Socioeconomic status is determined by several factors including income, level of education, employment status and occupation. On average, those from lower socioeconomic groups have a higher incidence of smoking, obesity and physical inactivity, which increases their incidence of cardiovascular disease, respiratory diseases and diabetes. People in lower socioeconomic groups are also less likely to use preventative health services. Heavy alcohol consumption is also more prevalent and mental health problems are more common in socioeconomically disadvantaged young people.

Overall mortality and disability rates are understandably higher in socioeconomically disadvantaged people. For example, males in the lowest socioeconomic group have a 37 per cent higher total burden of disease compared with those in the highest group. The level for females was 27 per cent higher (Australian Institute of Health and Welfare 1999). Mortality burden was worst in the 15 to 24 year age group, where male mortality was a staggering 70 per cent higher in the lowest group compared to the highest (Australian Institute of Health and Welfare 2000). Motor vehicle accidents and suicide are the commonest causes of death in young males.

Improving the health of socioeconomically disadvantaged people mainly involves changes to public health and social policies, including:

- The provision of adequate social welfare to ensure financial disadvantage does not impact too significantly on quality of life.
- The provision of adequate low-cost housing to long-term disadvantaged people.
- The provision of affordable primary health care.
- Health promotion campaigns targetting disadvantaged people, especially preventative health initiatives.
- The provision of adequate public facilities such as schools, hospitals etc.
- The creation of employment opportunities.

Further information

For people in rural and remote communities

Rural Health
Website: www.ruralhealth.gov.au

National rural health alliance
Website: www.ruralhealth.org.au

Farmsafe Australia
Website: www.farmsafe.org.au

National agricultural safety database
Website: www.cdc.gov/nasd/ (click on and locate by topic)

For non-English speaking Australians
A good source of health information in other languages is provided by the NSW Department of Health.
Website: www.mhcs.health.nsw.gov.au

The problem—achieving change

The aim of this book is to help you live a longer and healthier life. Achieving this aim involves adopting healthier lifestyle options. Most Australians are well aware that such options would benefit them. Many, however, do not apply this knowledge to their own lives. The issues underlying such behaviour are complex with most being mental rather than physical in nature. Inadequate knowledge is one reason for this behaviour, although this will obviously not apply to the people who read this book!

To some people, the recommendations made will seem too restrictive and appear to signal the end of many of life's pleasures, such as a night's drinking with friends, smoking, or regular high-fat meals. They may accordingly take the view that they would rather enjoy themselves while they're here and take the consequences when they come. The obvious problem with this argument is that relying on a hopefully favourable family gene pool is a risky business and the consequences often come much sooner than planned. The other problem is that these 'life pleasures' are not the things that bestow happiness and some, such as excessive alcohol, are the cause of much suffering. Happiness comes from loving relationships, enjoying the company and support given by true friends, and successfully planning and achieving meaningful goals in life.

Moderating lifestyle factors, such as food and alcohol consumption, will augment success in relationships and life goals and thus improve happiness. And there will still be room for indulgences from time to time for good measure.

Chronic illness can make achieving lifestyle change difficult. Such illness may be physical in nature, for example disability from an accident. However, mental illness, especially depression, can have an equally profound effect on your ability to bring about change. Depression, which is a very common problem, has a profound impact on a person's ability to make decisions about their health, both present and future.

Depression

There are numerous people in our society who suffer from significant depression for much of their lives and many more who have occasional, significant bouts of depression. About 20 per cent of the population become significantly depressed at some stage in their lives.

Depression is caused by a chemical imbalance in the brain. It is beyond the scope of this book to deal with the treatment of this condition in detail; however, there are medications and counselling techniques that work well in treating this chemical imbalance. Treatment can mean the difference between an enjoyable, fulfilling life, and a life of unhappiness for the sufferers and their families.

If you are concerned that depression is affecting your life or the life of a relative or friend, you should seek help from your doctor immediately. It is an unfortunate fact that only about 50 per cent of depressed people have their disease diagnosed and treated.

All GPs see many depressed people and most are well skilled at treating this condition. However, they can only help when they know there is a problem. (See the section on depression for more infomation.)

Probably the most significant problem associated with changing lifestyles is that it is very difficult. Many of the patterns that require changing have evolved with you throughout your life. They are complexly interwoven into your daily routines. They are part of you. The behavioural patterns that are important to your overall health include:

- eating patterns
- physical activity levels
- alcohol consumption and other drug use (including caffeine)
- cigarette smoking
- sleeping routines
- attitudes towards health prevention issues (i.e. Pap smears for women) and towards regular visits to your GP for check-ups
- attitudes towards relationships with your partner, family and friends
- stress management at home and at work.

These are the important areas that need to be addressed if you are to become and remain physically and mentally healthy and all of them are expanded upon later in this book. However, as stated above, changing entrenched behavioural patterns is difficult. It requires adequate motivation and the allocation of adequate time, energy and resources to plan and implement change. Many individuals find getting through day-to-day life hard enough, let alone aiming for improvement. Living in an unhappy home (or work) situation is a relatively common cause of emotional stress and is often difficult to fix. It always helps to address such problems and GPs are a good place to start. Even if they are not able to help with counselling themselves, they will be able to direct you to someone who can.

Many of the lifestyle changes you need to make will involve all members of your family, especially your partner. Your partner's involvement will provide extra insight into your problems and increase the likelihood of successful change for yourself and the whole family.

Behavioural patterns that make change difficult

Some of the detrimental behavioural patterns mentioned above make any sort of lifestyle change difficult because they reduce your level of motivation to change and also your resolve when attempting change. Prime examples of these behavioural patterns are:

- excessive stress or coping poorly with stress
- anxiety or depression
- insomnia
- alcohol and other drug abuse, including illicit drugs and caffeine. (Caffeine causes insomnia—and thus tiredness—and anxiety.) Drug abuse is often difficult to alter and almost always requires the help of a health professional.

If any of the above issues are significant problems in your life, then they should be given priority when deciding on lifestyle changes. Sorting out these issues first will improve your life, both physically and mentally, and maximise your chance of successfully modifying other important lifestyle problems.

What can lifestyle change achieve?

A longer life: A significantly improved life expectancy enables you to live a longer and fuller life with your partner, family and friends and provides more time to spend doing the things you enjoy. Neither of my children had the chance to meet either of their grandfathers.

A healthier life: The disabilities that accompany disease can often be avoided or delayed by a healthy lifestyle. For example, the psychological and physical trauma that accompany coronary by-pass surgery are not trivial matters. Neither is living with the diabetic complications of blindness or kidney failure.

A financially wealthier life: Avoiding illness enables you to avoid the expenses that accompany illness, such as payment for expensive treatments and medications and the significant loss of time from work, or even the loss of your job, that can accompany long-term illness.

A sense of achievement: This comes from doing something worthwhile for yourself and will positively influence all aspects of your life.

Improved fitness: Without a doubt, an improved level of fitness enhances your general feeling of well-being.

New activities and friendships: Increasing physical activity can introduce you to a new range of enjoyable activities, such as sports or an appreciation of Australia's natural environment through bushwalking, and with these new activities comes the chance to make new friendships.

Helping family and friends by setting a good example: By showing that you care about your own physical and mental well-being, you are acting as a good role model for friends and family. You can also actively teach those around you these good habits. Helping others is probably the most beneficial thing you can do for your own feeling of self-worth. And, in the end, self-worth and a 'meaningful and fulfilling life' are one and the same thing.

Finally, remember that an active, healthier lifestyle is a journey, not a destination. To be successful, it is important that the journey is a pleasant one! With all the above benefits, how could it be anything else!

The stages involved in changing lifestyle behaviours

As stated in the beginning of this chapter, becoming healthier means changing detrimental lifestyle habits. These develop over many years and your challenge to achieve change should, therefore, not be underestimated. The best way to successfully change is to approach each individual lifestyle problem with a well-thought-out plan. It is important you are involved in the planning process, as just being told what to do by your doctor rarely translates into meaningful change.

Presented here is an overall plan to assist in achieving lifestyle changes. There are five stages to the plan and the sections on treating obesity, lack of exercise and smoking follow these five stages. They are:

- Recognising the problem.
- Understanding the causes of the problem.
- Planning solutions for the problem.
- Implementing change.
- Maintaining change.

Stage 1—Recognising the problem

The first stage in changing behaviour is to recognise your health problems and then to decide that changing these problems is an important priority of your life. Making this decision can take some time and involves learning all about the problems you face. Most of the common health problems confronting Australians today are covered in this book.

Stage 2—Understanding the causes of the problem

Having recognised that you have a problem, it is essential you understand all the possible causes of the problem. For example, with regard to weight, the possibilities include lack of exercise, poor eating habits, medical problems that cause obesity etc. Whatever your problem, you will have your own set of causes for it. Identifying possible causes involves looking carefully at your lifestyle and your body. Such an analysis is often complicated and is best done with the help of a health professional.

Stage 3—Planning solutions for the problem

Having defined the causes of your health problem, your next task is to determine the behavioural changes necessary to overcome this problem. Often the required behavioural changes are obvious from the cause itself. For example, a sedentary lifestyle requires increased physical activity. However, there are often numerous ways of achieving such 'generalised changes'.

When changing your behaviour, you need to focus on the behaviour and not specific outcomes. This may seem obvious, but many people fall into the trap of concentrating on an outcome rather than the way to achieve it. For weight loss, it is important to concentrate on an overall change in dietary and exercise habits and not on a specific weight goal.

Your planned behavioural changes need to be both appropriate for your lifestyle and sustainable in the long term. There is no point implementing a behavioural change that will be too difficult to continue for many years. In order to do this, it is necessary to look closely at your lifestyle so you can decide which solutions will best fit your goals.

Your goals need to be significant enough to make a difference. Having said this, an acceptable balance needs to be achieved between worthwhile achievement and goals becoming a detrimental obsession. For example, becoming obsessive with regard to weight loss could become a detrimental influence in your life should you develop, say, anorexia.

STEP-BY-STEP GOAL SETTING

Your optimum behavioural change is often best achieved by setting a series of goals. This has the benefit of reducing the chance of initial failure and the associated guilt and loss of self-esteem/self-confidence. Some goals need to be addressed gradually. For example, if you do not exercise at all, it is important to increase your exercise level in stages.

As well, not all goals need to be addressed at once. You will probably have multiple issues requiring attention and addressing all your problems at once is often a recipe for failure. On the other hand, successfully addressing a single initial problem will greatly assist subsequent outcomes. For this reason, you should try to avoid treating the most difficult problem first. Some behaviours, such as excessive use of alcohol or tiredness due to lack of sleep, make change difficult. These problems should therefore be given priority when planning lifestyle change.

PLANNING YOUR TIME

When setting goals, you should remember they often need a significant period of time to be achieved. Do not set unrealistic time limits for your goals; this is not helpful. Be patient. Beneficial change usually occurs slowly and the changes that are needed are for the long term.

Once you have become sufficiently motivated to achieve a change, the allocation of adequate time is probably the most important factor restricting your ability to change. For most people, time is limited and must be rationed according to daily commitments.

One way of generating more time is to reduce the relative priority you give to some areas of your life and allocate this time to healthier activities. For example, you can reallocate some of your passive leisure time, such as watching television, to active leisure time, such as walking. Extra time can also be gained by doing necessary tasks more efficiently. Finally, you can gain time for healthy activities by changing the nature of your present commitments—rather than doing administrative work for your child's sporting team, try being the team coach.

The allocation of time to healthier options does not mean that, in the end, you lose time for other activities. Adopting a healthy lifestyle usually adds several years of quality time, free of physical incapacity, to your life. You'll live longer by being healthier!

COMPROMISE IN GOAL SETTING

Deciding on achievable goals requires a compromise between the lifestyle changes you require for optimal health and the resources you have to achieve your goals. For example, an optimum exercise routine should entail 30 minutes of exercise each day. This time will not be available to many people, so a compromise of 20 minutes each day may be an achievable option. To decide on these compromises, a fairly detailed assessment of your day-to-day life is required so the areas where change may be achieved can be identified.

You need to accurately assess your time and other resources when setting goals, otherwise you may end up being too optimistic about your planned changes. This could lead to giving up because you feel guilty about not achieving your set goal. On the other hand, being too pessimistic will just reduce the benefit you can achieve.

GETTING HELP

Most people require the assistance of health professionals, such as GPs or dietitians, to achieve and maintain their desired changes. Remember that change is difficult and you should not be afraid to seek help, especially if you have previously been unsuccessful in achieving change. Your friends can be a source of support. Behavioural change is often achieved more easily when family and friends also participate in the change. Quitting smoking, for instance, is often much easier with a 'quitting partner'. In this way, both of you benefit from the change and from the support you provide each other.

Stage 4—Implementing change

Do not just start a behavioural change when you think of it. Behavioural change requires careful planning if it is to succeed. Setting a specific day to start your change in behaviour enables you to allocate enough time to prepare properly for the change. Choose a low-stress day that is not too far away.

In order to reduce the chance of failure, you need to understand the potential problems likely to arise and develop strategies to avoid them. For example, weight gain is often a problem when stopping smoking and gaining prior dietary counselling will help avoid this problem.

Try not to waver from your behavioural change objective as this can reduce your resolve and is often the cause of failure. Failure is most common in the early stages of behavioural change so you should be especially vigilant during this period. However, please remember that a single departure from the plan does not always cause failure. You can learn from the mistake and avoid it next time. You should be aware that alcohol tends to reduce your resolve when implementing change so consumption should be carefully watched and perhaps reduced for the first few weeks.

It is important to reward yourself regularly during this initial period of change. Go to the pictures or buy a new CD. Also, remind yourself regularly why you want to change your behaviour and the advantages you will gain. Such reminders can be displayed at work and at home. A picture of your partner, children or grandchildren will remind you that you will be with them longer because of your change!

Stage 5—Maintaining change

Having implemented a change, you need a program for assessing your progress. Remember, this should be an assessment of the behavioural change rather than a specific outcome. Performing these assessments regularly, preferably with the help of a health professional, will give positive reinforcement where success is occurring, identify areas where the plan is failing so appropriate changes can be made, and allow discussion of appropriate modification of your plan, if needed.

Behavioural changes should not be 'cast in stone' and should be modifiable. Your 'lifestyle plan' is unlikely to be perfect and even if it is, personal circumstances continually change and these impact on your ability to achieve the behavioural goals you have set. Therefore, don't be afraid to change your behavioural goals, both up and down.

The risk of failure reduces with time. Those with an increased risk of failure include people who cope poorly with life stresses, drink excessive amounts of alcohol or use other drugs, or suffer from excess stress or tiredness. Remember, these problems are best addressed before attempting other behavioural change.

Assessing medical information

In Australia, medical advice is available from a variety of health professionals. Many of these practitioners provide conflicting advice regarding diagnosis and treatment, so deciding on what is right for you and your family is not always an easy task. It is, however, a very important task. Your upbringing, the experiences of family and friends and the media are just some of the influences that help you decide on your medical direction.

Hopefully you will not often have cause to question the medical advice you receive. However, if you are worried about the advice you receive or you get conflicting opinions or you just wish to know more, you will need to stand back and accurately assess the medical advice and treatment being offered. To do this, you require information about some basic issues, as outlined below.

Can your practitioner provide quality treatment that works?

Your practitioner's field of expertise needs to be one that provides quality care that works. The best way to identify fields providing quality care is to ask the following questions.

- Does the government regulate or recognise the field? Most health treatments that benefit patients are supported and encouraged by government health services.

- Do well-recognised educational institutions, such as universities, regulate the education of practitioners in the field?
- Is there a broad-based community acceptance of treatments by practitioners in this field?
- Is there a well-recognised professional body that represents most of the practitioners and coordinates their initial and ongoing professional training?

  Such well-recognised fields include traditional medical practice, physiotherapy, dental surgery, occupational therapy, optometrists, social workers, dietitians, psychologists etc.

If the field is less well-recognised, it does not mean that it cannot contribute to quality health care in the community. However, it does mean their profession is less well regulated, both by government bodies and by the profession itself, which may affect educational standards. Also, the knowledge base for both professional education and treatments may be less well researched, leading to treatments based on less accurate information and a greater variety in the treatment practices offered by practitioners in the field. This can lead to inappropriate treatments and it means that you need to be more careful in assessing the accuracy of advice given.

It is important to ensure the person providing the information is adequately trained in their field. Where did they obtain their medical education?

Conflict of interest

Also worth considering is whether your provider of medical care has a conflict of interest in the advice or treatment being given. While all providers of medical care make their living from seeing patients, some can obtain additional financial benefits on top of their fee. For example, they may also supply medications and other treatments for which they receive payments. For this reason, it is illegal for most doctors to sell medications. Also, they may receive benefits for referring patients for other forms of care or treatment. For instance, they may be financially associated with practitioners to whom they refer patients. Some practitioners may have a financial interest in medical facilities, such as hospitals, that might be used in your care.

Such conflicts do not mean the care you receive will be less than optimum. It just means that interests other than your best health are involved and you should be careful.

A reasonable fee for the consultation

As stated above, all health professionals earn a living by seeing patients. They have generally studied for numerous years to attain their qualifications and are entitled to a reasonable financial reward for their labours. They also have to cover the considerable expenses of running their practice.

For these reasons, you should be suspicious of any practitioner who receives no fee at all for their consultation time. It means they are either very generous or aim to make their money from the treatments or medications they advise or sell.

The problem with paying for the treatment and not the consultation is that to avoid going broke, they have to treat you for something whether you need it or not. (If they don't, it means the next patient is kindly paying for your treatment; a highly unlikely event!) Also, if they wish to continue receiving remuneration for seeing you, you will need to continue receiving treatment that is perhaps unnecessary.

What evidence is there that the treatment is beneficial?

'If a lot of cures are suggested for a disease, it means the disease is incurable.'

Anton Chekhov (1860–1904)

If you are unsure about the advice you are receiving and wish to know more, it is quite reasonable to ask for information about the advised treatment. This information then needs to be assessed as to its true worth. Asking the following questions will help ascertain this.

- Does the information come from a well-respected source that is not financially associated with selling treatments? (Those selling cures will obviously tell you that it does.)
- Does the information come from well-conducted research? (For information about this subject, see Appendix 2.)
- Is the treatment being advised available from a wide range of practitioners? Beware of treatments that only a few practitioners can provide. If a treatment works, it is usually readily available. (The converse, of course, is not necessarily true.)

There is nothing more upsetting to a practitioner than being unable to help a patient. When this occurs, it is natural for the patient to seek other opinions, often from practitioners working in different medical fields. Please be wary of practitioners offering cures for difficult problems. Ask for the evidence! There is no point wasting time, energy and money in the hope that something might happen.

In the past few years, there has been a strong move in traditional medicine to base all treatments on well-founded medical evidence. This has not always been the case. This strategy for medical care is termed 'evidence based medicine' and this subject is covered in detail in Appendix 2.

The fact that there is more money for research in areas of traditional medicine gives it a research advantage over some other areas of health care. However, the onus is on all practitioners to justify their treatments. Treatments should not be based on poorly conducted research or assumptions/unproven beliefs. Such beliefs can be long held and may sound reasonable but if they haven't been proven, be careful. Treatments based on the past experience of a single practitioner are not good enough in modern medicine. Practitioners using unsubstantiated treatments are really just experimenting on patients. Remember: if you are in doubt about a treatment, ask more questions. It is your right.

The best place to access medical information and advice based on quality evidence is the Cochrane Institute. Information regarding a multitude of health topics can be gained from its consumer oriented site at: www.cochraneconsumer.com

Those wishing even more detailed information can visit the Cochrane Library itself at: www.cochranelibrary.com

Medication labels

All medications should be properly labelled with an accurate description of the contents. If it is good enough for all our food products to have their contents disclosed, it is good enough for our medications as well.

In the case of medications provided directly by the health professional rather than a pharmacist, it is worthwhile asking about their source. Can the practitioner 'guarantee' the reliability of the source and the contents? This is very important in areas such as herbal medicines as regulations are far less strict and there is thus more room for medication error or dosage inaccuracy.

Part 2

Mental health

Functioning in our society

Relationships—an integral part of mental health

Relationships in Australia today are far more diverse than they were 30 years ago and include a complicated mix of conventional marriages, defacto relationships and gay and lesbian relationships. While each group has its own unique characteristics and problems, it is true to say that the behaviours that encourage successful relationships are similar in all. The statistics and information presented in this section regarding relationship breakdowns and how to avoid them were compiled from studies of heterosexual couples. However, much of the advice is general in nature and applies for many homosexual relationships also.

Gay and lesbian relationships do have some unique problems to deal with, such as discrimination, lack of social supports, recognition issues for non-biological parents and, in some cases, isolation from family and friends. Those wishing information specific to maintaining and improving their gay or lesbian relationship should consult the references mentioned at the end of this section. There is also helpful reading material for heterosexual couples.

Accessing counselling

People often delay addressing relationship problems because they do not know how to access good quality counselling. There are numerous counselling services operating in Australia. Here are some suggestions:

Local community health services

Counsellors associated with community health services can be accessed by phoning the health service (or mental health service) in your area. If you can't find the number, your GP or local hospital should be able to help.

Psychologists in private practice

To ensure that you access a well-qualified psychologist, try to find a member of the Australian Psychological Society. (Members are well qualified to help in relationship counselling and in the treatment of mental health problems such as anxiety, depression, eating disorders, etc.) All members have a degree in psychology; full members have a minimum of six years training and associate members have at least four years. Your GP will probably have psychologists that he/she deals with regularly and can recommend. The Australian Psychological Society operates a service throughout Australia to help you find a suitable counsellor in your area. (They also have lists of psychologists able to speak languages in addition to English.)

Relationships Australia

Relationships Australia operates counselling services, including telephone and face to face counselling. Its counsellors have qualifications in family or couple therapy and past experience in counselling. There are 88 branches throughout Australia.

Relationships Australia also runs short group programs (about 4 to 8 sessions each) on various relationship issues. Topics include pre-marriage issues, building better relationships, managing conflict, couple communication, step families, self esteem and after separation.

Gay and lesbian counselling services

Gay and Lesbian Counselling and Community Services of Australia offers telephone counselling for gay and lesbian relationship and sexuality issues and can organise face-to-face counselling. Branches are located in each state except the Northern Territory and Tasmania. (This service's website details other suitable contacts in these areas.)

Most trained psychologists are also well qualified to provide help on gay and lesbian issues.

Your general practitioner

Many GPs have excellent counselling skills and often have the advantage of knowing the person or couple well already. For people needing more specialised help, GPs are usually in a good position to know the best psychologists practising in their area.

The importance of relationships

> 'More marriages might survive longer if the partners realized that sometimes the better comes after the worse.'
>
> Doug Larson

Having a good relationship with your partner is probably the most influential factor contributing to happiness and satisfaction in your life. It is also associated with feeling healthier, especially with respect to reduced stress levels, and provides a vital learning experience for your children and others around you.

With this in mind, the consequences of the 40 per cent failure rate of Australian marriages (and even more in defacto relationships) present a major social problem in modern life. Between 1990 and 2000, the proportion of divorced people in Australia rose by a staggering 63 per cent, with over 1.1 million Australians being divorced in 2000. Those involved suffer enormous emotional and financial hardship and it generally takes about two to three years for the couple to start re-establishing their lives.

Many would argue that those involved in relationships that break up are often incompatible and that the stress involved in breaking up is 'for the best' in the long run. This is undoubtedly true for many couples, especially those where abusive behaviour was present in the relationship. However, for many others, the evidence does not support this view. A survey conducted in 2001 by Relationships Australia showed that divorced/separated people were the least satisfied with their lives (38 per cent). On the other hand, people in long-term relationships (married/de facto) were found to be the most satisfied group (70 per cent).

Many people who separate from their partners regret their actions later. About 37 per cent of divorced people regret their divorce five years later and 40 per cent feel that their divorce could have been avoided. Many people in long-lasting relationships note that difficult periods are often transient. A difficult period is not necessarily a one-way street and making the effort to survive these periods can strengthen the bond between couples.

Successfully unearthing a second lifetime partner is also not that easy. Twice as many second marriages (66 per cent) break up as first marriages (33 per cent) and figures from 1994 show that these broken marriages lasted only an average of five years (Australian Social Trends 1999).

Thus, it is definitely worth examining preventative measures that can help or even save your relationship. Remember, your relationship is probably your most important asset. It is an integral part of who you are.

Who is at greatest risk of divorce/separation?

Breakdowns mostly occur early in relationships, with 43 per cent of divorces occurring in the first ten years of marriage. In marriages that end in divorce, the average length of time before separation is about eight to nine years. (Actual divorce occurs on average about three years later.) (Qu 2001). The 20 to 35 year age group is at greatest risk. There are several factors that indicate a relationship is in trouble. These include:

- Abandonment of shared activities and channelling energies towards interests outside the relationship.
- Recurring arguments that are never resolved.
- Feelings of dissatisfaction and unhappiness.
- Complaints of loss of affection.
- An affair.
- Problems at work.
- Substance abuse, especially alcohol.
- Domestic violence. Physical violence should never be tolerated and if you are a victim, you need to seek immediate help. As well as physical violence or sexual assault, domestic violence includes threatening or intimidating behaviour, verbal or psychological abuse, using children to manipulate the relationship, and the isolation of a partner by restricting activities or access to family and friends. As many as 10 per cent of women in relationships experience persistent emotional, physical or sexual abuse from their partner.

If you would like to gauge the health of your relationship, try doing the Relationship Australia relationship quiz. It can be accessed via the internet at: www.relationships.com.au/utilities/quiz/rate.htm

How you can improve your relationship

> 'Success in marriage is more than finding the right person. It is becoming the right person.'
>
> Anon.

Figure 2 shows the results of a recent survey conducted by Relationships Australia where Australians were asked to identify the principal issues that contribute negatively to their relationships. The rest of this section looks at these issues with a view to identifying ways to help your relationship. Remember, all relationships can be improved.

TIME TOGETHER

Lack of time spent together is a major factor harming relationships and is especially a problem in the 25 to 40 year age group. Allocating times each week to spend alone with each other can help reduce this problem, as can ensuring you encourage shared activities you both enjoy. Try resurrecting past common interests and developing new ones, especially those that can be continued throughout your lives together. In the end, finding more time is all about reviewing your priorities, and your relationship with your partner should be a major one.

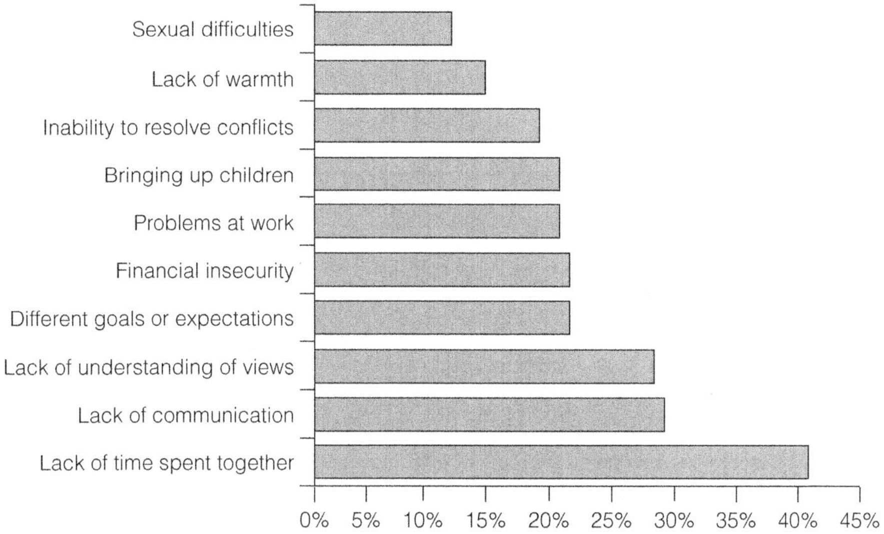

Source: Relationships Australia Incorporated, Survey 2001.

Figure 2 Aspects negatively influencing relationships

COMMUNICATION, UNDERSTANDING AND RESPECT

Communication is not something that comes naturally to many people and learning how to communicate well can help all aspects of your life. The following information can help.

Time: Part of your time spent alone together should be specifically allocated to communication. There will be topics every week that need to be addressed, such as issues relating to household duties, finances, children, planning activities, work, sex, family and friends.

Be happy to take the first step: Someone has to start the communication process and often your partner will be only too happy to participate. If you are not used to communicating regularly, be prepared to take things slowly at first but don't give up.

Become an attentive listener: Contrary to popular opinion, people do not instinctively know what their partner feels or is thinking. You need to listen carefully to your partner's views and respect them; there may be an issue you have not considered. Try not to be judgmental and make sure you are not twisting intended meanings towards your own views. If you find you are reacting aggressively, make sure you have not misunderstood what your partner has said. Good listening habits include: outwardly showing you are interested, such as by the use of hand gestures; sitting or standing at the same level as your partner and keeping relaxed eye contact; not fidgeting or doing other things while listening; and ensuring there are a minimum of other distractions about.

Express your views clearly: You need to make sure your views and feelings are expressed clearly and honestly and that they are understood and respected. Do not be afraid to tell your partner when you are unhappy about something. Remember, it is not just what you say, but how you say it and the body language you are using. The feelings you convey when speaking need to match your words. If you want to say something important, make sure you are looking at your partner directly, not wandering about.

Talk about your needs: Talk about what you want rather than what your partner should do. Use 'I would like' type statements. This will make your partner feel less threatened and reduce the likelihood of a defensive or aggressive reaction to your views.

Negotiate: You are in a partnership and an essential element of any partnership is compromise. You cannot have your own way all the time and need to find solutions that suit you both. Willingness to put your partner before yourself is strongly related to success in relationships, and practice at successfully achieving compromise will help when more difficult issues arise.

Be positive and don't complain excessively: Focusing on the positives in your relationship is integral to its success, with research showing that one positive act in a marriage can compensate for five negative acts (Parker 2001). Continued criticism just leads to contempt and defensiveness. A positive attitude is not possible if you always talk about problems when you are communicating. Spend time talking about your successes. Try to let trivial problems pass without mention. You should keep in mind the old saying, 'Change what you can, leave what you can't, and be wise enough to know the difference'. Also, try not to bring up old controversial issues that have already been dealt with. Concentrate on issues facing you now.

ENCOURAGE BEHAVIOURS THAT ARE GOOD FOR YOUR RELATIONSHIP

Don't be afraid to ask your partner for help: Gaining assistance helps you, and providing help will give your partner a great self-esteem boost. Showing you trust your partner also improves the respect you have for each other.

Share both the loads and the treats in your relationship: Hopefully everyone tries to share the work in the relationship, but make sure you also share the good things that you both like to do too, such as activities with your children.

Show appreciation for all kindness: Most people are appreciative of special actions, but try to occasionally show appreciation for the ones that are part of everyday life and taken for granted.

Try to do several special kind acts each week: This can be for your partner, your friends or your workmates. Think of it before going to bed. Write down your ideas for kind acts in a book so you can remember them for subsequent occasions. Your children should also be encouraged to do kind acts for their friends or teachers.

Make sure you give yourself some time: This should include time for rest and time for the odd thing you like to do by yourself.

Spend time welcoming and saying goodbye to your partner: When leaving or returning home, take a few minutes to talk to each other. Discuss the day's events and show empathy with problems that have arisen.

Rewards: Make an effort to reward yourselves when a difficult problem in your relationship has been resolved to your mutual satisfaction or when a plan you both devised to help your family has worked.

What are the qualities that maintain a healthy relationship?

- Supporting and respecting your partner.
- An ability to change and adapt to change.
- Accepting that some things cannot be changed (compromise). Don't expect perfection.
- A long-term commitment to the relationship and valuing the effort that maintaining a long-term relationship requires.
- Trust, honesty and fidelity.
- Shared values and interests.
- Balance in the relationship.
- Good sexual relations.

Difficult problems

Most relationships will have specific problem areas when it comes to communicating. These usually relate to matters where compromise cannot be reached or to behaviours or characteristics of your partner that make you unhappy. When this occurs, try to elaborate further on the issues involved. This will help ensure both your partner's and your views are not being misinterpreted and may also help you tease out hidden issues your partner might have difficulty discussing. Remember, these problems may have their source in unhappy past experiences and will often need to be handled delicately.

Sometimes trying new ways of communicating and problem-solving can help. Changing your usual communication situations may provide opportunities that are more conducive to achieving compromise or revealing hidden issues. This process may need the help of a counsellor.

Conflict without anger

Conflicting views are part of every relationship. They cannot and should not be avoided. If they are, it usually results in the problems remaining unresolved; they are left to 'fester inside'. What needs to be avoided is the hurt that can occur through expressing anger. Rather than acting angry by yelling etc., try saying you are angry. Try to talk about yourself and avoid using accusing statements that will make your partner feel threatened and want to retaliate. Rather, describe the feelings your partner's actions/views have brought about in you, such as sadness, neglect or disappointment.

If you or your partner are feeling too angry to discuss the problem reasonably, leave it until you have both calmed down; but don't avoid it.

If your partner is the one who is angry, try not to retaliate. Hear them out and acknowledge their feelings. Showing that you are taking your partner's feelings seriously will help calm him/her down, allowing the problem to be addressed reasonably.

Remember that physical violence is never acceptable and help should be sought immediately should this occur. Physical violence rarely occurs as an isolated event.

The art of ageing well—self-worth and achievement

> 'Successful ageing means giving to others joyously whenever we are able, receiving from others gratefully whenever one needs it, and being greedy enough to develop one's own self in between.'
>
> George Vaillant, 2002

Following the advice about disease prevention in this book will allow you to live longer. However, this does not necessarily mean you will age successfully. To age successfully you must live well in addition to living long. Part of living well is being free from physical disability and this book provides the recipe for achieving this. The other, more difficult part is being happy. While happiness is a very complex and individual concept, there are some general truths which are worth discussing.

Ageing is a combination of the benefits of maturity and the problem of increasing decay that leads to death. To be happy as you age, you need to maximise the first and achieve an acceptance of the second.

Maximising the benefits of maturity

> 'You can only perceive real beauty in a person as they get older.'
>
> Anouk Aimee (1932–)

In order to maximise maturity, you need to have a concept of what it is. George Vaillant in his illuminating book, *Ageing Well,* states there are six stages adults who 'age well' go through.

- Achieving your own identity.
- Learning to intimately love and live with another person.
- Achieving competence in your chosen vocation(s).
- Guiding the next generation.
- Preserving the meaning in your life, such as ethnic customs or the environment.
- Integrity in older age.

The first three goals are essentially aimed at establishing who you are. Necessarily, they are mainly self-centred in nature, and to maintain a well-balanced life, it is important they are approached in an altruistic manner by being considerate and helpful to those around you and by also pursuing activities that help others. A common problem in modern society is the single-minded pursuit of work-related, financial goals at the expense of developing and expanding relationships with partners, family and friends, and helping the general community.

Once you have successfully attained the above, you begin to lose the need for achievement and start to move away from these self-centred pursuits. You increasingly focus on helping others and share the wisdom you have gained through your years of experience. The more successful you are in mastering the initial three stages, the richer your range of experiences will be and the more you will be able to give to others. Thus, you start to guide the next generations, the people who will outlive you.

For many people, this process is initiated with the upbringing of children. One of the most important legacies you can leave is a family that has been loved and well supported. This caring process then leaves the home and spreads out to include assisting in the general community and at work, perhaps as an educator, a consultant or a coach. The handing down of knowledge and experience is an integral part of leadership roles that mature adults take on, both at work and in community organisations. For example, players become coaches or administrators in their sport.

Finally, the process evolves further into the role of preserving those things you have found important in your life. This often involves fundamental truths about your work and the world around you. Subjects that come to mind include environmental issues, your own family history, cultural traditions, ethical concepts such as freedom and equality, or important long-term issues associated with your vocation. Work in these areas is often done gratuitously and is thus ideally suited to those who have retired and have reduced monetary requirements. That is, people whose children have become self-supporting.

Confronting the process of decay—being positive

The final stage in adult maturity is 'integrity', which basically deals with how you confront the process of decay. This is a difficult task and one that gets progressively harder. Your ability to successfully address this task will depend on maintaining a positive attitude and using the resources you have developed during your life. There are many things to be positive about in old age.

You got there: The first and perhaps the most important positive aspect is that you got there. You should be proud of the achievements in your life; the person you are. Seeing older people who are happy and contented with their lifetime achievements is one of the best examples children, grandchildren and great grandchildren can be shown.

Activities: Continuing to be involved in activities and community causes which you enjoy or feel are important provides motivation for yourself and sets a great example once again for those younger than yourself. It is never too late to learn or to contribute.

Family and friends: Enjoying the company of your partner and friends is one of the great joys of old age. Making and keeping as many friends as possible should be a priority throughout your life. They will be a more important asset than your financial wealth. Make sure you remain active in your family and friendships and help where you can. With the majority of families having both parents in the workforce, minding the grandchildren can be a real help, both logistically and financially, to your children. There will also be many opportunities to assist friends. It is best to remember that care can go both ways in old age. Be prepared to give joyously and accept graciously.

Dignity in death: Finally, showing dignity in very old age and in death is once again a very good example for those younger than yourself.

Hindrances to successfully achieving adult maturity

The main hindrances to ageing well relate to mental rather than physical disease. Alcohol is a major cause of social problems in our community and its abuse compromises the lives of both problem drinkers and their families. Everyone who consumes alcohol, about 80 per cent of the population, needs to be informed about reducing harm associated with alcohol use. If you consume alcohol, please read the 'Alcohol use and abuse' section.

Having a positive attitude to life in general is a huge advantage in dealing with problems that inevitably arise. People with depression find adopting such an attitude difficult for much of the time. There are, however, methods of changing your thinking patterns if you are a 'half empty' rather than 'half full' person and these are outlined in the 'Mental illness' section. The major stumbling block is recognising the problem in the first place, with about 50 per cent of depressed people remaining undiagnosed. As 20 per cent of people will have at least one significant depressive episode in their life, everyone needs to become familiar with the signs and symptoms of depression.

Poor coping mechanisms are commonly used in adolescence to deal with problems. With time, most people learn better alternatives. Those people who continue using these immature coping mechanisms are less able to deal constructively with life's problems. Their natural development of a mature personality, as outlined in the section above, is stunted and their value to their family and their community is reduced. These poor coping mechanisms, such as always expecting the worst scenario, are also termed automatic negative thoughts and are discussed in the following chapter on 'Mental illness'.

Aids to successfully achieving adult maturity

> 'Only a life lived for others is a life worthwhile.'
>
> Albert Einstein (1879–1955)

Probably the most important aid to successful ageing is having a loving partner. The realisation that another person can accept and love you as you are is one of the strongest sources of self-esteem obtainable and the mutual support that such a relationship provides is of great assistance in getting through life's problems. Nourishing a warm extended family and network of friends provides similar benefits. Also of great significance is having a sense of meaning or purpose in life. Clear life goals, being dedicated to a cause, having values that transcend personal benefit, and possessing strong religious beliefs are a few of the attributes that provide such meaning.

Looking after yourself physically, including eating well, being physically active and not smoking, has numerous psychological as well as physical benefits.

While all coping mechanisms help deal with problems in the short term, the development and use of mature coping mechanisms helps deal with the problems constructively and is beneficial to your character in the long term. Some examples of good coping mechanisms include the following:

- Redirecting negative feelings to a problem you have endured so that they can be used in socially constructive or creative ways, such as preventing similar problems happening to others or helping others cope with similar experiences. An example would be helping counsel people with an illness that you also suffer from.

- Anticipating the problems associated with an unpleasant event so that you are prepared for them.
- Taking an appropriately positive attitude towards solving a problem rather than looking only at the negatives involved.

Finally, it is worth noting that, as long as basic needs can be comfortably met, wealth has little effect on happiness and ageing well.

Can you change the way you are?

There has been considerable debate over the years as to whether a person's nature can be fundamentally changed. The truth is probably that some aspects can and some can't. George Vaillant states that personality is the sum of two components—temperament and character. Temperament, which includes such factors as degree of extroversion and intelligence, is the component that tends to be constant. Shy children tend to become shy adults. Your character, on the other hand, does change.

Character is defined as the way you respond to life's challenges and it is profoundly affected by environment and maturity. Experience provides you with a greater variety of possible responses to challenges. Repeated exposure usually reduces the likelihood that you will be frightened or intimidated by a particular situation, and thus it permits more constructive responses to that situation. Such change can occur naturally as part of the normal maturing process. Individuals with psychological problems, including anxiety and depression, can be helped by therapy, especially regarding poor coping mechanisms. (See the following chapter on mental illness.)

Adolescent risk-taking

> 'I've never understood why people consider youth a time of freedom and joy. It's probably because they have forgotten their own.'
>
> Margaret Attwood (1939–)

Experiences, both good and bad, are the way we develop as a person. Identity cannot be gained from a book. Risk-taking is an integral part of this process. It starts in adolescence and continues throughout our adult lives. The reasons this process presents a problem in adolescence are twofold.

Firstly, adolescents have little experience in risk-taking and it is not easy for them to choose wisely. They cannot always sort out those risks worth taking, those that will help their development into a more capable and self-confident adult, from those that provide no such benefits. The second is that, although adolescents are still under the control of their parents, it is the time that parental influence is gradually being replaced by self-determination. This is a difficult adjustment for parents as they know they need to let go but they still feel they are responsible for all that happens to their child. If something goes wrong, not only does the parent suffer because their child is injured in some way, they feel guilty about it as well! Thus parents restrict, usually quite appropriately, their adolescent's behaviour. While setting limits is an important part of preventing inappropriate risk-taking and can act as a positive learning experience for the adolescent, the other outcome is the normal tension that develops between the adolescents and their parents.

In adolescence there are two types of risks. There are risks worth taking, those that help development of personality and add opportunity to life. These are often referred to as challenges. Good examples of constructive risk-taking include accepting the risk of possible failure, such as when taking on new activities or when performing a difficult task in front of one's peers, and making important life decisions, such as subject and career choices. Another is performing activities where the risk of physical injury is combined with the rewards of achievement and acquiring new skills that may be useful as a lifetime career or interest. These activities include contact sports or activities such as horseriding. Extremely adventurous adolescents may even take up activities such as mountaineering (under expert supervision). Mrs Hilary almost certainly had some anxious moments when her son was on top of Mt Everest, but she probably accepted over the years that such worry was part of being Sir Edmund's mother, and the knighthood was probably some compensation.

Other risks, however, have no overall benefit with regard to personality development and present the chance of harm to both the adolescent involved and those in his/her immediate peer group. These are the activities that all parents fear: illicit drug use, alcohol abuse, dangerous driving practices, unsafe sexual practices etc. Males are significantly more likely to partake in these behaviours, with those who tend to act impulsively and have poor self-esteem, depression and inadequate social skills being at greatest risk.

Preventing deleterious risk-taking

If all adolescents need to take risks, albeit to differing degrees, how can parents and teachers direct this need into constructive challenging alternatives? Here are some ideas.

Set a good example: This is a great start. If you are a constructive risk-taker, your children have the opportunity to watch you and learn. (Sir Edmund Hilary's son Peter also climbed Everest.) If you are a person who drinks and drives, they will also learn that type of behaviour. If you don't take any risks at all, your children will have to learn risk-taking skills by themselves or from someone else. Ensuring your children are brought up to consider the moral implications of adult decisions will help them make the correct choices later on. Discuss with them the moral implications of the important decisions you make and let them be part of family decision making. It's good practice.

Provide constructive risk-taking options: Adults need to make sure the adolescents they are responsible for have constructive risk-taking opportunities available to them. If they are not available, then there is a greater chance of detrimental alternatives being adopted. Try to find out what activities are available at their school. Encourage activities in primary school that can become a real challenge in adolescence. Adolescents are often reticent to act on suggestions, so it is not enough just to mention alternatives. Try introducing them to new activities on a family holiday or find out what activities their friends are doing and encourage those. Getting them involved in as many activities as possible, especially sport, leaves less time and energy for poor risk-taking activities. If a chosen activity involves the risk of physical injury, adults can help by finding the safest environment in which their child can participate. Finally, unhealthy activities, such as driving too quickly, can be turned into 'healthier' hobbies, such as professional racing.

Being there: Just being around and knowing what is going on in your adolescent's life is very important. You should know, as much as possible, where they are and who they are with. Try to keep a close eye on your adolescent's peer group as it is often the source of detrimental risk-taking activities. Encourage your children's friends to visit your home as often as possible, offer to take them to activities, and keep in regular contact with their parents. Most children expect and benefit from limits set for them, even if they don't tell you. When a problem has occurred because of an adolescent's risk-taking, make sure you discuss the issues involved with them without being condescending and saying, 'I told you so'. It will help them learn from the experience. You can even talk about similar mistakes you made.

Education: Both at home and at school, education is important in preventing risk-taking. Parents need to ensure their children gain appropriate information and understand this information. Sex education is a prime example. Be prepared to talk frankly with them about the consequences of their actions and never assume that a particular topic is not your concern because it will be covered in school.

The consequences of several risk-taking behaviours are mentioned in the sections on alcohol abuse and illicit drug use, and teenage pregnancy.

Preventing teenage pregnancy

> 'Contraceptives should be used on every conceivable occasion.'
>
> Spike Milligan (1918–2001)

By year 12 at school, about 50 per cent of males and females have had sex. Teenage pregnancy is a very important health issue in Australia with the potential to cause much long-term emotional suffering. Teenage parents are more likely to suffer from mental health problems. Teenage mothers experience three times the usual incidence of post-natal depression. They also have to deal with social problems that are the result of reduced opportunities for education and work, and a reduced standard of living. Further, a termination of a pregnancy can also be associated with significant emotional/mental health problems.

The rate of teenage pregnancy was 44 per 1000 teenagers per year in the year 1999 (i.e. 29 000 pregnancies). Overall about 30 per cent of Australian women will become pregnant in their teenage years. About 53 per cent of these end in termination. This termination rate of 24 per 1000 is one of the highest in the world and does not compare favourably with many other developed countries. Germany has a rate of about 3 per 1000. Of those giving birth, 90 per cent are unmarried and 60 per cent have no male partner.

With all this in mind, it will come as no surprise to learn that Australia, unlike many other developed countries, has no major teenage pregnancy prevention initiative. Until such a program exists, it is up to individual families and schools to educate their teenagers regarding the risks of pregnancy. Do not pretend the problem will not affect your family.

There is insufficient room in this book to provide extensive information regarding the many issues involved in pregnancy prevention. Details regarding this information can be sourced from your GP or perhaps your school. The information provided to adolescents should include the following:

- Accurate information about the risks of not using contraception. (About 50 per cent of first time intercourse occurs without contraception.) Issues that need to be addressed include pregnancy and sexually transmitted diseases. It needs to be emphasised that protection against becoming pregnant is not enough. Unless the couple is in a long-term relationship, barrier methods of contraception (usually condoms) need to be used with all intercourse to prevent infection with potentially dangerous diseases such as HIV/AIDS, herpes and chlamydia. One major problem is that many young couples give up condom use after a relatively short sexual relationship, sometimes as short as three weeks. Before stopping barrier protection, partners should consider being screened for common diseases, such as chlamydia. To make the cost and inconvenience of such screening worthwhile, condom use for much longer than three weeks is highly recommended.
- The provision of adequate access to contraception (in addition to condoms). This should include information about emergency contraception.
- Education about the issues involved in giving birth and bringing up children when young. (Interestingly, recent research has shown that some teenagers have little insight into the above issues and don't use contraception because they don't mind the idea of pregnancy.)
- Education about the importance of having a long-term partner to help with the child's upbringing.

- Measures to reduce the incidence of unwanted sexual activity, such as refusal skills and skills to prevent date rape. This should include education about the association of alcohol and other drug use with unprotected sexual activity and subsequent regret about sexual activity.

Sleep and tiredness

> 'Sleeping is no mean art; it is necessary to stay awake for it all day.'
>
> Friedrich Nietzsche

Sleep is a necessary period of rest and recuperation for the body that is regulated by your brain according to day–night cycles. There is no correct amount of sleep. The important issue is how you feel about the quality of your sleep during the night and whether you are tired the next day. Most people need about seven to eight hours sleep. The amount of sleep you need tends to decrease with age, with six hours being common among the elderly.

Problems associated with sleep deprivation include daytime sleepiness, fatigue, poor memory, poor concentration, delayed reaction time, irritability and mood changes. In short, your relationships and work suffer and you are at greater risk of accidental injury. Fatigue-related workplace accidents cost Australia $1 billion a year and 20 to 30 per cent of motor vehicle accidents are due to fatigue.

There are many causes of feeling excessively sleepy or tired including:

- Insomnia (poor sleep)—by far the most important cause and it is discussed further in this chapter.
- Mental illness including depression and anxiety, which are common causes of insomnia and tiredness.
- Drugs and medications—those causing most problems are alcohol, caffeine and antihistamines (sedating types).
- Medical problems, including an under-active thyroid, nocturnal asthma, chronic pain, anaemia etc.
- Shift work.
- Environmental factors, such as disruptions from other family members (crying babies) or neighbours, or a poor sleeping environment (too light, hot, noisy etc.).
- Other sleep disorders including sleep apnoea (a common problem, especially in men over 30 and in the obese), restless legs syndrome (where irritation is felt in the legs, especially the calves, and the person feels they have to regularly move their legs), and rare sleep disorders, including sleep walking and narcolepsy (a disorder where extreme tiredness causes involuntary napping during the day).

Many people with tiredness due to insomnia can be helped by improving their sleeping habits. However, if you have long-standing problems with tiredness, you will probably require help to exclude any underlying medical cause and gain assistance with techniques that will help improve your sleep. Your best sources of help are your GP or a clinical psychologist. (Your GP can probably recommend one. If not, contact the Australian Psychological Association or a specialist sleep clinic. These are usually attached to hospitals.) Specifically, you should get help when:

- sleeping problems are long-standing
- tiredness is interfering with work or home life
- you have had or almost had an accident or injury due to tiredness
- your tiredness is associated with excessive snoring, indicating that sleep apnoea may be a problem
- sleeping problems are associated with mood changes or other symptoms of depression/anxiety—early morning waking is common in depression
- pain or other medical symptoms, such as cough or shortness of breath, are the cause of your insomnia
- prescription medications are interfering with your sleep.

Insomnia

Insomnia is a common problem, regularly affecting 33 per cent of people from time to time and most people occasionally. Insomnia can be either short or long term. Short-term insomnia is usually associated with a specific cause, such as a stressful event, an illness, overseas travel, or taking stimulants, such as coffee. Chronic insomnia occurs when the problem persists for longer than one month. Most people (about 80 per cent) with chronic sleep problems have problems that result from worrying, either about problems they have in their lives or just about the fact that they can't sleep. This leads to anxiety and thoughts which can't be turned off at bed time, often racing about in the person's mind.

One reason that insomnia is so common is that it is not given adequate priority in people's lives. Sleep needs to be viewed positively as it is an integral part of preparing you for each day's activity.

Improving your sleep

Achieving a good night's sleep involves developing good sleeping habits and a regular sleeping routine. If you suffer from insomnia, successful treatment will require time and effort on your part to achieve these aims. Once you have adopted better sleeping habits, it takes about four to six weeks for noticeable improvements to occur. During this time you should try not to judge your sleep on a night-to-night basis. It will just make you worry more. Below is a plan to help you improve your sleeping problems.

1. Leading a healthy lifestyle is an important part of sleeping well. This includes eating well and exercising during the day. A good time to exercise is in the early morning sunlight as it helps strengthen normal sleep rhythms. Exercise before bedtime should be avoided as it can make you more alert. Also, avoid having large meals close to bedtime. You should cut down your general level of smoking and alcohol consumption. (To nil for cigarettes!)
2. Try to establish a regular sleeping routine, where you go to sleep and wake up at about the same time each day. This includes weekends.
3. Avoid sleeping in, even if you have had a bad night's sleep.
4. Do not take naps during the day. Stocking up on sleep in preparation for a late night does not help.
5. Avoid stimulants, such as drinks and foods containing caffeine (coffee, tea, caffeinated soft drinks and chocolate), cigarettes and alcohol, in the late afternoon and evening. Caffeine also makes you pass urine more often and this may make you wake up. If you try to reduce your total daily caffeine intake, do it slowly as a sudden withdrawal can cause symptoms such as headache, irritability and tiredness.
6. Avoid taking any fluids after dinner as the need to go to the toilet may wake you during the night. It is also useful to make going to the toilet part of your 'going to bed' routine.
7. Sort out your problems and your schedule for the following day well before going to sleep. You should not have to plan for tomorrow with your head on the pillow.
8. Ensure you have a good sleeping environment that is quiet, dark and well ventilated.
9. Try to establish a 'going to bed' routine. Make the time immediately before going to bed relaxing by doing a relaxing activity, such as having a bath, meditating or listening to relaxing music. Try not to read an exciting book or watch a stimulating TV program.
10. Go to bed only when you feel sleepy and when your partner is ready for bed. This may mean going to bed later.
11. Activities done in bed should be restricted to sleep and sex. Do not watch TV in bed and you should also avoid reading in bed (especially work-related reading). It is also best not to read or work in bed during the day.
12. A common problem is that people keep themselves awake worrying about their sleep. If you can't get to sleep in roughly 20 minutes, get up, go into another room and do something relaxing until you feel sleepy again.
13. Finally, you should avoid judging your sleep on a day-to-day basis.

For most people, adopting the above measures will be enough to cure their sleeping problem. However, if after giving the above plan a genuine try you are still having problems, there are likely to be other issues in your life that you need to deal with. The most important of these is worry/stress. Solving these problems can be a more difficult task which is likely to require the assistance of a doctor or psychologist, especially if the problem has existed for a long time.

Techniques often used to reduce stressful thoughts include relaxation techniques. Focusing on a relaxing image or phrase whenever you feel stressed can help and, if your body is tense, sit quietly and try to relax the affected muscle groups. This often involves the neck and head muscles. While doing either of the above, you should try to concentrate on slow but not deep breathing. These techniques are best learned with the help of a doctor or psychologist and should be practised four or five times a day as well as when you are feeling tense or anxious. They can then be used in bed when you feel stressed. Techniques, such as repeating a song in your head or even counting sheep, are effective in taking your mind off persistent thoughts. Thinking pleasant thoughts can have the same effect.

Stress can be due to committing yourself to an unrealistic amount of work/activities. As stated above, if you are going to solve your sleeping problems, they have to be made a significant priority in your life. For overcommitted people, this will mean prioritising your work/activities and then either delegating or deleting your less important work/activities. Another alternative is to become more efficient with your use of time if that is possible. Remember, working right up to the time you go to bed is a recipe for sleep problems.

Another technique used by therapists to help difficult cases of insomnia is sleep restriction therapy. This therapy actually restricts the time spent in bed by a small amount so that a greater percentage of time in bed is spent asleep. Sleep is restricted for a couple of weeks and then time in bed is gradually lengthened again, the whole process taking about four to six weeks. The wake-up time remains unchanged and time in bed should never be less than 5 hours. The aim is to promote rapid sleep onset and to achieve sleep for a minimum of 85 per cent of the time spent in bed.

Sleeping tablets

Sleeping tablets are not a solution for sleeping problems. They do not help in restoring good sleeping patterns or improve quality of life. They also increase the risk of both work-related and motor vehicle accidents and the risk of falls in the elderly.

Sleep apnoea

Sleep apnoea is an important cause of daytime tiredness, occurring in about 5 per cent of Australians. It is a condition where relaxation of throat and tongue muscles causes an obstruction in the throat above the voice box, resulting in regular episodes where the person stops breathing for short periods. Each time this happens, the brain wakes the person just enough so that the person takes a breath, often as a snort or a gasp. The person then falls back to sleep, usually unaware that they have woken. In this way, sleep is continually disrupted, sometimes up to hundreds of times, during the night.

The severity depends on the number of interruptions, with less than 5 per hour being normal and over 50 per hour indicating severe sleep apnoea. Snoring is a common symptom in people with sleep apnoea. Its presence in association with day-time tiredness suggests that sleep apnoea may be occuring and that investigation is needed. Physical indicators of sleep apnoea include structural abnormalities in the upper airway, a small mouth opening and obesity. (A waist measurement greater than 127cm or a neck/shirt measurement/size greater than 43cm indicate a high risk of sleep apnoea.) Men over 30 years of age are more commonly affected.

The tiredness and reduced nocturnal oxygen supply that sleep apnoea causes create numerous health problems, including a high incidence of motor vehicle and other accidents, intellectual impairment, memory loss, personality changes and cardiovascular problems such as abnormal heart rhythms, hypertension, coronary artery disease and heart failure.

The causes of sleep apnoea include:

- Excess weight—this is a very important cause and even a small weight loss can dramatically improve the problem.
- Alcohol, especially in the evening, causes the throat muscles to relax, worsening the problem.
- Conditions that block your upper airway, such as enlarged tonsils, nasal obstruction, or a large thyroid goitre.
- Medications, including sedatives and sleeping tablets.

Treatment includes weight loss, reducing alcohol consumption, machines that assist with breathing by providing continuous positive airways pressure (CPAP machines), mouth splints and, occasionally, surgery to correct upper airway blockages.

Stress

Stress will often be a factor in your life and can cause significant distress. It may come from home or work or any other activities that you undertake. If you become upset while under stress, learning how to manage it well will play an important part in making your life more successful and enjoyable.

With respect to achieving your goals for lifestyle improvement, the ability to cope with stress often determines whether you will relapse into detrimental old behaviours. For this reason, you should address the problem of coping with stress before you attempt other behavioural change, such as improving eating habits, and have a framework for addressing stress ready for when it occurs.

Coping with stress

Avoiding unnecessary stress is an important strategy. Try to anticipate problems that might occur while they are still avoidable and make sure you learn from your mistakes. Spend a little time each evening (not just before bed) to plan your activities for the following day. Scheduling your more stressful tasks for times when you are fresher and better able to cope, for example in the morning, can help considerably.

If your problem cannot be avoided, then take note of the age-old advice: change what you can, accept what you cannot, and be wise enough to know the difference! You will be wasting your time and effort worrying about problems that can't be changed or that would cause 'World War III' in doing so.

If you can't change the situation, then put it to one side and forget about it for the time being. Try to focus on the positive things that are happening in your life. The situation may change to your advantage later on. For example, some situations are stressful because you are unable to perform a required task as well as you would like. Further education and experience may enable you to approach the problem from a new perspective. If, on the other hand, you can change things for the better by facing the problem, then it is usually better to do so. Letting it simmer will only cause you more anxiety and often your worries about the outcome will have been exaggerated anyway.

Enlisting the help of others who are similarly affected by the problem, a common occurrence in work-related stress, can be of great assistance. The effects of stress can also be lessened by having family and friends close at hand to share your problem. As well as lending a sympathetic ear, they may be able to suggest alternative strategies to solve the problem. Do not take out your work stress on those at home. Talking about it is much better. Try to ensure you have time each day to talk with your partner.

Alcohol and other drugs are not a constructive way to cope with stress. Their effects on your personality can often make stress worse and they also worsen your self-esteem and resolve.

In the workplace (and most other places), communication is the main issue. If you manage people at work, ensure you make time to meet with them regularly to discuss any problems they are facing. It will improve workplace relations and assist in anticipating problems before they occur. Having a stress management policy and, if possible, a human relations manager, will assist in this process. Taking into account the personal lives of employees when deciding on hours of work, holidays etc. will make everyone happier.

WAYS TO FEEL BETTER WHEN STRESSED

Regular exercise helps reduce stress. It should be enough to get you a bit puffed and needs to be done several times a week. Equally important is relaxation time. Give yourself time to relax each day, especially with people whose company you enjoy and who make you feel good. Meditation and yoga are also often beneficial.

Everybody becomes more stressed when tired and a good sleep routine is an important part of stress management. Similarly, consuming nourishing food with lots of vegetables and fruit makes you feel well. Remember that caffeine-containing foods, such as coffee, chocolate, tea and caffeinated soft drinks, can cause stress symptoms, including agitation, palpitations and tremors. Alcohol should be avoided as a remedy for feeling stressed as there is a significant risk of drinking to excess and developing alcohol dependency.

Concentrating on the positive things in your life, such as activities that you enjoy and are good at, is also beneficial. Be helpful to those around you as this will increase your self-esteem.

Getting help

Stress that continues for too long can lead to chronic anxiety conditions and depression. If you are finding problems caused by stress are not resolving quickly, you are feeling stressed for no obvious reason, or you just cannot cope, you should see your GP (or other appropriate health professional) to obtain help. Everyone can benefit from treatment. However, the longer you leave the anxiety problem, the worse you will feel and the longer it will take you to improve with therapy. Anxiety disorders and depression are dealt with in the next chapter. Many of the comments regarding cognitive behavioural therapy for the treatment of anxiety and depression also apply to dealing with stress. And most people would benefit from learning about this therapy and applying it to the stresses in their live (see page 72).

Further reading

Relationships
D. Schnarch, *Passionate Marriage: Love, sex and intimacy in emotionally committed relationships*, W.W. Norton, 1997

H. Hendrix, *Getting the Love You Want: A guide for couples*, Pocket Books, 1993

John Gottman, *A Couple's Guide to Communication*, Research Press, 1976. (John Gottman has also published a more recent book called *The Seven Principles for Making Marriage Work*.)

D. Jansen & M. Newman, *Really Relating*, Random House, Sydney, 1989.

B. Montgomery & L. Evans, *Living and Loving Together*, Nelson, Melbourne, 1995.

Ageing well
George Valliant, *Ageing Well*, Scribe Publications, Melbourne, 2002.

Adolscent risk-taking
Dr Janet Hall, *Sexwise*, Random House, Sydney
What every young person and parent should know about sex. Dr Hall empowers her readers by telling them the facts and giving it to them straight.

Bronwyn Donaghy, *Unzipped*, HarperCollins, 2001
A book that deals frankly and sympathetically with the crucial role that love and emotions play in every aspect of adolescent sexuality.

For other books on puberty and adolescent sexuality see the Children's Hospital, Westmead, website at www.chw.edu.au/parents/books. Both books listed above are recommended by staff at the hospital.

Sleep and tiredness
T.J. Sharp, *The Good Sleep Guide*, Penguin Books, Ringwood, 2001

Stress
Sarah Edelman, *Change Your Thinking*, ABC Books, Sydney, 2002
A good book on cognitive behavioural therapy, a subject everyone should understand and put into practice.

Further information

Counsellors
Australian Psychological Society
Ph: 1800 333 497; website: www.aps.psychsociety.com.au

Relationships Australia
Ph: 1300 364 277; website: www.relationships.com.au

Gay and Lesbian Counselling and Community Services of Australia
Ph: 1800 184 527 (between 7.30 pm and 10 pm local time); website: www.glccs.org.au

Ageing well
National Ageing Research Centre
Ph: 03 8387 2148; website: www.nari.unimelb.edu.au

Adolescent risk-taking
The Resource Center for Adolescent Pregnancy Prevention
A good source from the United States that provides information and skills for both adolescents and educators about preventing unwanted teenage pregnancies.
website: www.etr.org/recapp.

Gay & Lesbian websites
www.glccftl.org/library/couples
www.buddybuddy.com

Mental illness

Of all the illnesses you may face, mental illness is probably the most debilitating. It has the potential to compromise your ability to achieve happiness and contentment, your ability to achieve your full potential in your home and work environments, and your ability to pursue the goals needed to achieve optimum physical health.

Approximately one million Australians (5 per cent) suffer from significant mental illness with 50 per cent of these being affected long term. With the inclusion of substance abuse (mainly alcohol), it accounts for about 20 per cent of Australia's disease burden. Figure 3 shows the incidence of mental illness by age in Australia.

Mental illness is primarily suffered by younger people, with the onset usually occurring in mid-to-late adolescence. The illnesses tend to become chronic, affecting future psychological development and compromising the most important and productive period of people's lives. The fact that people in this age group are responsible for the care of young children is especially important, as it means these children are adversely affected by their parents' mental illness. They are also likely to learn the inappropriate behaviours of their parents. For this reason, parental mental illness needs to be diagnosed and treated as early as possible. Parents need to be given all the support they can get from family members and friends, especially when they are exposed to the extra stress of bringing up very young children.

The major mental health problems in Australia are depression, anxiety disorders, schizophrenia and substance abuse, particularly alcohol. Mental illness is more common in

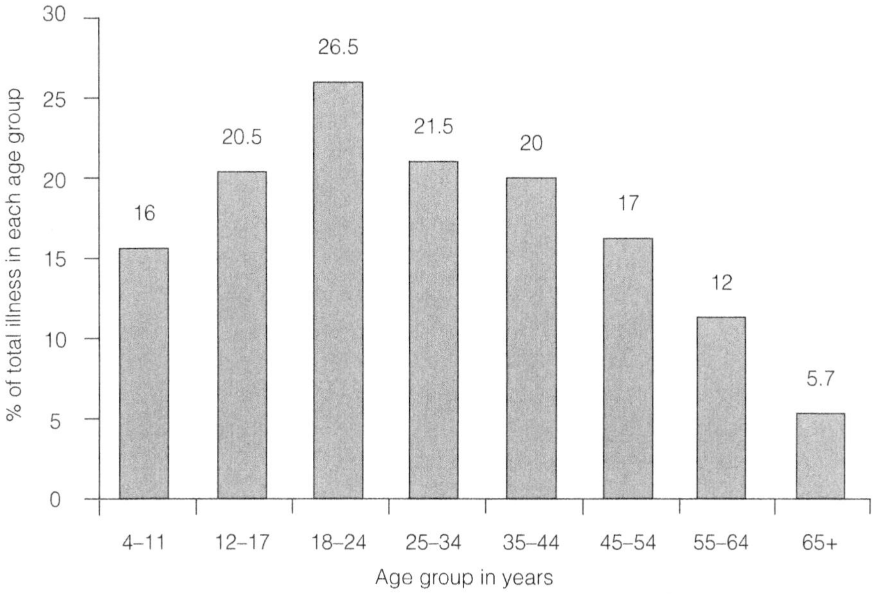

Source: Australian Institute of Health and Welfare 2000.

Figure 3 Age incidence of mental illness in Australia

people who are separated/divorced (25 per cent), in people who have not been married (over 20 per cent), in those living alone, and in those who are unemployed.

Of those chronically affected, only about 40 per cent seek help and receive treatment. If mental disease affects you or a close friend or relative, make sure you seek help from your family doctor or community mental health worker. Unfortunately, despite being such a huge health problem, only about 5 per cent of the Australian health budget is at present spent on mental illness. This means that treatment resources are sometimes 'thin on the ground' and makes the additional support that you, as a friend or relative, can provide vital in caring for the mentally ill.

Anxiety disorders

Anxiety is a normal response to a stressful life situation such as illness, job loss, relationship breakdown, imminent danger etc. At these times, it is normal to feel tense and irritable and sometimes even to panic. These feelings are often accompanied by physical symptoms such as palpitations, sweating, chest tightness, tremors, difficulty in breathing, hot and cold flushes, nausea, difficulty swallowing, diarrhoea, headaches and muscle tension.

Anxiety disorders, on the other hand, are associated with persistent feelings of high anxiety that are inappropriate for the person's situation and are significant enough to interfere with daily life activities. These disorders are common and affect about 5 per cent of the population at any one time. Like most mental illnesses, they are chronic in nature.

Anxiety symptoms usually develop during early childhood and anxiety conditions are at least as common in childhood as they are in adults. Up to 25 per cent of 8-year olds and 15 per cent of teenagers experience anxiety conditions. These children have a significantly increased likelihood of developing adolescent depression and substance/alcohol abuse, and they are much more likely to become anxious and depressed adults.

The exact cause of anxiety disorders is still unclear. However, in most cases there are both inherited and learned (environmental) components present. The learned component has mostly occurred by the time adulthood is reached. The good news is that there are many good programs for the management of anxiety which have strong evidence of their benefit. Stress management can also be learned in childhood by using programs such as FRIENDS (see page 66) and good parenting techniques.

There are various types of anxiety disorders.

Generalised anxiety: People with these disorders worry inappropriately about all manner of things, such as finances, health and relationships.

Agoraphobia: These people have a fear of places or situations that may trigger a panic attack or from which escape is difficult if a panic attack occurs. This is a very common disorder, especially in women, and is usually experienced in crowded situations, such as lifts or public transport. Hence sufferers often tend to stay at home.

Panic disorder: These people experience extreme panic attacks, often with the fear that they will lose control or even die.

Specific phobia: Sufferers are inappropriately fearful of a specific situation or thing, such as mice.

Social phobia: These people feel their character is flawed and that other people will think badly of them in some way. They fear public scrutiny and thus avoid social gatherings. It is a very common anxiety disorder.

Obsessive compulsive disorder: These people inappropriately worry about specific thoughts, such as cleanliness, and often develop rituals to placate these thoughts. These beliefs and rituals occur in a highly repetitive and stereotyped way.

Post-traumatic stress disorder: These people have unresolved anxiety associated with a particular traumatic event in their lives.

Separation anxiety disorder: This disorder occurs primarily in children. They focus on a fear of being separated from caregivers due to injury or illness. It is usually associated with a refusal to go to school, friends' homes etc.

Preventing and addressing anxiety disorders in children

As anxiety disorders (and the depressive disorders they are associated with) are often well established by late adolescence, the only realistic prevention strategy is to address the problem during childhood and adolescence.

Recognition and treatment of early symptoms in children is vital. Many children at increased risk of developing significant anxiety disorders can be identified early and treated effectively (Renner 2001). Children at increased risk of developing anxiety disorders include those that:

- are shy or withdrawn and have negative feelings, especially towards themselves
- show symptoms of depression
- have a family history of anxiety disorders
- have overprotective and overly critical parents with unrealistic expectations for their children
- have a predominantly 'negative' relationship with their parents
- have suffered from neglect.

Identifying anxious children is not always easy. They are often very well behaved at school and don't bother anyone. Thus they are often missed. They will often only show their fears by avoiding the situations that worry them, such as performing in public, participating in class discussions, or engaging in unfamiliar activities. This avoidance behaviour often occurs on Mondays or at the beginning of school terms and can include pretending to be sick, with headaches and stomach problems being common complaints.

At school, anxious children usually require constant reassurance, ask many unnecessary questions, and get upset when they make mistakes. Some are perfectionists with a pessimistic attitude to tasks, thinking they will never produce work that is good enough. They are often loners or have only a few friends. They may refrain from social activities, such as birthday parties, and have difficulty separating from parents. Problems with sleeping are not uncommon.

The best treatment for these children revolves around building their ability to cope with problems constructively and improving their self-esteem. Encouraging children to become self-reliant can be achieved by promoting the development of good problem-solving and social skills, increasing 'success experiences' by encouraging hobbies/interests, and providing opportunities for the child to become independent. Challenging fears in a step-wise fashion through exposure to graded anxiety-provoking situations is also helpful. All non-anxious behaviour should be rewarded.

Parental attitudes can significantly influence the anxiety levels of their children. Some attitudes that provide a good example for children have been previously mentioned but are worth repeating here. They are:

- planning for the future and maintaining a sense of purpose in the home
- developing trusting and loving family relationships
- maintaining an optimistic outlook when dealing with family problems
- maintaining a flexible outlook towards problem solving and trying to maintain control of the situation when solving problems
- showing how to learn from mistakes
- anticipating and planning ahead for stressful situations
- taking care of yourself and appreciating yourself, including keeping yourself healthy by exercising and eating well.

Parents with anxiety problems expose their children to inappropriate behaviours which the children can easily adopt. Treating these problems by improving the mental health of the parent and by increasing the parent's awareness about how their inappropriate behaviours may be influencing their children will help reduce this exposure. For example, it is not uncommon for anxious parents to actually reward anxious and avoidance behaviours in their children. Such interactions need to be identified and changed.

Where the child's (or parent's) anxiety problems are significant or not improving, help should be sought from a GP, school counsellor, or local community health centre. The Child and Adolescent Anxiety Clinic at Macquarie University in Sydney runs several anxiety treatment programs covering all child age groups and includes a home-based course, called COPA-K, for rural and remote families (including those from other states and overseas) with anxious children in the 6 to 12 age group. The courses run for about 12 weeks. (See Further Information on page 80.) The book *Helping Your Anxious Child* was written by staff at this unit and it is a very helpful resource. *Treating Anxious Children and Adolescents: An evidence-based approach* is a companion book for health professionals involved in the treatment of anxious children. There are also several school-based programs, including the FRIENDS program (see the box below), to help prevent anxiety in children.

The FRIENDS program

The FRIENDS program is an Australian-developed school-based program to help children cope with and manage anxiety and depression, both now and in later life. It is conducted by teachers and takes only ten class periods. The program aims to promote self-esteem, problem-solving skills, psychological resilience, self-expression, and positive relationships with peers and adults. It does not involve individual child assessment and does not discuss specific topics such as suicide, drug abuse, depression or violence.

For further information about the FRIENDS program and how to go about running it at your school, see the FRIENDS website at www.friendsinfo.net

Treating anxiety disorders in adults

The treatment for anxiety disorders is often similar to the treatment of depression. In many cases, the two conditions co-exist. The approach taken depends on the type of disorder present. Treatment in most cases involves a counsellor and uses a form of cognitive behavioural therapy. A brief outline of the principles of this therapy are given in the section on treating depression (pages 71–5). Antidepressant medications can also be of assistance in the treatment of anxiety cases.

CONTROLLING HYPERVENTILATION

An important aspect in the treatment of many anxious people is the control of the physical symptoms that occur when a person is in an anxiety provoking situation. The most frightening of these symptoms, including shortness of breath, chest tightness, light-headedness or feeling faint and tingling feelings in the hands and lips, are due to over-breathing or hyperventilation. The average person requires about 10 to 12 breaths of normal depth per minute. This normal breathing rate and depth increases when you are anxious, resulting in a reduction of the carbon dioxide level in your blood. This causes the above symptoms. Whilst this is not dangerous, it is frightening and acts to heighten the anxiety levels being felt, making the situation even worse.

Over-breathing can be identified by counting your breathing rate when you feel normal and comparing it to when you are anxious. The use of 'controlled breathing' helps avoid over-breathing. This technique is performed as follows.

1. Take a medium breath and hold for six seconds.
2. Exhale and say the word relaaaaaaaaaax to yourself calmly.
3. Breathe in and out slowly, taking three seconds to breathe in and three seconds to breathe out. (A second can be counted by saying 'one hundred and one . . .') Make sure you do not take breaths that are too deep.
4. After one minute hold your breath again for six seconds and repeat the process.

This technique should be practised regularly when you are not feeling anxious so that it becomes second nature and is easy to use when symptoms are likely to occur or are occurring.

Depression

Depression is the most common mental illness in Australia, with 3.4 per cent of males and 6.8 per cent of females reporting the condition in 1997. It is also the fourth most common reason for GP consultations. Significantly, depression does not just affect the sufferer; their whole family is usually intimately involved. It is an illness that is on the increase and will be one of the major health problems of this century.

Depression is also a disease more prevalent in the young. Generally it is considered to be a greater problem in females. However, as figure 4 shows, when the burden of disease from suicide and depression are added together, males actually suffer more from these conditions.

A major concern surrounding this disease is that only about 50 per cent of people with depression are diagnosed and receive treatment. A more realistic estimate of the incidence is about 20 per cent of the population will suffer a significant bout of depression at least once in their lives. There is also a 50 per cent chance of recurrence after an initial

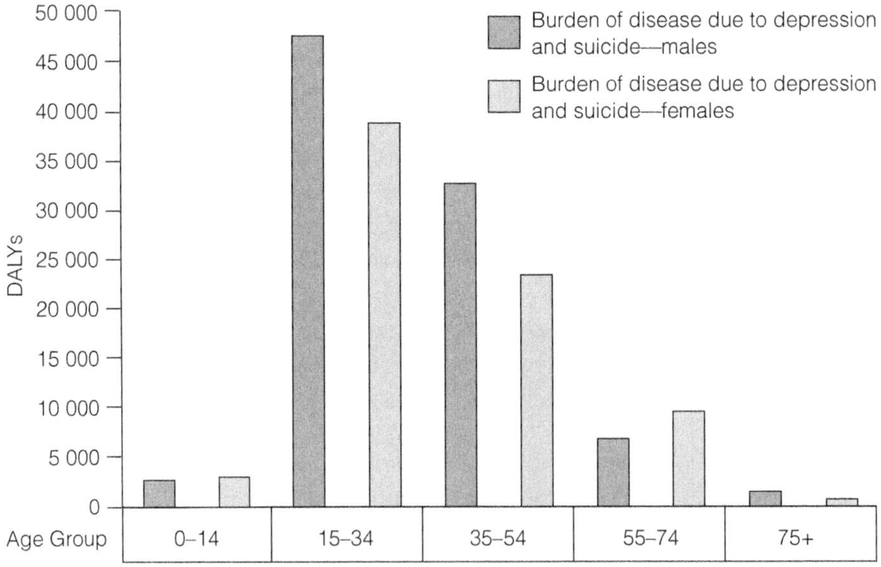

Source: Adapted from Australian Institute of Health and Welfare, Mathers, 1999.

Figure 4 Years of life lost due to disability and mortality (DALY) from both depression and suicide (1996)

episode. Overall, it is likely that most Australians will be closely affected by depression, either directly or through a family member or close friend, at some stage during their lives. Depression is also often associated with anxiety and their causes and treatments are similar. Adolescents with anxiety and/or a problem with substance abuse are particularly at risk.

Psychological, biological and environmental factors can all cause depression and any combination of these can be present in one person. Psychological causes relate primarily to early life experiences, inappropriate parenting and learned negative thoughts. The prime biological factor is genetic predisposition and this is a major cause in many depressed people. Depression often runs in families. Other biological causes include chronic illness, hormonal changes and some medications. Biological (and perhaps psychological and environmental) factors work by reducing the levels of chemicals that assist in nerve cell transmissions in the brain. These substances are called neurotransmitters, the principal ones being serotonin and noradrenalin. Drugs used in treating depression act to alter the levels of these chemicals in the brain. Environmental factors relate to causes of significant stress, including relationship problems, work-related stress (or job loss), bereavement and traumatic events.

Prevention of depression

Most people with depression develop their problem during childhood, usually as a result of childhood anxiety problems. As with the prevention of adult anxiety, the prevention of adult depression really requires the development of good coping skills during childhood. You can accomplish this by ensuring you practise good parenting techniques and that your child's school has programs to improve self-esteem.

Diagnosis of depression

Depression is diagnosed when at least five of the following nine symptoms, including at least one of the first two symptoms, are present for at least two weeks.

- Depressed mood or sadness for most of the day.
- Loss of interest or pleasure in all or most activities for most of the day.
- Difficulty concentrating, indecisiveness or deteriorating school performance.
- Lack of energy, enthusiasm, motivation or feeling slowed down.
- Changes in sleeping patterns, including insomnia or excessive sleeping.
- Large increases or decreases in appetite with significant weight loss or gain (5 per cent or more).
- Feelings of guilt or worthlessness.
- Withdrawal from friends, family and previously enjoyed activities.
- Suicidal thoughts or actions.

Substance abuse and medical conditions, such as hypothyroidism, need to be excluded as causes of the above, as does recent bereavement.

Other questionnaires for diagnosing depression are available on the 'beyond blue' website at www.beyondblue.org.au. Click on *depression information*, located at the top of the 'topic column' on the left hand side of the screen, then click on *Do I have depression?*.

Some signs to look for in friends, relatives or yourself include an increase in any of the following: alcohol and drug use, social withdrawal, irritability or moodiness, and time missed from school or work. Being awake through the night, unnecessary risk taking and loss of interest in pleasurable activities such as food, sex or exercise are also common.

It goes without saying that most people who commit or attempt to commit suicide are depressed. Factors that increase the risk of suicide include the depth of depression, suicide ideation, a past history of self-harm, a family history of suicide, male gender, increasing age, and co-existing illness or alcohol abuse.

It is common for chronic lack of sleep to cause depression. This is a very significant factor in post-natal depression. Instruction on how to reduce insomnia can, when successful, also improve this associated depression. Sometimes the reverse is true; the depression is causing the insomnia. If this is the case, then the depression needs treatment.

Screening people for depression

While there are no guidelines (yet) for screening specific groups for depression, it should be considered in all people at increased risk. These include:

- Teenagers, especially if involved with alcohol or drug abuse. In all, about 5 to 8 per cent of this group are depressed (Rey 2001).
- People over 65 years of age, especially those with dementia, a chronic illness or pain (depression is six times more common in this group), and those who are socially isolated, for example after the death of a spouse or when ceasing driving.
- Anyone with a chronic illness or chronic pain. About 50 per cent of depression sufferers have a related physical problem.
- Women who have recently given birth or who are pregnant.
- Those experiencing significant life events, such as the death of a relative or friend, separation from partners or job loss.
- People with a past history of depression or an anxiety disorder.
- People who abuse alcohol or other substances.
- People with sleep disorders.
- People with eating disorders.
- People with attention deficit/hyperactivity disorders.

Recognising and preventing depression in pregnancy

Depression is a well-recognised problem after delivery, with 10 per cent of new mothers becoming depressed. Recent research suggests depression is just as common during pregnancy and you need to be aware of this problem to help recognise symptoms in friends, relatives or yourself. The most important risk factor is a past history of significant depression, with these women having a 50 per cent chance of developing depression associated with their pregnancy.

Anxiety is a common feature, especially when there is conflict with the partner or there are other significant family stresses, such as a death in the family. Other associated features include lack of social support, especially if the woman has other children, and ambivalence about continuing the pregnancy.

Prevention of depression in pregnancy relies on maximising family support and providing time for relaxation, especially if this is not the first child. Sleep deprivation and over-working need to be avoided as well. Programs aimed at identifying women who are at risk of or who have post-partum depression are starting to be introduced in Australia.

How can I help a depressed friend or family member?

- Tell them that you've noticed a change and are worried.
- Encourage them to get professional help, help them find that help and accompany them on visits to health professionals involved.
- Make an extra effort to remain in contact with the person and include them in your social network/activites.
- Encourage other friends and family to be similarly supportive.
- Also read the section on page 78 entitled, 'Helpful intervention by family and friends'.

Treatment of depression

The most important issue in treating depression is recognising it in the first place. This is especially the case with adolescents and males. If you fit the above criteria, do not disregard your feelings—they are adversely affecting both you and your family. Seek help! If a friend or relative is the sufferer, discuss it with them and encourage them to seek medical help. All GPs see many depressed patients and most of them are well skilled at treating this condition. They really can help, but only when they know there is a problem. Tell them!

The majority of patients can be successfully treated with medication and/or psychotherapy (usually cognitive behavioural therapy). Both are equally effective in treating mild to moderate depression but more severe depression requires treatment with medication. It is important that the treatment chosen is one that the sufferer feels comfortable with and will thus comply with. Increased physical activity should also be an important part of treatment in most people.

All medications seem equally effective, but different medications are beneficial for different people. As it is not possible to tell beforehand which medications are likely to succeed, some trial-and-error may be necessary to find the most effective medication. If the initial drug does not work, it is worthwhile trying several others before giving up. However, medication often works quickly, with benefits being seen in a couple of weeks. Untreated, depression usually lasts for six months or more. For this reason, treatment usually needs to be maintained for a period of about 12 months. Antidepressant medication can also be effective in the treatment of anxiety in some cases.

The most important part of treating depression is consistent long-term follow-up by the treating practitioner. People requiring treatment with drugs or psychotherapy need treatment for at least a year, and those suffering more severe or recurrent symptoms will need follow-up for up to three years.

PSYCHOTHERAPY AND OTHER SOLUTIONS FOR DEPRESSION AND ANXIETY

In the past, psychotherapy for depression and anxiety focused on trying to identify the underlying causes for problems that people faced in their everyday lives. These causes are often deep-seated and often commenced in the person's distant past. The psychoanalysis therapy used to uncover these causes and to reverse their effects was very time-consuming (and therefore expensive) and required great patience from both patient and therapist.

Cognitive Behavioural Therapy

Over the past ten years, psychoanalysis techniques have been largely replaced by cognitive behavioural therapy (CBT), which works equally well for treating depression and anxiety. With the help of a trained therapist, people learn ways of dealing with their psychological problems so they can manage their problems by themselves. They learn to become their own therapist. CBT focuses on addressing the actual problems the person is facing rather than their deep-seated causes. Once problems are identified, solutions can be sought through the following.

Education: People need to understand the nature of the problem they face. It is also important to explain the nature of acute anxiety symptoms, especially those that occur with panic attacks, and how they can be avoided.

Structured problem solving: Having identified a particular problem, the person is encouraged to write down possible solutions for the problem. All the solutions are then assessed, looking at their individual advantages and disadvantages. The one the patient feels is most likely to be successful is then chosen and a plan to put it into practice is made. A review of progress occurs at the next consultation.

Challenging automatic negative (unhelpful) thoughts: Most people with depression and/or anxiety have negative thoughts that automatically come into their heads many times each day. They may occur in association with a specific problem, such as one particular anxiety causing situation, or with most of the activities the person does, as is often the case in depressed people. They develop over many years and become as second nature as cleaning your teeth. Without consciously thinking of them, they actively shape responses to the daily problems the person faces. Such thoughts fall into the following broad categories:

- catastrophising—where people take the worst possible scenario as the only possible outcome
- all or nothing thinking—everything is seen as either black or white and no middle ground exists
- setting unrealistic expectations—where only the best (usually unachievable) outcomes are seen as satisfactory and anything else is seen as failure
- over-generalising—a problem associated with a specific activity is seen as applying to other present and future activities
- loss of perspective—a person unrealistically focuses on negative aspects of an activity, ignoring other more positive aspects
- inappropriately blaming oneself or others for problems that are unavoidable.

The anxiety that these thoughts cause leads to unhelpful responses, such as avoidance behaviours and obsessive/compulsive behaviours, and ultimately to depression. Helping to identify the existence of these negative thoughts and challenging their validity allows people to recognise and challenge such thoughts when they occur in real life situations. They are then able to make more appropriate and beneficial responses.

Activity scheduling: Most depressed people have significantly reduced the activities they are involved in. Encouraging increased participation in both new and old activities is a significant benefit in improving mood. Often involvement of the person's partner can assist significantly.

Exercise: Almost all people with anxiety or depression benefit from increasing regular physical activity.

Graded exposure: This technique is used in people who have adopted avoidance behaviours due to their anxieties, such as avoiding crowded places. The anxious person grades (out of ten) a variety of related situations according to their ability to provoke anxiety. The person then exposes themselves to the least anxiety-provoking situation. Once this is mastered, the next situation is challenged and so on up the list until the problem has been overcome.

Often cognitive behavioural therapy can be used alone. However, in more severe cases, medication also needs to be added; usually for short periods.

Under the supervision of a trained practitioner, all the above techniques have been shown to help in the majority of depressed or anxious people. However, success depends on the sufferers taking on the major role as they practise their newly learned techniques in real life situations. The therapist's role is to act as a guide. As with almost all the lifestyle changes suggested in this book, motivation is the key to success and the person must be ready to start therapy.

Another form of therapy being increasingly used to help psychological problems is interpersonal counselling. The techniques used are similar to those of cognitive behavioural therapy, but the emphasis is on improving relationships.

Interpersonal counselling

Not uncommonly, counselling is needed to help with relationship problems. A form of therapy being increasingly used to help psychological problems is interpersonal counselling (Robertson 2002). The techniques used are similar to those of cognitive behavioural therapy, but the emphasis is on improving relationships.

Relationships with family and friends are an integral part of day-to-day life and problems with these relationships account for many of the psychological problems people face. They lead to disruption of the social support networks that are very important in providing support and encouragement during challenging and stressful times. This lack of support can lead to more serious problems such as depression.

Interpersonal counselling attempts to identify and improve existing relationship problems and increase the person's social network by helping establish new friendships. These improved and new relationships then assist the person in coping with other current life stresses, such as job loss or bereavement.

To assist with therapy, interpersonal counselling attempts to separate the reasons for the problems into three categories. These are grief, interpersonal disputes and role transitions. Often several problems exist at once and problems can fall into more than one category. For example, the death of a spouse will cause both grief and role changes.

Grief can be any loss, such as death, job loss or injury, experienced by a person. While grief is a normal part of experiencing loss, excessive grief is inappropriate and will affect a person's ability to communicate with partners and friends. Rebuilding these relationships and establishing new ones, often through establishing new interests, helps in overcoming the grieving process.

Interpersonal disputes develop when people communicate poorly or have unrealistic expectations of their relationship. Therapy requires assessment of whether the disputes are capable of resolution. If they are, then compromise needs to be the aim. Reassessing expectations and improving communication and problem-solving skills are integral parts of this process. Unsalvageable relationships need help so a peaceful dissolution that minimises further psychological stress can occur.

Role transitions occur when changing life circumstances cause changes in the functions the person has to perform. For example, divorce will drastically change a person's family roles. Therapy needs to promote adaptation through emphasising the positive aspects of new roles and the negative aspects of old ones, and encouraging the person to develop new skills that will enable them to replace old roles with new ones.

Some people have characteristics that make it difficult for them to establish and maintain lasting quality relationships. The issues here are often complex and require more specialised counselling before interpersonal therapy can be of benefit.

Interpersonal therapy usually requires only about six sessions. The initial session of about an hour assesses current relationship problems and how these are affecting the person's coping ability. More serious problems, such as significant depression, that need other treatment modes are also identified. The following shorter consultations attempt to probe the person's perception of the problem, identify possible effective solutions, slowly implement these solutions and review progress. This is similar to the approach taken in cognitive behavioural therapy.

Suicide prevention

Suicides and attempted suicides are tragedies that haunt families and communities for many years after they occur. In 1998, 2683 Australians (2150 males and 533 females) died from suicide. This is similar to the number of people that die on our roads. For each person who dies, many more attempt suicide. In contrast to suicide deaths, the rates for attempted suicide are greater for females. There were about 20 000 hospital admissions for suicide attempts and self-harm injuries in 1997/98.

The rates for actual suicide are highest for young males and have increased threefold in the 30 years up to 1990. Since then the rate for 15 to 19 year old males has remained unchanged but the rate for 20 to 39 year olds has continued to rise.

People at risk of suicide

People at greatest risk of suicide include young men in rural areas, older men, homeless people, people with alcohol or drug abuse problems, people in custody and, as would be expected, people who have attempted suicide previously, especially if this episode was in the past 12 months. Up to 50 per cent will make a repeated attempt at suicide. People with mental illness are especially at risk, particularly those recently discharged from psychiatric units. Most people who attempt suicide, especially young people (about 90 per cent), have mental health problems, particularly depression. In 1998, approximately 33 per cent of those who died from suicide and 40 per cent of those who attempted suicide were receiving psychiatric treatment before the event.

While suicide and depression are often linked together, it is important to note that 10 per cent of people with schizophrenia commit suicide and 40 per cent attempt suicide. This rate is up to 12 times that of the general population. Most of these suicides occur within the first ten years of their illness.

Figure 5 shows that suicide incidence increases with increasing isolation. The reasons for this include isolation from people in general, reduced access to help for mental illness, poorer economic conditions in rural areas, and increased access to firearms. Young men in these locations are particularly at risk. Older farm managers also have a high incidence, with financial problems being a significant factor. Having said this, Australia is an urbanised society and most suicides still occur in the cities.

Preventing suicide

As stated above, most people who commit or attempt suicide are depressed; suicide rarely happens without warning. As about 50 per cent of depressed people go undiagnosed in

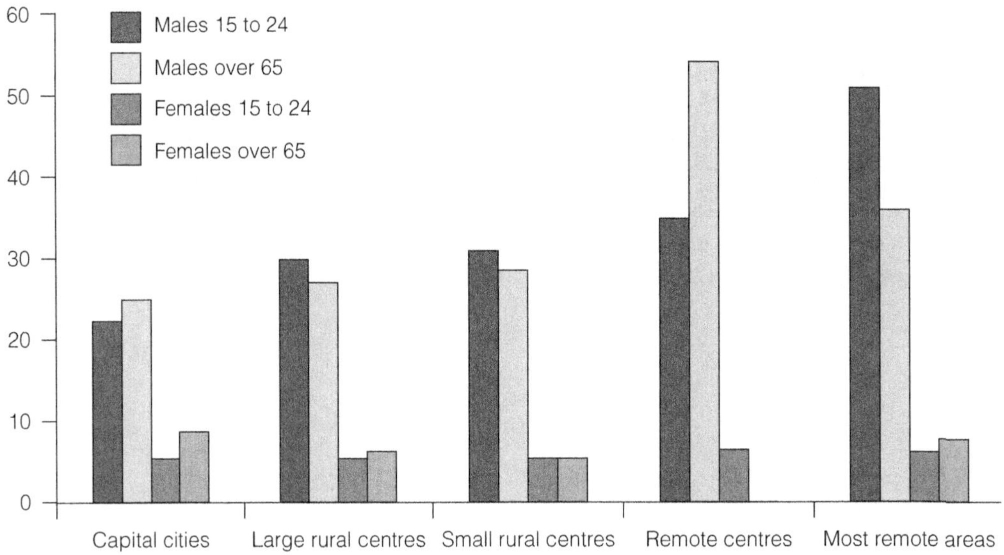

Source: Australian Institute of Health and Welfare, 2000.

Figure 5 Suicide death rates in high-risk age groups according to location (per 100 000 population)

Australia, particularly males, it is important you are aware of the symptoms of depression and look for them in those around you. Anyone displaying symptoms should be encouraged to seek medical help as soon as possible. Young males with depression are far less likely to be diagnosed and treated as this group has more difficulty in expressing emotions and therefore seek help less often.

When a person with undiagnosed and untreated depression has their condition exacerbated by a stressful event or life crisis, a suicide attempt may well follow. The stresses involved typically include recent losses, such as loss of an important person through death or separation, the recent suicide of a friend or relative, or breaking up with a boyfriend/girlfriend. Feared or confirmed pregnancy, trouble at school or with the police, family conflict or domestic violence, being a victim of sexual or other abuse (present or past), and drug abuse can also precipitate suicide.

Youth suicide warning signs

- Statements showing suicidal ideas or thoughts such as 'I wish I was dead', 'No one cares if I live or die', 'Does it hurt to die?'. Death or suicide themes dominating written or creative work need to taken seriously.
- Planning self-harm, especially when thought has been given as to how effective the plan might be.
- Expressing feelings of hopelessness and worthlessness (letting parents and others down).
- A decline in schoolwork and attendance.
- Giving away personal possessions and withdrawal from friends.
- A relatively high level of impulsiveness.
- A poor level of social support from parents, friends etc.

HELPFUL INTERVENTION BY FAMILY AND FRIENDS

If you are concerned that a person is at risk of committing suicide, you should always discuss your concerns with your GP or mental health worker without delay. Suicide conselling is a difficult area and is best co-ordinated by health professionals. However, you may be the only person the at-risk person trusts and you may therefore have to play an integral role in helping this person seek help and in their on-going management. At-risk people will often ask the people they confide in not to inform others. This is not a reason for not seeking help and it is important not to promise to keep secret any threat of self-harm. You should also be prepared to help the person make and keep contact with professional help.

Be prepared to bring up the subject of self-harm and when self-harm/suicide is discussed, address the issues seriously with the person and suggest the person receives help as soon as possible. Discussing suicide is likely to reduce the risk of a suicide attempt, not increase it. Be honest about concerns and feelings and try to discuss them calmly. Allow the person time to talk about their feelings/situation and avoid offering too much advice, being judgmental or trivialising the person's concerns. If the person is evasive and denies suicide and you are still worried, go with your gut feeling and seek help anyway.

Presenting alternatives to suicide and affirming the self-worth of a person can assist them to feel less alone and hopeless. Be supportive and stay with the person if you think there is an immediate risk of self-harm. People with suicidal ideas, a plan, and the means to implement their plan, are particularly at risk. Where possible, it is appropriate to limit access to means of self-harm, such as firearms, while help is being sought or treatment is in progress. Ensuring they avoid all alcohol use is also very beneficial, as alcohol can reduce inhibitions and increase the risk of a suicide attempt.

Some people contemplating suicide may also have thoughts about harming others, especially the parents of young children. If you feel others are at risk, seek help immediately and, where possible, provide support while help is coming and during treatment.

Finally, it is worth noting the obvious: maintaining good social connections with families and friends is the best way to prevent people being at risk of suicide.

Some questions for doctors to assess the risk of suicide in patients

- Are things so bad you sometimes wish you won't wake up in the morning?
- Have you had any thoughts of harming yourself?
- Have you thought about ways of harming yourself?
- Have you made any plans to harm yourself?
- Have you thought about when you might do this?
- Have you ever done something to harm yourself?

If you are going to try to bring up the topic of self-harm, it is very important to simultaneously acknowledge their revelations, express empathy, and reassure them that their feelings are due to depression which can always be cured. This will require some time on your part. You then need to help them seek professional help and do all you can to ensure they are safe until this help is at hand.

Schizophrenia

Schizophrenia is a group of mental disorders of varying severity that are characterised by disturbances of thought and perception, where people lose touch with 'outside' reality (e.g. delusions). It is often associated with reduced social activity or decreased emotional expression and occurs in about 1 per cent of the population. Onset is usually gradual and commonly occurs in late adolescence. Schizophrenia is inherited in some cases. (A person with a first-degree relative with schizophrenia has about a 7 per cent chance of developing the disease.) While it is unfortunately not really preventable, it is mentioned here for several reasons.

Firstly, people with schizophrenia have a high incidence of significant depression and are at risk of committing suicide. This often occurs in the early years of the illness. Depression needs to be anticipated and treated early.

Secondly, it is thought that the severity of the disease can be reduced by early diagnosis and treatment. As the onset is often insidious, this can be difficult and relies on being on the look out for early symptoms. These symptoms include suspiciousness, depression, anxiety, irritability, restlessness, change in appetite, social isolation/withdrawal, marked impairment in role functioning, markedly peculiar behaviour, vague or digressive speech, odd or bizarre ideas, unusual perceptive experiences, a marked lack of energy or interest, and a sense of alteration in one's self, others or the outside world. While many of these symptoms are non-specific, they are made more relevant if associated with the following characteristics: persistent, marked and unexplained changes in behaviour; increasing severity of symptoms; and a family history of psychosis/schizophrenia (Keks and Burrows 1998).

Illicit drug use, particularly cocaine and amphetamines, is occasionally associated with experiences that can closely resemble episodes of schizophrenia. Also, some people with underlying schizophrenia have their first episode (and subsequent episodes) while under the influence of illicit drugs. These facts have two implications. Firstly, underlying schizophrenia should be thought of in those who have such episodes, although treatment for the episode should not occur unless the diagnosis of schizophrenia is fairly certain. Secondly, people with schizophrenia or a family history of the disease should avoid taking drugs wherever possible.

Further information

Mental Health Branch of the Department of Health and Aged Care
Ph: 1800 066 247. Their website www.mentalhealth.gov.au provides information about crisis supports and contacts, general mental health information, mental health information brochures/publications about specific topics such as depression, anxiety, information about suicide prevention etc.

Beyond Blue: The National Depression Initiative
Website: www.beyondblue.org.au

National General Practice Youth Suicide Prevention Program
Website: www.iinet.au/~suicide

Lifeline
Lifeline provides an immediate counselling service for all people. Ph: 13 1114; website: www.lifeline.org.au

Kids Help Line
A national 24-hour counselling service for children and young people. Ph: 1800 551 800; website www.kidshelp.com.au

The Clinical Research Unit for Anxiety and Depression (CRUfAD)
CRUfAD is a group of researchers and clinicians concerned with anxiety and depression. It is a joint facility of St Vincent's Hospital and the University of New South Wales, Sydney. The self-help section of the website has useful information about both anxiety and depression for the general public; Website: www.crufad.com

Macquarie University Child and Adolescent Anxiety Clinic
This unit runs 12-week courses for anxious children in the 6 to 12 year age group; Website: www.psy.mq.edu.au/muaru

Further reading

R. Rapee, S. Spence, V. Cobham and A. Wignall, *Helping Your Anxious Child: A step by step guide for parents*, New Harbinger, 2000.

R.M. Rapee, *Overcoming Shyness and Social Phobia: A step by step guide*, Lifestyle Press, Sydney, 2001.
Deals with social phobias and shyness.

Susan Tanner and Jillian Ball, *Beating the Blues*, distributed by Tower Books, Sydney.
A good book for issues dealing with the treatment of depression.

Andrew Page, *Don't Panic: Overcoming anxieties, phobias and tensions*, Liberty One Media, Sydney, 2002.
Deals with panic disorders, phobias and anxiety.

Sarah Edelman, *Change Your Thinking*, ABC Books, Sydney, 2002.
A good book on cognitive behavioural therapy.

Alcohol and illicit substance use and abuse

'Drunkenness doesn't create vices, but it brings them to the fore.'

Seneca (4 BC–AD 65)

While the overall consumption of alcohol per person has decreased from 9.7 litres per year in 1981 to 7.6 litres per year in 1997, many Australians still put themselves at risk of harm through alcohol abuse. Over 45 per cent of men and 33 per cent of women who consume alcohol are at increased risk from their drinking with the highest levels occurring in both males and females in the 15 to 24 year age group. About 50 per cent of the population over 14 years of age drink at least once a week, and 80 per cent at least a few times per month.

Harmful effects of alcohol

Alcohol is the main drug of abuse in Australia and it is responsible for 2.2 per cent of the nation's total disease burden. This figure is made up of two components: harmful effects (4.9 per cent) due to the conditions stated below and beneficial effects (2.7 per cent), which arise from a reduction in vascular disease. One is subtracted from the other to achieve a net harmful effect of 2.2 per cent.

This subtraction simplifies the true situation somewhat because the beneficial and harmful effects occur at completely different ages. The harmful effects occur mostly in younger people and are the cause of tremendous amounts of death and disability in this group. (Almost 3 per cent of the total disease burden of the whole country!) The beneficial effects are due mainly to the reduction in vascular disease (especially heart attacks) that occurs in older, low-risk alcohol consumers.

Alcohol caused an estimated 3700 deaths in Australia in 1997 and this figure is on the rise. (It may be as high as 6000.) The main causes of alcohol-related deaths are road accidents and liver disease. Alcohol is involved in over 40 per cent of driving fatalities. There were 96 000 hospital admissions due to alcohol in 1998 and over 33 per cent of Australians reported being abused, either verbally or physically, by someone under the influence of alcohol. Ten per cent reported being victims of alcohol-related property damage or theft.

The significant social disharmony that alcohol causes in many families imposes a huge cost on society that is frequently underestimated. Even 'mild' abuse that may not be obvious to those outside the family will, over a long period, permanently scar many relationships. All people who consume alcohol should regularly question whether their family relationships are being adversely affected by any behavioural changes that accompany their drinking. The impact of long-term personality changes and changes in brain 'thinking' function is also often underestimated by those involved and society at large.

The economic costs, to both the nation and the families involved, of impaired work performance and alcohol-related accidents at work are huge. The contribution of the above to the illness burden caused by alcohol is shown in Figure 6.

Physical effects of alcohol on the body

The National Health and Medical Research Council states that only small amounts of alcohol are beneficial to health. One to two standard drinks per day is maximal (10 to 20 grams of alcohol). Any intake above two standard drinks per day (20 grams) has no overall beneficial effect, either physically or mentally.

This does not mean that people who do not drink should be encouraged to take up drinking as alcohol is associated with numerous health problems and there is no guarantee that problems will be able to be avoided.

Alcohol and liver disease: Drinking large amounts of alcohol over a prolonged period progressively destroys liver cells and can lead to liver cirrhosis and death. It is especially a problem in people with other chronic liver disease, such as hepatitis B or C. The incidence of liver cancer is also greatly increased in those consuming large quantities of alcohol.

Alcohol and gastrointestinal tract cancer: As well as liver cancer, alcohol is responsible for a significant increase in cancers of other areas in the gastrointestinal tract, including the lips, mouth, throat, larynx and oesophagus, and perhaps the stomach and pancreas. There is also evidence of an association between alcohol and colon cancer.

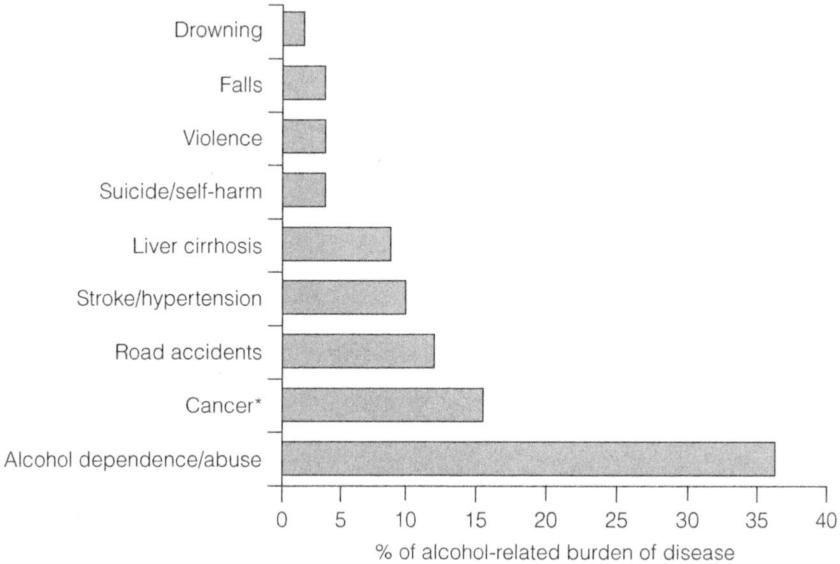

* The main cancers caused by alcohol are breast, colorectal and cancer of the mouth, pharynx, larynx and oesophagus

Note: Low-risk alcohol consumption (i.e. two drinks per day or less) causes a reduction in disease burden in older age groups due to a reduced incidence of vascular disease.

Source: Adapted from Australian Institute of Health and Welfare: Mathers, 1999.

Figure 6 Distribution of burden of disease caused by alcohol (1996)

Alcohol and breast cancer: Alcohol also causes an increase in breast cancer, with the risk increasing linearly with increasing alcohol consumption. In one comprehensive review paper, women who drank three to four glasses a day were calculated to have a rate of breast cancer 35 per cent greater than that in women who did not drink. This figure rose to 67 per cent with the consumption of more than four drinks per day (NHMRC 2001). There is evidence this effect is more prominent in older women. Reducing alcohol intake in middle (and later) life is likely to reduce this effect. The rise in breast cancer is thought to be due to alcohol increasing the production of oestrogen and this increased oestrogen level is responsible for an increased incidence of breast cancer. The rise in body acetaldehyde levels that accompanies alcohol consumption may also have a causal effect.

Alcohol and vascular disease: There is good evidence that low-level alcohol consumption has beneficial effects with respect to vascular disease, especially when the alcohol is taken with food. Alcohol on its own increases HDL cholesterol, perhaps decreases LDL cholesterol, and produces a slight reduction in blood pressure when taken in small amounts (20 grams per day or less), all of which help reduce vascular disease. Higher intake levels increase blood pressure and the incidence of strokes. Red wine has the added benefit of possessing antioxidants (polyphenols and anthocyanins). These antioxidants are the red pigments from the grape skins and may play a role in helping reduce vascular disease by preventing the oxidation of LDL cholesterol. One negative factor with regard to vascular disease that concerns all alcoholic products is that they exacerbate obesity. This occurs because alcohol provides the body with large amounts of energy.

What is a standard drink?

A standard drink is one that contains 10 grams of alcohol. Unfortunately, the alcohol content shown on bottles is not expressed in weight (i.e. grams) but in percentage by volume. The weight of alcohol contained in a glass varies depending on the percentage alcohol content of the drink and the volume in the glass.

A very important observation that can be made from Table 5 is that a normal Australian serving of beer, wine or spirits can, and often does, contain more than one standard drink (i.e. 10 grams of alcohol). As an example, if you were to drink a full-bodied Australian red wine with an alcohol content of 14 per cent (quite common these days), one standard drink would equal about 90 ml of wine. If you measure this out you will see that this is a small glass of wine! All alcohol products state the number of standard drinks that they contain.

Table 5 Alcohol content of typical Australian drinks

Beverage	*% alcohol content*	*Volume of a normal serving*	*Alcohol content of serving*	*No. of standard drinks in a normal serving*	*Volume in a standard drink with 10 grams of alcohol*
Beer (normal strength)	4.5	350 ml ('stubbie')	12.4 g	1.24	280 ml
Beer (light)	2.8	350 ml	7.4 g	0.74	450 ml
Beer (extra light)	0.9	350 ml	2.4 g	0.24	1410 ml
Wine	11.0	150 ml	13.0 g	1.30	115 ml
Wine	13.0	150 ml	15.0 g	1.50	98 ml
Wine	15.0	150 ml	18.0 g	1.80	85 ml
Spirits	40.0	30 ml ('nip')	10.0 g	1.00	30 ml

Safe and problem alcohol consumption in Australia

Unfortunately, many Australians do not consume alcohol at safe levels. Nine per cent of both males and females are at risk from long-term harmful alcohol consumption and about 46 per cent of males and 33 per cent of females are at risk from short-term alcohol consumption.

The National Health and Medical Research Council guidelines on safe alcohol consumption (NHMRC 2001) and short-term and long-term low-risk alcohol consumption are outlined in Table 6. They indicate the levels of consumption that pose a risk to your health and you should study them carefully. Where do you fit in? In addition to the guidelines shown in this table, there are numerous groups specially mentioned in their guidelines.

Young people (up to 18 years): All young people should be encouraged not to drink. If they have the opportunity to drink alcohol, they should be supervised by a responsible adult and keep consumption to a minimum. If you are organising a party for young people, monitoring or excluding alcohol is your responsibility. Parents are also responsible for gradually introducing their children to safe drinking habits, if the child and parent wishes. There is evidence that the risk of harmful alcohol use developing is increased by starting alcohol use early and by frequent use. People in this age group should never drink to become intoxicated.

Young adults (18 to 25 years): This group is the most likely to be harmed by alcohol and should keep strictly to (or drink below) the low-risk levels. In particular, they should not consume alcohol at all before undertaking risky activities, such as driving or swimming. Alcohol should not be taken with other drugs that affect mood and behaviour.

Performing skilled or risk activities: You should not consume any alcohol before or while doing an activity that requires skill or involves risk, such as flying, driving, water sports, skiing or operating machinery.

Problems with alcohol already: People with a health or social problem that is made worse by alcohol should preferably stop consuming alcohol for good (especially if they have developed severe alcohol dependence or have a severe health problem worsened by alcohol) Stopping for at least several months, and then perhaps reintroducing alcohol gradually under medical supervision, is an option for those with minor alcohol related problems. (They should ensure that they drink at low levels.)

Pregnant women (or women who might soon become pregnant): Women having a baby should consider not consuming alcohol at all. If they choose to drink, they should not exceed a maximum of seven standard drinks per week, have no more than two drinks in any one day, and never become intoxicated. The risk to the foetus is highest in the early stages of pregnancy.

Table 6 Guidelines for assessing alcohol consumption risk level

	Low risk (standard drinks per day)	Risky (standard drinks per day)	High risk (standard drinks per day)
	Risk of harm in the short term		
Males (on any one day)	Up to 6 but no more than 3 times per week	7 to 10	11 or more
Females (on any one day)	Up to 4 but no more than 3 times per week	5 to 6	7 or more
	Risk of harm in the long term		
Males (on an average day)	Up to 4	5 to 6	7 or more
Males (overall weekly level)	Up to 28 (should include some alcohol-free days)	29 to 42	43 or more
Females (on an average day)	Up to 2	3 to 4	5 or more
Females (overall weekly level)	Up to 14 (should include some alcohol-free days)	15 to 28	29 or more

Notes:

1. These levels assume that alcohol is consumed at a moderate rate to minimise intoxication, i.e. for men, no more than two drinks in the first hour and one drink per hour after that and for women, no more than one drink per hour.
2. These guidelines apply to men over 60 kg and women over 50 kg. Smaller people should drink less.
3. These levels do not apply to people who:
   - have a condition made worse by drinking
   - are on medication
   - are under the age of 18 years
   - are pregnant
   - are about to engage in activities involving risk or a degree of skill (e.g. flying, driving, water sports, skiing, operating machinery)
   - have a family history of alcohol-related problems.

Source: Adapted from NHMRC, *Australian Alcohol Guidelines*, 2001.

(Table based on *International Guide for Monitoring Alcohol Consumption and Related Harm*, World Health Organisation, Geneva, 2000.)

Family history of alcohol problems: If you have a first- or second-degree relative with alcohol-related problems, you are at a significantly increased risk of developing similar problems. and should be especially careful about how much you consume. You should also be sure to have alcohol-free days to reduce the likelihood of dependence developing. Not consuming alcohol at all is an option that should be seriously considered.

Mental health problems: If you have a mental health problem, you also need to watch your alcohol consumption carefully and keep to the low-risk guidelines. Another option is to give up altogether, especially if alcohol has already exacerbated your mental illness.

Older people: If you are older, you should consume less alcohol as you will attain higher blood alcohol levels than a younger person.

Taking medications: Many medications interact with alcohol and may require a reduction in alcohol intake. You will need to check.

People who choose not to drink: You should support people who choose not to consume alcohol. They often have a good reason for their decision and are likely to be healthier for it.

Alcohol consumption and driving

It is an unfortunate fact that many people, especially young adults, drive while under the influence of alcohol. Thirty-seven per cent of male road injuries and 18 per cent of female road injuries are attributable to alcohol. The best way to stay below the 0.05 per cent blood alcohol limit is as follows.

For males: A maximum of two standard drinks in the first hour and then one drink per hour after this.

For females: A maximum of one standard drink in the first hour and then one drink per hour after this.

The speed you are able to break down alcohol in your body is solely determined by the speed that your liver can process the ingested alcohol—nothing you do will speed this up. The reason that females should drink less initially is that they have relatively less water content in their bodies for the ingested alcohol to 'dissolve in'. (Women have a higher body-fat content and alcohol does not dissolve in fat.) Because of this, their blood alcohol level is raised more quickly, even though their liver is still able to break down alcohol as quickly as a male's liver; a rate of 10 grams per hour.

The following groups may need to consume less alcohol than stated above to stay under 0.05:

- people with a small build (due to relatively less body water)
- people in poor health (due to poorer liver function)
- people who are overweight (due to relatively more body fat and less body water).

Drivers who need to stay below a blood alcohol level of 0.02 per cent should not consume alcohol at all as even one drink will put them over this level. If you ride a bicycle, you also need to refrain from drinking alcohol completely as just one drink raises the risk of a fatal or serious injury fivefold. This is because riding a bike requires alertness and considerable co-ordination skills.

Alcohol and the young

Alcohol use by young people is a great concern in Australia, with about 66 per cent of their alcohol use posing a short-term risk of harm. Consuming alcohol in a manner that poses short-term harm occurs in 69 per cent of males and 52 per cent of females in the 18 to 24 year age group, with most of this being high-risk drinking. The fact that 52 per cent of alcohol-related, serious road accidents occur in the 15 to 24 year age group (and 75 per cent in the 15 to 34 year age group) is a potent reminder of the consequences of this behaviour.

In keeping with the above recommendations, young people should make a special effort to reduce harm from alcohol by adopting the following behaviours.

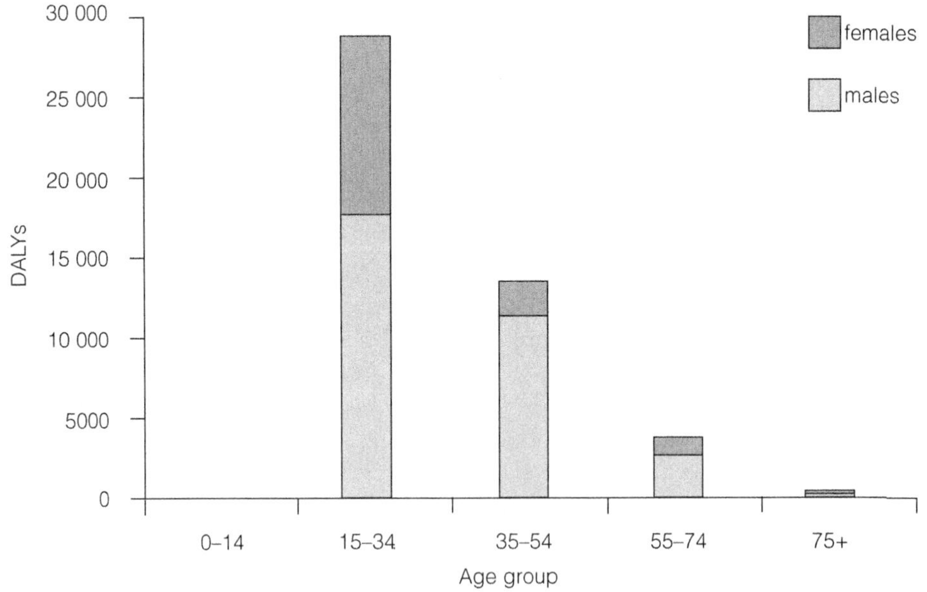

Source: Adapted from Australian Institute of Health and Welfare, Mathers, 1999.

Figure 7 Age related years lost due to disability and death (in DALYs) from alcohol abuse (1996)

- *Avoid loading doses of alcohol.* Loading doses refers to the rapid intake of alcohol, usually at the beginning of a period of alcohol consumption. Drinking cocktails is a good example. Loading causes loss of control, changes your personality and increases the likelihood that you will indulge in risk-taking behaviours, such as combining alcohol consumption with driving.
- *Drink with food and use non-alcoholic drinks to slow down alcohol consumption.* If you consume alcohol with food, you will slow down your alcohol absorption and this helps reduce your peak blood-alcohol levels. Drinking non-alcoholic drinks also helps. Try to drink some water before consuming any alcohol so that alcoholic drinks are not used as thirst quenchers.
- *Restrict number of drinks in a period of alcohol consumption.* In a short drinking session (four hours or less), drinking five drinks (50 grams) or more (binge drinking) is hazardous as it increases risk-taking behaviours, such as being driven by a person under the influence of alcohol or sexual practices that may lead to regret, unplanned pregnancies and increased exposure to sexually transmitted diseases. At high intakes, alcohol may lead to acute physical problems such as fitting, loss of consciousness and even death.
- *Avoid drinking in hazardous situations.* You should avoid consuming alcohol when driving, when pregnant, while operating vehicles, boats or machinery, when swimming and when in charge of children.
- *Avoid mixing alcohol with other drugs, such as cannabis.*
- *Alcohol should be reduced or avoided in those with mental illness.* It may exacerbate anxiety, depression and the risk of suicide.
- *Alcohol should be reduced in those who experience adverse changes in behaviour with its consumption.* Such changes include aggression and inappropriate loss of inhibitions that may cause public drunkenness, violent behaviour at home and in the general community, relationship problems due to inappropriate behaviour with your partner, inappropriate attitudes to work, and later regretted sexual activity.

For the parents of young people, drug avoidance/harm minimisation strategies taught in schools need to be reinforced at home. This should include problem-solving skills, self-care and safety skills, assertiveness training and peer-support skills. You need to provide information about safe alcohol consumption and discuss safer consumption strategies, such as avoiding loading drinks and consuming alcohol with food. Other issues relating to risk reduction include contraception and the importance of condoms to avoid sexually transmitted diseases and strategies to avoid driving with someone who has been consuming alcohol. It is also a good time for you to bring up the subject of other drug use.

DRINKING ALCOHOL IN THE PRESENCE OF CHILDREN

As well as avoiding hazardous and excessive alcohol consumption, it is important to adjust your consumption habits according to the occasion, especially when children are present. You should consider not drinking at all if you are in charge of the safety of young children (especially if swimming is at all likely). It is important to moderate your alcohol consumption if you will be interacting with children or teenagers. They can tell if you've consumed too much and will appreciate your company less. Alcohol consumption habits are often learned at home and your habits should act as a good model for your children. If your children wish to start consuming alcohol when they are old enough, allowing them to drink responsibly at home is an excellent way to learn responsible alcohol consumption habits.

Recognising problem drinking

Any of the factors mentioned below indicate that a problem probably exists.

- Recognition at any time that you are unable to control your alcohol consumption.
- Recognition that your behaviour is significantly altered by alcohol consumption. (It is always worth asking a friend or your partner what they think.)
- Comments by others (at any time) that your alcohol consumption is a problem at home, socially, or at work.
- Failure to fulfil social or work obligations due to alcohol.
- Regular intake at levels that deleteriously affect your health.
- The presence of any of the harmful physical or mental effects of alcohol.
- Binge drinking.
- Consuming loading doses of alcohol.
- Unhealthy alcohol consumption habits, such as persistent drinking alone, early drinking, or drinking with others who abuse alcohol.
- Drinking alcohol to control nerves.

There are several screening questionnaires used by medical practitioners to help identify people with alcohol problems. One of the most common, the AUDIT questionnaire, appears in Table 7. What is your score?

Alcoholism is a difficult concept and there is much controversy regarding the use of the term. It is perhaps best defined as a disorder that evolves slowly over several years and involves frequent or regular alcohol consumption. This use often involves problems such as recurrent use of alcohol in hazardous situations, legal problems in relation to alcohol, and failure to fulfil occupational or social obligations.

Over time this dangerous alcohol consumption pattern leads to the development of the symptoms of dependency. Tolerance to alcohol occurs, so that more alcohol is needed for the same effect, and chronic alcohol-related problems emerge, such as deteriorating behaviour and impaired performance and skills. The desire to drink becomes persistent and recurrent attempts to cut down are unsuccessful. Coping skills diminish and guilt and a sense of

Table 7 AUDIT Questionnaire (developed by the World Health Organization)

Question	*Score for each response below*					*Your score (0 to 4)*
	0	*1*	*2*	*3*	*4*	
1. How often do you have a drink containing alcohol?	Never	Monthly or less	Once a week or less	2 to 4 times a week	5 times or more a week	
2. How many standard drinks* do you have on a typical day when you are drinking?	1	2	3 or 4	5 or 6	7 or more	
3. How often do you have six or more standard drinks on one occasion?	Never	Less than monthly	Monthly	Weekly	Daily or almost daily	
4. How often during the last year have you found that you were not able to stop drinking once you started?	Never	Less than monthly	Monthly	Weekly	Daily or almost daily	
5. How often during the past year have you failed to do what was expected from you because of your drinking?	Never	Less than monthly	Monthly	Weekly	Daily or almost daily	
6. How often during the last year have you needed an alcoholic drink in the morning to get you going after a heavy drinking session?	Never	Less than monthly	Monthly	Weekly	Daily or almost daily	
7. How often over the past year have you had a feeling of guilt or regret after drinking?	Never	Less than monthly	Monthly	Weekly	Daily or almost daily	
8. How often over the past year have you been unable to remember what happened the night before because you had been drinking?	Never	Less than monthly	Monthly	Weekly	Daily or almost daily	
9. Have you or someone else ever been injured because of your drinking?	No		Yes, but not in the last year		Yes, during the last year	
10. Has a friend, doctor or other health worker been concerned about your drinking or suggest you cut down?	No		Yes, but not in the last year		Yes, during the last year	

Total score out of a possible 40

A score of 7 to 12 in males or a score of 6 to 12 in females:	The person is drinking too much or the person has or has previously had problems with drinking. Physical dependence on alcohol is unlikely.
A score 13 or more:	The person has problems with drinking and is likely to be dependent on alcohol.

* A standard drink is defined on page 84.

Source: Adapted from National Preventive and Community Medicine Committee: Guidelines for preventive activities in general practice, *Australian Family Physician* 2002, 31(5): SI59–SI61, the Royal Australian College of General Practitioners.

helplessness sets in. In Australia, about 5 per cent of males and 2 per cent of females are dependent on alcohol.

This pattern can occur in people as young as 20 as well as in older people.

Alcoholics Anonymous

Alcoholics Anonymous (AA), the most successful program for helping people with chronic alcohol problems, has been running for over 60 years. At present there are over 100 000 AA groups with about 2 000 000 members worldwide. Members come from a broad cross-section of the community and the degree of their problem with alcohol also varies significantly.

AA does not solicit members. Nor does it try to control its members. Rather, it is for people who are ready to admit that they have a problem with alcohol use and wish to stop drinking. AA is a program of total abstinence and anyone with a drinking problem who wishes to stop drinking is welcome. It attempts to achieve sobriety through sharing the experiences of its members, mainly at AA meetings. There is also a 'sponsorship' system, where each new member is assigned an existing member to help them. The main focus is to stay sober 'today' and take each coming day as another challenge.

There are several types of meetings. Open meetings can be attended by anyone, whether they have an alcohol related problem or not. They are an ideal way to find out more about AA. Closed meetings are for people with an alcohol problem who are current or prospective members of AA. 'Step' meetings are meetings that discuss one of AA's 'twelve steps' to achieving sobriety. All members remain anonymous and no case history or membership records are kept.

AA is not affiliated with any religious, political or other group and does not provide medical facilities or treatments. Membership is voluntary and there are no fees.

Al-anon is an organisation for the families of people with alcohol problems. Meetings give them a chance to discuss the difficulties arising from living with a person with an alcohol problem.

You can find out more about AA by attending one of their open meetings or from their website.

Addressing alcohol abuse

The first issue in dealing with an alcohol problem is to ensure the affected person realises the problem exists. This may come in the form of self-awareness or the person involved may need to be told. If you have identified a personal problem with alcohol from the above, you should discuss it with your GP. If a friend or relative has a problem then you need to discuss it with them. This is not always easy, and if you do not feel comfortable discussing the problem with the affected friend or relative, it is worthwhile discussing the matter with your GP, a drug counsellor or a social worker to decide on the correct strategy.

You should act on problems early as this is the best time to correct the problem. As with any entrenched behavioural pattern, alcoholism is difficult to treat in the chronic stages. Education regarding alcohol and its problems is the cornerstone of treatment for anyone with an alcohol problem.

Reducing alcohol intake can be achieved by avoiding exposure to situations likely to lead to alcohol consumption, such as after work, having alcohol-free days, setting maximum daily alcohol intake levels, ceasing binge and loading drinking, and avoiding abnormal consumption patterns, such as morning drinking and drinking alone.

The risk of short-term harm needs to be minimised, including avoiding mixing alcohol with driving or swimming, avoiding alcohol-related sexual behaviour problems, and avoiding situations where alcohol-related violence may occur.

Addressing work, social, and relationship problems that have evolved due to the alcohol problem and encouraging support from family members and friends are important priorities.

Intervention needs to be tailored to the person and there are two broad treatment groups. People with less-severe alcohol consumption problems who are reasonably motivated to change can be treated with help from their GP, with initial treatment involving breaking the present alcohol cycle. This can be accomplished either in hospital or at home. Relapse is quite common and people often blame this on a craving that accompanies withdrawal. This craving can be reduced by the use of medication.

People with alcohol dependence usually require more specialised care in a drug and alcohol centre. Treatments include detoxification and rehabilitation with psychological intervention. Abstinence is the preferred goal as this group has not been able to control their drinking previously and fewer than 10 per cent of people with alcohol dependency achieve controlled consumption. Two drugs, naltrexone and acamprosate, can assist with the maintenance of abstinence.

Referral to Alcoholics Anonymous is recommended for all those wishing to stop alcohol use.

Illicit substance use and abuse

The use of mood altering drugs has been taking place for thousands of years and is common practice in Australia today. Many people use these drugs on an occasional basis without significant long-term or short-term harm, although this is dependent on the type of drug being used and it should be emphasised that there is no safe level of drug use. It is also worthwhile remembering that alcohol and tobacco use cause far more harm than illicit drugs in both adults and adolescents.

Both short-term and long-term drug use can cause serious health problems and the problem of addiction can occur with most drugs. Drug use causes about 1 per cent of the total burden of disease in Australia.

Risk factors for substance abuse include adolescence, antisocial behaviour, being male, childhood physical/sexual assault, lack of social bonding, poor school performance, early age of first use, associating with substance abusing peers, high stress and lack of coping mechanisms, and poor quality family relationships and parenting skills (Kang 2002). The difficult task of reducing adolescent risk-taking behaviour is discussed earlier in the section on mental health.

A problem with drug use should never be viewed in isolation. It is always important to look at all possible issues including:

- The reasons a person is taking drugs.
- Underlying medical problems that may precipitate use, such as depression.
- Medical problems associated with drug administration. The mode of drug administration is responsible for significant illness, not the least of which are viral diseases, such as hepatitis B and C and HIV, which may occur with injecting drug use.
- Medical problems caused by the drug. Psychiatric illness, such as depression or psychosis, occur in some people who abuse drugs. Multiple drug use can make these problems considerably more likely.
- Problems with drug overdose. It is often difficult to know how much of a particular drug is present in the substance purchased. Many drug users feel that once they are experienced in taking a drug their risk of overdose is reduced. In fact, the opposite is the case because more frequent users have a greater chance of occasionally getting a higher dose than normal and are more complacent about the risks involved in drug taking. Thus, it is wise to never use drugs on your own and to ensure that at least one person with you is a non-user.
- Social/environmental problems associated with drug use. These include crime, financial problems, violence, employment and relationship problems, legal issues, and poor living standards. While these problems are more common in chronic dependent users, some, such as violence and legal issues associated with drug use, can occur with infrequent users also.
- Harm from increased risk taking.
- Harm from the use of drugs while pregnant. It is not wise to use any drugs when pregnant or possibly pregnant.

Harm minimisation is an integral part of reducing morbidity due to drugs. The following information gives a brief outline of some of the drugs in common use in Australia at present. However, drug use is constantly changing and if this health issue affects you or a member of your family, you will need to continually update your knowledge. The websites at the end of the chapter are excellent resources, as is your GP. You can also discuss any drug related problem by contacting the Alcohol and Drug Information Service in your state.

Cannabis/marijuana

Cannabis is a central nervous system depressant that is usually smoked, although it also can be eaten when added to cakes or biscuits. Cannabis generally makes you slow down and feel sleepy and its effects can last up to 12 hours. It is widely used in Australia, with approximately 33 per cent of Australians over 14 having used the drug. (Up to 70 per cent of young Australians have tried cannabis.) Most people are infrequent users and do not experience short- or long-term harm from the drug. However, dependence does develop in about 10 per cent of users. These people are usually very frequent users and are at risk of long-term harm from their use. There have been no reported deaths from the direct effects of cannabis.

The most significant problems are associated with mental illness. Acute or short-term effects include an increase in psychotic symptoms such as delusions, especially if a pre-existing psychotic illness is present. Thinking ability and memory may be impaired, and problems with coordination affect the ability to drive, operate machinery etc., especially if alcohol is used at the same time. Decreased inhibitions can lead to increased risk-taking behaviours, such as dangerous driving and unsafe sex. Some people can become anxious when taking cannabis. Simultaneous use of other drugs can worsen these effects.

Chronic, long-term effects include impaired thinking and motivation, reduced educational achievement and chronic bronchitis. Pre-existing mental illnesses are often made worse by cannabis use, especially in those with psychoses and anxiety disorders. These effects are particularly marked in adolescents. Cannabis use is common amongst people admitted to psychiatric hospitals.

People who have developed a dependence on cannabis should be encouraged to reduce or cease its use. Withdrawal is associated with symptoms that include anxiety, depression, irritability, lethargy, cravings and insomnia. It is best achieved through counselling although a short course of benzodiazepine sedatives or antidepressant drugs may be useful. Information about quitting can be gained from the Alcohol and Drug Information Service in your state. (See the further information section at the end of the chapter.)

HARM REDUCTION

- People with pre-existing psychiatric illness should be discouraged from using the drug.
- The drug should not be used when pregnant.
- You should not drive or operate machinery etc. when using the drug.

- Use with other drugs such as alcohol should be avoided as the effects of the drug increase.
- As with all illicit drugs, possession is a criminal offence that attracts severe penalties, especially if you possess more than you would realistically use yourself.

Heroin use

Heroin is a narcotic derived from the poppy plant. It acts as a central nervous system depressant and is mostly administered through injection, although it can also be smoked. It is hard to estimate heroin use but it was thought that there were about 60 000 (and perhaps up to 120 000) Australians using this drug in 1997. Dependence occurs in somewhere between 25 and 50 per cent of users, which means that at least half those using the drug are occasional users.

There are both short- and long-term problems with heroin use. Short-term problems include vomiting, constipation, tiredness and, most significantly, shallow breathing. With overdosage, breathing can stop altogether, resulting in death. Long-term problems include an increased likelihood that overdosage will occur, an increased likelihood of contracting serious viral infections (HIV and hepatitis B and C), vein damage, skin infections, constipation and pneumonia. There are also significant social problems surrounding heroin dependence, including illegal behaviour to finance heroin purchases.

HARM REDUCTION

Harm prevention is of paramount importance in assisting people using heroin. The main aim should be to minimise the risk of death due to overdose and infection with HIV and hepatitis B and C.

It is important that safe injecting procedures are used. These strategies for the herion user include:

- Choosing a safe place to inject and NEVER injecting alone.
- Cleanliness to reduce infection. This includes washing hands well before commencing, cleaning the utensils to be used, cleaning the area where you are mixing before and after use, and cleaning the injection site before and after drug use.
- Never sharing needles or any other materials used for mixing or administering heroin.
- Using needles and syringes only once.
- Recapping your own needle.
- Never recapping another person's needle
- Disposing of contaminated materials in a safe manner that will not endanger others.
- Never using heroin at the same time as other drugs, especially alcohol or tranquillisers, as this increases the risk of overdose.

Heroin is usually mixed with other compounds and varies in strength. To avoid overdosage, you should buy heroin from a regular, trusted dealer. If you are using heroin from a new supplier or you are a new user or are starting use again after even a short break, you are at increased risk of overdose and should use a small amount first to test the strength.

HEROIN USE IN PREGNANCY

Heroin use can affect the baby both while in the uterus and after birth and every effort should be made to avoid use during pregnancy. Problems include an increased incidence of foetal deaths, stillbirths, infections such as hepatitis B and C and HIV, and sudden infant death syndrome.

HOW TO HELP A PERSON WHO HAS OVERDOSED

The signs of overdosage include very slow breathing, cold skin, a slow heart beat, muscle twitching, blue tips of fingers, slowness to respond or unresponsiveness, and a gurgling sound in the throat. The following actions can help save a life.

- Phone an ambulance immediately.
- Stay with the person and try to keep them awake by talking to them.
- If the person looks like they're about to lose consciousness, put them on the floor on their side.
- If the person is unconscious:
  - Put them on their side in the recovery position.
  - Assess their breathing, clear their airway, and do mouth-to-mouth resuscitation if needed.

You should never place somebody who has overdosed in the shower to 'wake them up', inject them with anything else (unless by a health professional), or place anything in their mouth.

OUTCOMES FOR HEROIN DEPENDENT PEOPLE

Most people who are dependent on heroin are between the ages of 20 and 40. About a third of these people are able to quit, another third continue to use intermittently, and a final third continue severe dependence behaviours, end up in goal or die. There are various treatments for heroin dependence, the main ones being supervised withdrawal and methadone. Treatment is best conducted by a specialised drug rehabilitation unit.

Amphetamines (Speed)

Amphetamines are a group of drugs that stimulate the central nervous system. They are either sniffed, injected, or taken in tablet or capsule form and are being increasingly used in Australia. The drug is not supplied in a pure form, but is mixed with a variety of other substances that can have harmful effects.

Amphetamines make you more energetic, alert and excited, which can lead to feelings of aggression and anxiety/panic and increased risk-taking behaviour. They also cause your blood pressure to rise, your heart to beat faster, faster breathing and problems with sleeping. These effects can last from a few hours to a few days. Large amounts can bring on headaches, dizziness, shaking, feelings of power and hostility and may even lead to psychosis, a condition associated with experiencing delusions (seeing things or hearing voices that are not there).

Long-term use may result in dependence, significant depression, repeated violent behaviour and recurrent episodes of psychosis. Dependent people may also have social problems related to relationships, finances and employment.

Anyone using the drug can overdose and even small amounts can cause overdose symptoms in sensitive people. Overdose symptoms include psychosis, heart attack, stroke, a very high fever and can result, although rarely, in death.

Withdrawals in dependent users are associated with cravings, tiredness and prolonged sleep, anxiety and significant depression. Such symptoms usually last for short periods.

HARM REDUCTION

- People already suffering from mental illness, particularly anxiety, depression or schizophrenia, should not use this drug as it may make symptoms worse.
- Take heed of advice from others regarding any deterioration in behaviour when taking the drug and avoid further use if there are problems.
- Amphetamines should not be mixed with other drugs as this increases the risk of overdose. Sleep is a particular problem for regular users and they often need to take other drugs, such as alcohol and sedatives, to help them sleep, initiating a perpetuating cycle of drug use.
- The method of administration can also cause harm. The dangers involved with injecting drug use and advice regarding harm minimisation were covered in the section on heroin use. The effects of long-term nasal use are difficult to prevent.
- Amphetamines should not be used during pregnancy as they increase the risk of miscarriage, premature births and low birth-weight babies. Babies may also suffer from drug withdrawal.
- Increased risk-taking activity associated with using amphetamines means that you should not drive or use machinery when taking the drug.

Ecstasy

Ecstasy is a central nervous system stimulant that is available as tablets or powder that can be snorted, injected or dissolved in a drink. Like amphetamines, ecstasy is not usually sold in a pure form, rather it is mixed with substances such as amphetamines or ephedrine. Ecstasy is chemically related to amphetamines and has similar effects on the body. It also gives a feeling of closeness to others. Unwanted effects include sweating, feeling hot with a risk of overheating, dehydration which causes significant thirst (dry mouth), jaw clenching, nausea and anxiety. There is also a possible link to liver damage. High doses can produce hallucinations, irrational behaviour, vomiting and convulsions. Deaths have occurred due to overheating and dehydration. Ecstasy can also produce a hangover effect with symptoms such as insomnia, depression and muscle aches.

HARM REDUCTION

- It is important to keep sipping water to prevent dehydration. However, drinking too much water has led to serious fluid overload in some people. To prevent problems with dehydration, anybody using ecstasy should be accompanied by a non-user and a reduced dose should be taken by people not used to the drug. Adverse reactions should be treated in hospital emergency departments.
- Preventing complications associated with administration is an issue with injecting users.

Hallucinogens (including LSD)

Hallucinogens are a group of drugs that work on the brain to cause hallucinations (seeing, hearing, smelling and tasting things that are not there). These substances occur naturally in trees and fungi ('magic mushrooms'), or can be made synthetically, an example being LSD. Some other drugs, such as ecstasy and cannabis, can cause hallucinations when taken in high doses.

LSD (Lysergic Acid Diethylamide) is the most commonly used hallucinogen. It is taken orally, usually as a tablet. Effects occur about 30 minutes after ingestion and can last up to 12 hours. Visual hallucinations are quite common, such as colours becoming very bright and distortions of space. Other effects include floating sensations, emotional swings from intense happiness to profound sadness, strange body sensations and changed thoughts. Sometimes the hallucinations can be frightening (bad trips) and cause extreme anxiety or fear, paranoia, panic attacks and feelings of losing control. Aggression and self harm can very occasionally accompany these episodes. LSD psychosis, lasting up to months, can occur, although rarely and usually when large, cumulative doses are taken by susceptible people.

There are no long-term side effects although flash backs of sensations experienced during use can occur for months to even years after taking the drug. They are more common in regular users, can last up to several minutes and can occur without warning. Addiction to LSD is very rare and there are no withdrawal symptoms.

HARM REDUCTION

- People who have not used the drug frequently should not take it alone. They should have a non-using friend with them to help them through possible 'bad trips'.
- Users should not drive, operate machinery or perform other similar tasks.

- Adverse reactions need to be treated in hospital emergency departments.
- People with a psychological disturbance or a family history of schizophrenia should not take LSD.
- Pregnant women should not take LSD as it causes contractions of the uterus.

Cocaine

Cocaine is a central nervous system stimulant. It can be taken nasally, by injection or by smoking. As with many other drugs, it is not sold pure and is mixed with a variety of other substances, some of which are harmful. Its effects include becoming more excited, alert, confident and aggressive, all of which can lead to increased risk taking. Your heart beats faster and you move more quickly. Larger doses can cause dizziness, headaches, violent behaviour, difficulty concentrating, convulsions, heart attacks and psychosis (imagining things such as voices). Long-term use can lead to dependence, aggressiveness, and home, financial and work related problems. It is not uncommon for other drugs such as sedatives, alcohol and marijuana to be used, all of which help overcome the insomnia caused by cocaine.

Overdosage can cause breathing problems, heart failure, strokes and even death and is more likely with multiple drug use. Dependence and withdrawal symptoms occur in some people. These symptoms are usually short-lived and include cravings, nausea and vomiting, shaking, tiredness, hunger, depression and even feelings of suicide.

HARM REDUCTION

- Problems associated with drug injecting use need to be avoided (see the section on heroin).
- Cocaine should not be used during pregnancy as it increases the risk of miscarriage, premature births and low birth-weight babies. Babies may also suffer from withdrawals.
- Increased risk raking means that you should not drive or operate machinery when using the drug.

Further information

Centre for Education and Information on Drugs and Alcohol (CEIDA)
CEIDA's website has useful information for medical practitioners, parents, students and practitioners working in the fields of drugs and alcohol. Also available are specific information leaflets about most types of drugs.
Website: www.ceida.net.au

Alcohol and Drug Information Service
The drug and alcohol information services in your state will provide information and/or advice regarding problems with drugs and alcohol. They can also refer you to health professionals who can help you personally regarding alcohol and other drug problems.
Ph: ACT 6205 4545; NSW 9361 8000 or 1800 422 599: NT 8981 8030 or 1800 422 599; Qld 3236 2414 or 1800 177 833; SA 1300 131 340; Tas. 1800 811 994; Vic. 9416 1818 or 1800 136 385; WA 9442 5000 or 1800 198 024. (Check directory assistance if these numbers have changed.)

Australian Drug Foundation
Another good general site regarding drug use. Easy to access information about most types of drugs.
Website: www.adf.org.au

Family Drug Support 24-hour hotline
Ph: 1300 368 186 (throughout Australia)

Australian National Council on Drugs
Website: www.ancd.org.au

Alcoholics Anonymous
Website: www.alcoholics-anonymous.org

Part 3

Nutrition and illness prevention

What's in your food?

Nutrient groups in your diet

The nutrients in food are divided into two main groups: those present in large amounts, called macronutrients, and those in small amounts, called micronutrients. The macronutrients consist of carbohydrates, fats, fibre and protein, while the micronutrients consist mainly of vitamins and minerals. Table 8 indicates the energy content and functions in the body of each of these groups. The roles nutrient groups play in causing and preventing illness in Western society are discussed in detail throughout this book. It needs to be emphasised that the majority of Australian diets are not nutrient deficient. In fact, the opposite is the case; a reduction in excess fat and energy intake would benefit many Australians. There are, however, a few groups of people who are likely to have micronutrients deficiencies. This issue is discussed in the sections on micronutrients, vegetarian diets, and osteoporosis. The role of antioxidants in disease prevention is also discussed later in this section.

Body energy imbalance—a major health dilemma

One of the major problems associated with our modern, technology-based society is that it has dramatically altered our body's energy balance, unfortunately for the worse. We are doing less physical activity and have less time to prepare nutritious foods, relying instead on prepared

Table 8 Function and energy content of nutrient groups

Nutrient	Foods	Energy content		Function
		cal	*kJ*	
Fat Fatty acids	See tables 9 and 10	9	37	Mostly stored as fat for later energy use by the body when needed. Also an integral part of all cell membranes.
Fat Cholesterol	Lambs' brains, liver, eggs and some seafoods			Synthesis of body compounds including cell membrane and body chemicals, such as steroid hormones.
Alcohol	Alcoholic beverages	7	29	Used for energy. Alcohol is not converted to fat but is metabolised to provide energy before fat and thus reduces the rate of fat breakdown.
Protein	Meats, fish, poultry, eggs, milk products, cereals, nuts and legumes, including soy beans, lentils, beans and peas	4	17	Mostly used in the synthesis of body components. Only rarely used as an energy source, such as in starvation.
Carbohydrate Starches (complex) Carbohydrate Sugars—sucrose, glucose, fructose, lactose (simple)	Pasta, potato, breads, cereals, fruit, legumes Fruit, honey and other sweet syrups	4	16	Provides energy for the body's functions and some energy storage. It is usually stored as glycogen in the liver (and the muscle) but may be converted to fat if consumed in excess. (Glycogen is just many glucose molecules joined together.) The sugar that circulates in the blood and provides energy for the body is glucose. The brain relies almost solely on this glucose for energy and thus it is very important for blood glucose levels to be maintained.
Fibre	Bread, cereals, vegetables, fruit	0	0	Fibre keeps the bowel functioning normally and has a role in the protection of the bowel from cancer-causing substances. Soluble fibre can reduce blood cholesterol levels.
Vitamins and minerals	A wide variety of foods is needed, especially vegetables, fruit, low-fat dairy and lean meat	0	0	Essential for the synthesis of many body components, especially enzymes. These nutrients have no significant energy function. Some are also important antioxidants.
Water	Fluids, fruit and vegetables	0	0	70% of the body is composed of water.

food that usually has a high energy content. This combination of using less energy and consuming more means many people have an energy intake in excess of their needs. This excess energy intake is stored as fat.

The contribution made by the different nutrient groups to this energy imbalance varies according to their energy content and their use in the body, with dietary fat being the main culprit. Table 8 shows that fat and alcohol have significantly higher energy contents than carbohydrate and protein. In addition to having a lower energy content, carbohydrates use up more body energy in the processes of being digested, stored (as glycogen in the liver), and released for use in the body than fat does. For these reasons, an increase in dietary fat is far more likely to increase body fat stores than a proportionate increase in carbohydrate intake.

It is an easy and efficient process for the body to store excess energy from dietary fat as fat in the body. The equivalent of only about 3 per cent of the energy provided by dietary fat is used in its storage as body fat. Carbohydrates can also be converted to stored fat if taken to excess. However, the body prefers not to do this as it is a less efficient procedure, with the equivalent of about 25 per cent of the energy contained in the carbohydrate being lost in its conversion to stored fat.

While alcohol is not stored as fat, the energy it provides means less dietary or body fat is needed for the body's immediate energy demands, resulting in increased fat storage. Protein is rarely used to supply body energy. (Starvation is an exception to the rule.)

In an optimum diet, carbohydrate, mostly in the form of starch, contributes about 50 to 60 per cent of dietary energy intake and fat about 25 to 30 per cent. The other 15 to 20 per cent comes from protein. The contribution from alcohol varies according to consumption. Unfortunately, in modern Western diets the energy contribution from fat is more in the region of 35 per cent and the overall energy intake from all nutrients is excessive.

Reversing this energy imbalance is a major preventative health dilemma facing many Australians. It is dealt with in Part 4, Obesity and Physical Inactivity. The next two sections outline the facts you need to know when making food choices based on fat and carbohydrate content.

Fat—the danger in our diets

Problems associated with the fat content of our diets cause significant disease in Australia, mainly through increasing the incidence of vascular disease and obesity. As stated above, excess total fat contributes significantly to the high-energy content in our diet and this is one of the main reasons for the obesity epidemic that is occurring in both adults and children. Excess saturated fat is a major cause of elevated blood cholesterol and is therefore responsible for a considerable proportion of the vascular disease that kills many Australian men and women each year. Recommendations for a healthy dietary fat intake are:

- Restrict your total fat intake to about 25 to 30 per cent of total energy intake. The Australian average at present is about 35 per cent and reducing total fat intake is important for all people who are overweight. You can calculate your recommended total fat intake by using the table on page 160.
- Minimise your saturated fat intake. It should be a maximum of about 30 per cent of total fat intake and not more than 10 per cent of total energy intake. This is an important issue for all Australians.
- Increase the proportion of omega-3 polyunsaturated fats and monounsaturated fats in your dietary fat allowance. Again, this is important for everyone.

These recommendations and the role of fat in obesity and vascular disease are discussed in detail in later sections of this book. Here we will look at the two main types of fat in our diets: fatty acids and cholesterol.

Fatty acids

Fatty acids are the principal type of fat used by the body. They are simple compounds made up of a chain of carbon atoms with an acid group at one end. The number of carbon atoms varies, with the most common ones having between 12 and 20. The type of bonds joining the carbon atoms together determine whether a fatty acid is saturated or unsaturated. Saturated fatty acids have single bonds joining all the carbon atoms. Unsaturated fatty acids, which include monounsaturated and polyunsaturated fatty acids, have a double bond between one or more pairs of adjacent carbon atoms.

Triglycerides are made up of three (tri-) fatty acids joined together by a small compound called glycerol. They are the form in which most fatty acids are consumed in the diet and transported in the blood. There are many types of triglycerides, depending on the combinations of fatty acids that they are made from.

While many fatty acids can be made by the body, a few cannot and they must be consumed in the diet. They are called essential fatty acids and are discussed later.

A list of the foods that have a high fatty-acid content and a table comparing the types of fat present in oils and spreads appear in Appendix 3.

SATURATED FATTY ACIDS

Saturated fatty acids do not have any double bonds between their carbon atoms. (This means they are saturated with hydrogen, hence the name.) These are the fats being referred to when mention is made of lowering dietary saturated fats.

Saturated fats are the main dietary cause of raised blood cholesterol (see Appendix 14) and it is important that all Australians take measures to restrict their saturated fat intake. Table 9 provides a list of the sources of saturated fats.

Table 9 Food sources of saturated fatty acids*

Animal sources (About 60% of total saturated fat intake)	*Vegetable sources (About 40% of total saturated fat intake)*
• Fatty meats (about 43 to 50%*)—those with especially high total fat levels include: – sausages – normal mince – lamb (chops and legs etc.—50%*) – salami – other processed meats – any meat that is not lean and has not had all visible fat removed. • Chicken (31%*)—lean chicken with skin removed has little fat. • Dairy products (about 65% to 75%*)—the only dairy products with no fat are some no-fat milks and yoghurts. These no-fat dairy products are excellent food choices. • Takeaway foods cooked in animal fat. • Biscuits and pastries prepared with animal fat.	• Biscuits/savoury crackers • Cakes and pastries • Takeaway foods—almost all of these foods are cooked in saturated fat of either vegetable or animal origin. • Crisps • Potato chips • Confectionery, especially chocolate • Coconut milk, oil or cream (90%*) • Palm oil (51%**) • Palm kernel oils (84%**) • Solid vegetable oils used in commercial frying*** • Margarines (about 12 to about 25% of their total fat content is saturated. This saturated fat is added to these products to make them solid at room temperature). • Copha (98%*)

Trans fatty acids

Most trans fatty acids that occur naturally in foods are not harmful and some are beneficial. However, the trans fatty acid called elaidic acid, which is formed during the processing of food, is harmful, having similar effects to saturated fatty acids (i.e. raising LDL and total cholesterol and lowering HDL). It also increases the potentially harmful lipoprotein (a). Elaidic acid is found mostly in fats produced for use in deep frying (takeaway foods) and in processed foods such as margarines.

Most margarines are now available with reduced (1 to 2%) or no trans fatty acids.

* All fat containing foods have both saturated and unsaturated fats present. The foods in this list have a large component of saturated fat in their total fat content. The percentages mentioned indicate the percentage of saturated fat in relation to the total fat content of the food. They do not indicate the overall fat content of the food.

** These oils are often used in processed foods and in commercial frying as they do not go off as quickly as unsaturated oils.

*** Unsaturated vegetable oils are often modified so that they become more saturated and do not go off as quickly. This process removes some of the double bonds in the fatty acids, thus increasing their hydrogen content (i.e. they become increasingly saturated with hydrogen). These oils are also used in processed foods and in commercial frying.

Traditionally, saturated fats came mainly from animal products. In modern Australia, however, a significant proportion comes from vegetable sources. The main sources are palm oil, coconut oil and unsaturated vegetable oils that have been modified to give them a much higher content of saturated fats. Such modified oils are easier to use in making processed foods, such as cakes, pastry and biscuits. They are also often used in the deep-frying of takeaway foods, such as fish and chips, as they taste better than unsaturated oils, which go off when repeatedly heated. Thus, while these oils are vegetable in origin, they are bad for your health. Signs saying a product contains 'no cholesterol' or 'only vegetable oils' are no reassurance that the product is healthy.

Dietary recommendations to lower fat in your diet

- Eat red meat that is lean and trimmed of all fat. Two to three servings a week is optimal. Servings should be about the size of a pack of cards or weigh about 80 grams.
- Eat lean servings of chicken with the skin removed.
- Use unsaturated oils for cooking. Oils should preferably have a saturated fat content of not more than 15 per cent and a large monounsaturated fat content. (Extra virgin olive oil is a good choice as it contains numerous antioxidants and other nutrients and contains mostly monounsaturated fat.)
- Do not use coconut or palm oils.
- Try to reduce your use of spreads or don't use them at all. Most margarines have a saturated fat content of about 20 to 25 per cent of their total fat content. Butter has a lot more!
- Use reduced-fat or low-fat dairy products. Do not eat butter or cream at all and watch carefully your intake of cheese.
- Do not eat fried takeaway foods and do not fry foods at home. (If you must occasionally fry at home, most oils should be used only once. This is because heating oxidises them, producing harmful free radicals. Olive oil can be used a few times.)
- Eat minimal amounts of biscuits, cakes and pastries. Low-fat (check the label!) muffins, cakes etc. are often relatively high in energy and are thus still bad for you. Additionally, people tend to eat a greater quantity when consuming 'low fat' foods, worsening the situation.
- Eat minimal amounts of processed snack foods such as potato crisps, chocolate bars etc.
- Eat fewer shop prepared foods/takeaway food. Prepare more foods at home.

UNSATURATED FATTY ACIDS

Monounsaturated fats have one double bond and polyunsaturated fats have more than one double bond between their carbon atoms. Polyunsaturated fatty acids are divided into two main groups, the omega-3s and the omega-6s, according to the position of the double bonds.

Some polyunsaturated fatty acids cannot be made by your body and must be consumed in your diet. They are called essential fatty acids and include linoleic acid, alpha-linoleic acid and arachidonic acid. The body can use these essential fatty acids to make the numerous other fatty acids it also requires but would otherwise not be able to produce. Some of these can also be found in foods, especially omega-3 fatty acids such as eicosapentaenoic acid and docosahexaenoic acid.

These essential fatty acids (and their derivatives) are vital for your health for two reasons. Firstly, they are important components in the structure of the membranes that surround body cells (especially in the retina of the eye and the brain). Healthy cell membranes are very important for proper cell and thus body functioning. Secondly, they are used in the production of substances called eicosanoids. These substances, which include prostoglandins, thromboxanes and leukotrienes, help control blood clotting, blood pressure, inflammatory reactions and the reproductive cycle. There are two types of essential fatty acids, the omega-6s and the omega-3s. Preventing problems such as high blood pressure, a worsening of inflammatory diseases such as arthritis, and an increase in the tendency to clot, which can worsen vascular problems such as coronary artery disease, requires an intake of adequate quantities of both omega-3s and omega-6s and the correct balance between both types. For example, excess omega-6s relative to omega-3s can actually increase blood clotting and worsen inflammatory diseases.

As the body can produce all other fatty acids by itself, the main aim of the fat component of your diet should be to ensure an adequate intake of these essential fatty acids. Good sources include nuts, legumes, soy beans, fish (the best source of omega-3s), breast milk, lean meat, vegetable-based oils and margarines, and even vegetables. Animal fats (including milk fats and formula milks used in place of breast milk) and fats used in processed foods are poor sources, another good reason for avoiding them. An ideal diet is one that includes about 25 per cent of energy as fat, minimises saturated fatty acid intake, promotes monounsaturated fatty acids and includes a good balance of omega-6s to omega-3s.

The balance between dietary omega-3s and omega-6s

With the increased use of polyunsaturated margarines and oils there has been a rise in the consumption of omega-6 fatty acids, altering the balance between omega-6s and omega-3s. This is a problem as it is the omega-3s that help reduce blood clotting, blood pressure and inflammation in the body. At present, the ratio of omega-6 to omega-3 fats in the diet is typically about fourteen to one. This figure should be about six to one. A high omega-6 intake is also a problem because it can act to reduce the amount of vegetable-sourced omega-3 that can be modified for use in the body. Vegetable-sourced omega-3s must be converted to other omega-3s before they can be used in the body and they compete with omega-6s for a particular enzyme in one step of this modification process. Excess omega-6s mean less of this enzyme is available for use by the vegetable-sourced omega-3s and thus less can be used.

Omega-3s sourced from fish are different from those sourced from vegetables. They are not affected by omega-6 metabolism and can be used directly by the body.

Luckily, the increasing popularity of olive oil and canola-based margarines, which contain a higher content of monounsaturated fats in place of omega-6s, is making this imbalance less of a problem. The imbalance can also be improved by using monounsaturated oils, such as olive oil, instead of polyunsaturated oils; using products made from linseeds, especially breads; and consuming more vegetables and especially more fish. Having said all this, omega-6 fats are healthy and should be part of your normal diet. Just not too much.

Unlike saturated fats, unsaturated fats are not responsible for raising blood cholesterol and in fact help to do the opposite. (These advantages of unsaturated fats are discussed in the section on lowering blood cholesterol through diet in Part 5.) Unsaturated fatty acids should represent at least 70 per cent of your total fat intake. Most Australians have a relatively low intake of omega-3 fats and their contribution to total fat intake should be increased. On the other hand, people who consume lots of margarines and oils containing predominantly omega-6s may have relatively too much of this type of fat. Dietary sources of theses fats are shown in Table 10.

SOURCING OMEGA-3 OILS—A PREFERRED FATTY ACID CHOICE

Fish is by far the best source of omega-3 oils for two reasons. Firstly, its omega-3s are different from those found in plant foods, the main ones being eicosapentaenoic acid (EPA) and docosahexaenoic acid (DHA). These omega-3s can be used directly by the body, especially the brain, whereas plant omega-3s (mainly alpha-linolenic acid) need to be converted to DHA to be useful. As stated above, an enzyme involved in this conversion is also used by omega-6 fatty acids and its presence can reduce the benefit gained from plant omega-3s. Secondly, fish generally has a higher level of omega-3s than plant sources. The exception is linseed, which has 57 per cent of its total fat content as omega-3s.

Two servings of fish per week provides an adequate amount of omega-3s. Traditionally, oily fish, such as salmon, were thought to be the best source. However, it is now recognised that all fish are good sources.

A new source of omega-3s is low fat milk with omega-3s added. A 250ml glass will contain about 200mg of omega-3 fats. It needs to be stressed that there is little evidence proving that such supplements provide the same benefits as omega-3s found naturally in fish. Other sources are shown in Table 10.

While nutrients gained from fresh food are always best, fish oil capsules can be used as a source of omega-3s. Be sure to purchase capsules produced by reputable companies as all omega-3s are unstable and can easily oxidise if not handled carefully. This is why fish goes

Table 10 Food sources of unsaturated fatty acids

Monounsaturated fats	
Chicken (56%)	Canola oil (63%)
Game meats	Macadamia nut oil (61%)
Fish	Peanut oil (46%)
All nuts except walnuts and coconut	Sunola oil (made from sunflowers bred to have mostly monounsaturated oils) (85%)
Olive oil (76%)	Some soy-bean oils are being genetically modified to contain more monounsaturated fat
Avocado (67%)	

Polyunsaturated oils	
Omega-6 types	*Omega-3 types*
Corn or maize oil (54%*)	Human breast milk
Grapeseed oil	Fish (fresh, frozen or canned—all fish count as good sources, although oily fish such as salmon, tuna, sardines and mackerel have more than white fish such as bream and whiting).
Sesame oil	Linseeds (or flaxseed) (about 54% of fats in linseeds are omega-3s and thus it is a good source of these fats. Linseed oil goes off quickly and the best source is breads containing linseeds).
Sunflower oil (66%*)	Walnuts and walnut oil (73%*)
Wheatgerm oil	Soy-bean oil (62%*)
Cottonseed oil	
Soy-bean oil (62%*)	
Walnuts and walnut oil (73%*)	
Peanut oil (35%*)	

* Fat content percentages relate to total polyunsaturated fat content (including both omega-3s and omega-6s).

Notes:

1. The percentages mentioned indicate the percentage of the particular type of fat in relation to the total fat content of the food. They do not indicate the overall fat content of the food.
2. Some foods are mentioned in two places. This is because they contain significant amounts of both types of fatty acids.

off more quickly than most other fresh foods. It is also the reason that linseed oil, which has a high omega-3 content, is not used very often. (Oxidised omega-3s smell off.) To help prevent oxidation, all sources of omega-3s should be kept in the fridge.

Omega-3s have numerous benefits regarding vascular disease prevention, including lowering your blood triglyceride levels, helping prevent blood clotting, and reducing the likelihood of harmful irregular heart rhythms occurring. They also help reduce high blood pressure. In addition to these benefits, Omega-3s are thought to be important for maintaining optimum brain function in both adults and children and may help in the prevention of illnesses such as depression. (Studies are under way to substantiate any such benefit.)

EXTRA VIRGIN OLIVE OIL—ANOTHER PREFERRED FATTY ACID CHOICE

Olive oil, like most oils, is about 90 per cent fat. About three quarters of this is monounsaturated fat with the other quarter being made up of equal amounts of saturated and polyunsaturated fats. Being low in saturated fats and high in monounsaturated fats, olive oil helps reduce vascular disease and assists in reversing any omega-3/omega-6 imbalance. Another important vascular disease benefit is its high antioxidant content. There is some evidence to suggest that olive oil may also help in lowering blood pressure and in reducing clotting.

Olive oils are classified according to how the olives are pressed to extract the oil. In times past they were pressed several times. Today they are usually pressed once only. However, the oil that comes out at the beginning of the pressing is different from that which comes out at the end. Initial pressings are called 'extra virgin olive oil'. It is generally darker in colour and contains many more flavour compounds. (To be called extra virgin, the oil must meet certain flavour criteria.) Many of these flavour compounds, such as phenolics, are antioxidants. There are over 35 antioxidants in extra virgin olive oil and they are thought to protect against vascular disease. Later pressings are called 'light olive oil'. It is a lighter colour, and contains less flavour compounds and less antioxidants. Light is not lighter in fat content, and it needs to be stressed that all olive oils contain the same amount of fat and the same energy content (i.e. the same number of kilojoules or calories). Thus, extra virgin oil is preferable to other forms both in taste and health benefits. However, as it is almost all fat, it should be consumed in moderation as part of your daily fat allowance.

Cholesterol

Dietary cholesterol accounts for only about 2 per cent of the total fat we eat, with the rest being made up of fatty acids. The body can make all the cholesterol it requires. However, the body typically produces about 75 per cent of our cholesterol needs with the rest coming from our diet.

Cholesterol is the fat that is deposited in artery walls, causing vascular disease such as coronary artery disease. For this reason, it is often viewed as a compound that is harmful to the body. However, this is the case only when it is in excess. Cholesterol is in fact an essential component of many important body structures, including the protective membrane that surrounds all cells, vitamin D, all steroid compounds (e.g. steroid hormones), and bile salts, which are produced by the liver to help digest dietary fat.

The two components of your diet that can increase your blood cholesterol level are your saturated fatty acid intake and your cholesterol intake, with your saturated fatty acid intake being the significantly more important factor. Thus, from a fat-content point-of-view, stating that a food is cholesterol-free does not mean that it is good for you. To be good for you the food should also have a low total-fat content, especially a low saturated-fat content. (Beware of foods stating that they are low in just cholesterol.)

While dietary cholesterol is less important than saturated fatty acid in determining blood cholesterol levels, restricting your cholesterol consumption still makes a significant contribution to lowering your blood cholesterol. This is important in those with risk factors for vascular disease or those who already have vascular disease. Foods especially high in cholesterol include lambs' brains, offal, tripe, liver, pâté, fish roe and egg yolks. (Prawns, lobster and squid also have a relatively high-cholesterol content, but their low total-fat and high-protein content makes this relatively unimportant.) Other foods that contribute to dietary cholesterol are similar to those that contribute to saturated fat intake. (Mainly meats and to a lesser extent full-fat dairy foods.)

GOOD AND BAD CHOLESTEROL—LIPOPROTEINS AND CHOLESTEROL TRANSPORT

Lipoproteins are used to transport fats in the blood because their outer coating makes them soluble in water. Fats, such as cholesterol (as cholesterol esters) and triglycerides, are generally not water-soluble and thus cannot be transported easily in blood on their own (as blood is mostly composed of cells floating in salty water). A lipoprotein consists of a central core of mainly cholesterol (as cholesterol esters) and triglycerides surrounded by a membrane (a phospholipid monolayer). Because they contain many fat molecules, lipoproteins are much larger than the fatty acids or cholesterol they contain.

There are several types of lipoproteins and these vary according to their size, the type and amounts of the fats they contain, and their actions in the body. They are generally divided into two groups that have been termed 'good cholesterol' and 'bad cholesterol', depending on their effect on vascular disease. These terms are unfortunate as they incorrectly imply there are different types of cholesterol itself. This is not true. It is the structures that the cholesterol is carried in, the lipoproteins, that are different. The 'good' or 'bad' grouping depends on whether the lipoprotein decreases (good) or increases (bad) cholesterol deposits in arteries (i.e. decreases or increases vascular disease).

The term 'good cholesterol' refers to high-density lipoproteins (HDL). These carry cholesterol from your body back to your liver. In doing this they actually reduce the amount of cholesterol in your artery walls and thus reduce blockages in your arteries. Bad cholesterol refers to several types of lipoprotein, the main one being low-density lipoprotein (LDL). These are formed from another bad lipoprotein called very low-density lipoprotein (VLDL), which is made in the liver. The LDL formed in the blood through changes to VLDL takes cholesterol to other tissues, such as muscles. As it travels through the arteries to get to these tissues, some is deposited into your artery walls. The higher the level of LDL, the more your vessel walls are exposed to cholesterol deposition.

When your blood cholesterol measurement is determined, it usually includes your HDL, LDL and total cholesterol levels. The total cholesterol is made up of HDL, LDL and other cholesterol sources.

Appendix 12 summarises the metabolism of cholesterol in the body and Appendix 9 shows how diet and other factors can alter blood cholesterol and vascular disease.

FOODS CONTAINING PLANT STEROLS

Plant sterols (and stanols) are compounds that are chemically similar to cholesterol. They occur naturally in small amounts in some foods. Unlike cholesterol, the body absorbs sterols only in very small amounts. Thus, almost all sterols are excreted in the faeces.

Sterols act to reduce blood cholesterol by reducing cholesterol absorption from the small intestine. This is accomplished by the sterols competing with cholesterol for absorption sites on the bowel surface. The effect of sterols on blood cholesterol is in addition to the reduction in blood cholesterol achieved through reducing dietary cholesterol intake or by taking cholesterol-lowering medication.

Sterols are found in soy beans, leaves, nuts, vegetable oils, corn and rice. A normal Australian diet contains about 200 to 400 mg per day of these compounds. (Vegetarian diets may contain higher levels, up to 600 to 800 mg.) These dietary levels do not have any significant effect on reducing cholesterol levels in the blood. To achieve its cholesterol-lowering effect, sterol intake needs to be about 3 grams per day. You can achieve dietary intakes of 3 grams per day by eating about 25 grams of sterol-enriched margarine. (This equates to about one and a half tablespoons of margarine or the amount needed to cover four slices of bread.)

Plant sterol products reduce the absorption of some fat-soluble vitamins and carotenoids found in fruit and vegetables, which are thought to give protection against numerous diseases, including cancer. For this reason, it is recommended that children and pregnant or lactating women not use these sterol-containing products. If you use plant sterol products, you should eat extra fruit and vegetables (i.e. more than the recommended five to seven servings per day). The intake of plant sterols should not be greater than 3 grams per day as a greater intake is no more beneficial and it reduces the absorption of these nutrients further. Sterols should not be used as a substitute for a low-fat diet.

Avoiding deficiencies in low fat diets

Low-fat diets have the potential to provide an inadequate intake of calcium, iron and zinc unless food choices are made carefully. Many people significantly reduce their intake of dairy products when reducing the fat content in their diet and thus greatly reduce their calcium intake. This is not necessary as low-fat milk products are a healthy substitute for full-fat dairy products, containing virtually no fat.

Red meat, and to a lesser extent chicken and fish, are still valuable sources of iron in low-fat diets. Iron can also be obtained from plant foods but this iron is less well absorbed. (The absorption can be improved by eating foods rich in vitamin C at each meal.) A list of iron-containing foods is provided in Appendix 5. Excess iron intake can be harmful and it is important not to take iron supplements unless blood tests have shown you have an iron deficiency or you are advised to do so by your doctor.

Zinc is important in enzymes and helps immune system maintenance. As intake can be low in people on low-fat diets, foods containing zinc should be encouraged and a good diet can supply all that is required. (Excess intake from supplements can be harmful.) Zinc is available from oysters, lean red meat, wholegrain cereals and legumes. A list of zinc-containing foods is provided in Appendix 5.

Children under five are growing quickly and need lots of energy. A strict low-fat diet is not appropriate in this group as they require some good quality foods that contain fat. One really good source is whole milk and this should be used in preference to low-fat varieties in this age group. Others are cheese, lean meats, peanut butter, yoghurt and eggs. (Nuts, especially peanuts, should not be given as they can cause choking.) Poor quality fatty foods, such as crisps, chocolate and takeaways, should still be omitted or used as an occasional (not daily) treat. Otherwise, poor eating habits that will be hard to break later on will be established.

Carbohydrates and low-glycaemic index foods

The dietary advice advocated in this book centres on a low-fat intake, especially low saturated fat, and a moderate to high intake of carbohydrates and fibre. Reducing fat is covered in Part 4. This section deals with choosing which carbohydrates you should include in your diet. Carbohydrates are divided into two groups: sugars, which are simple compounds, and starches, which are more complex compounds made up from simple sugars. Together, they should provide about 50 to 60 per cent of your dietary energy intake and the vast majority of this should come from starches.

Starch is the main carbohydrate found in cereal grains, root vegetables and pulses, so it is the main constituent of our breads, pasta and cereals. It is broken down to simple sugars (mostly glucose) in the intestine and absorbed into the blood stream. Dietary sugars include sucrose (found in white and brown sugar, golden syrup, maple syrup, molasses and many fruits), fructose (found in ripe fruits, honey and some vegetables), lactose (found in milk), maltose (formed from the breakdown of starches) and glucose (found in sweet fruits and some vegetables).

The sugar that circulates in the blood to provide energy to the body is glucose. This mainly comes from the breakdown of carbohydrates consumed in the diet or the breakdown of glucose that is stored in the liver as glycogen. (You have enough glucose stored as glycogen to provide energy for about 90 minutes of exercise. Then your body burns fat stores.) Glucose is the brain's source of energy and for this reason the body regulates its level in the blood very carefully.

When choosing carbohydrates, several factors are important, including:

- Energy content
- Nutrient content, especially vitamin and minerals
- Fibre content
- Glycaemic index.

In the past, complex carbohydrates have been advocated as being beneficial for your health. This has been found to be not necessarily the case. The preferred way to classify all carbohydrates with regard to their health benefits is according to their glycaemic index (GI). The GI is a measure of how a particular carbohydrate-containing food raises your blood sugar (glucose) level after being consumed. It takes into account the degree to which it is raised and the duration of the rise. A high-GI food is digested relatively quickly, thus raising your blood glucose quickly and to a higher peak level. A low-GI food is digested more slowly, giving a slower, more sustained rise in blood glucose with a lower peak level. Foods are given a GI rating from 0 to 100. The food that gives the maximum overall rise in blood glucose is glucose itself and it is given a score of 100. The blood glucose responses of other foods are then compared to this level and given an appropriate score.

Your body's response to a rise in your blood sugar is to increase the level of the hormone insulin. Insulin acts to move the sugar into your cells (to be used later to provide energy) and thus reduces the sugar level in your blood. The important factor to note is that the amount of insulin needed to reduce your blood sugar after a high-GI food is greater than the amount needed for a low-GI food. Therefore, people who eat a high-glycaemic load diet (i.e. a diet containing foods with high GIs) have a higher insulin requirement than people who eat a low-glycaemic load diet (i.e. a diet containing foods with low GIs). People who cannot produce enough insulin to cope with this additional requirement have glucose intolerance and may develop diabetes.

The increased insulin secretion associated with a diet containing a high-glycaemic load also increases the risk of developing the metabolic syndrome, which includes problems such as obesity, coronary artery disease, hypertension and adverse changes in blood lipids.

In addition to reducing the likelihood of diabetes and the metabolic syndrome, the low, prolonged rise in your blood sugar caused by low-glycaemic load diets also helps to suppress your feeling of hunger longer, helping to reduce snacking and thus obesity. All this translates into the following health benefits for a low-glycaemic load diet:

- Weight loss
- Improved blood lipids
- Reduced glucose intolerance and reduced risk of developing diabetes
- Better control of diabetes in those with the disease
- Reduced risk of coronary heart disease (heart attacks).

It is important to note that, by necessity, GI figures are calculated when a single food is consumed. Meals are a combination of numerous food groups and the consumption of fats and proteins is likely to significantly affect the glucose response to carbohydrates. Thus, GI levels should be seen as a guide. Small differences in the GIs of foods are insignificant and need not affect food choices. However, choosing a food with a substantially lower GI than the alternative will be beneficial.

Achieving a low GI diet

The glycaemic index has been calculated for over 700 foods and is available for many common foods on the Glycaemic Index website www.glycaemicindex.com or in many publications.

The glycaemic index is also becoming commonly stated on food packaging. You should look for the 'GI Symbol', as this indicates that the GI value has been assessed by an accredited laboratory.

As a general indication, foods can be divided into three GI groups; low GI foods (GI value of 0 to 55), medium GI foods (GI value of 56 to 70) and high GI foods (GI value of 71 to 100). As stated above, it is important not to become too obsessed with GI values and to use them as a general guide to dietary habits.

All foods have some carbohydrate, but most of our carbohydrate intake comes from bread, cereals, potatoes, rice and pasta. Therefore, it is these foods you need to concentrate on when adding low GI foods to your diet. A food high in fibre does not necessarily have a low GI; for example, wholemeal bread. The best way to reduce the glycaemic load in your diet is to include a large portion of at least one low GI food in each meal and include as many other low GI foods as possible. Consuming smaller meals more often rather than a few large meals also helps.

When choosing your carbohydrates, please remember that the GI index is only one factor in your choice. Nutrient, fibre and energy content are equally, if not more, important considerations. A list of low GI foods appear in Appendix 6.

Appropriate food choices for a good low GI diet

- a low-GI breakfast cereal (that is also high in fibre), such as those based on wheat bran, barley and oats
- grainy breads made with whole seeds
- pasta, sweet potato or couscous instead of normal potato
- low-GI rice alternatives, such as Basmati, Doongara or wild rice, instead of higher GI rices, such as brown, calrose or jasmine rice
- barley, semolina, noodles and bulgar
- apples, oranges and pears instead of tropical fruit—less ripe fruits have a lower GI
- more acidic foods, such as lemon juice, vinegar-based salad dressings, and sourdough breads.
- less refined/processed foods.

Fibre in the diet

Fibre is defined as any food matter that passes through the small intestine undigested. Having gone through the small intestine unchanged, all but the lingin component of the fibre (the toughest part) is at least partially broken down (fermented) by bacteria in the large bowel. This process adds bulk to the faeces.

Dietary fibre can be divided into two types: soluble fibre, which can be dissolved in water, and insoluble fibre, which cannot be dissolved in water. Most fibre-containing foods have both types.

Insoluble fibre and the bowel

Insoluble fibre is beneficial for your bowel. Good sources of insoluble fibre include wheat bran (found in cereals and wholegrain breads and also sold as unprocessed or natural bran), brown rice and vegetables. Insoluble fibre helps reduce several bowel diseases, including irritable bowel syndrome, diverticulitis and, most probably, bowel cancer. The effect on cancer arises by several mechanisms, including favourably altering the bacteria in the bowel, which enables a better breakdown of ingested cancer-causing chemicals, and the binding of fibre to some cancer-causing chemicals, which aids in their excretion. Also, the extra faecal bulk added by fibre acts to dilute any ingested cancer-causing chemicals, helping to reduce exposure of the bowel wall to these chemicals. Fibre also assists with the production of butyric acid, a compound that can slow cancer-cell growth. This is produced as part of the fibre breakdown process in the bowel.

Evidence supporting fibre as a factor in reducing bowel cancer incidence has been brought into question by some data from recent studies. It has been suggested the protective effect of foods high in insoluble fibre is due to other compounds found in these foods, such as antioxidants, rather than the fibre component. However, there is still a large body of evidence showing that fibre is protective. More research is being done on this topic.

Soluble fibre and cholesterol

Foods rich in soluble fibre reduce plasma cholesterol levels by binding to cholesterol in the gut. This prevents the cholesterol from being reabsorbed back into the body from the small intestine as it is excreted in the faeces attached to the soluble fibre. Foods containing soluble fibre include oat bran, barley bran, rice bran (less than oat and barley bran), lentils, dried beans, fruit and vegetables. Insoluble fibre, such as wheat bran, does not bind cholesterol, so it does not help reduce cholesterol levels.

High-fibre diets

A high-fibre diet requires at least 30 grams of fibre a day, preferably a mixture of soluble and insoluble fibre. This can be gained from a daily intake of all of the following:

- a bowl of bran cereal
- three slices of wholegrain bread
- two pieces of fruit
- three servings of vegetables
- a serving of beans.

Micronutrients and other useful compounds

Vitamins and minerals

Vitamins are a group of nutrients the body needs but cannot produce itself in adequate amounts. Thus, they must be obtained from the diet. All minerals need to come from the diet. As a general rule, Australians do not need to take vitamin or mineral supplements as their diet provides adequate amounts. The more common exceptions to this rule are as follows and, even in these situations, careful attention to diet will avoid the need for supplements in most cases.

- Folate supplements for women of child-bearing age. They may also prove to be beneficial in reducing coronary artery disease.
- Calcium supplements in those with a low-calcium intake, particularly in post-menopausal women.
- Iron intake in women (and men) with diagnosed (by blood tests) iron deficiency and no other underlying cause, such as blood loss from a cancer.
- Frail, aged people who eat poorly.
- Some vegetarians (see page 124).
- People with multiple food allergies or intolerances.
- Alcoholics who are likely to be deficient in vitamins (especially vitamin B1).
- People with diseases affecting their bowels, which reduce their ability to absorb vitamins and minerals from their diet. Such diseases are quite rare.
- Those with an inadequate diet due to poverty or bizarre eating habits.

Magnesium has also been in the news lately. Most people can obtain adequate magnesium from their diet. Foods rich in magnesium include green vegetables, nuts, legumes, wheat germ and wholemeal bread. Deficiencies can occur in chronic alcoholism and in association with some medications, such as some diuretics. Supplements should not be taken unless a deficiency has been proven by blood tests and they should be prescribed by a doctor as they can cause diarrhoea and can be toxic, especially in the elderly.

While vitamin deficiencies severe enough to cause disease are relatively rare in Australia, there is debate over whether less severe deficiencies can pose a health risk. At present there is little concrete evidence that this is the case. One exception is folate, where levels not low enough to cause the symptoms of classical folate deficiency are suspected to be responsible for raising the blood level of homocysteine. This in turn increases the risk of vascular disease. This relationship is still being investigated and it may be that the recommended daily intake of folate will need to be increased, at least in those at risk of vascular disease.

INAPPROPRIATE USES OF VITAMIN SUPPLEMENTS

All vitamins and minerals have been the subject of extensive study. The daily recommended intakes for vitamins and minerals advised by health authorities are based on all the well-researched information available. There is no reason for them not to be! They are therefore the most reliable guide to vitamin and mineral intake you will find.

These levels can be maintained in most people by adhering to their usual varied diet. Despite this, many Australians continue to purchase vitamins that are of no benefit. Some common reasons for this practice are as follows:

- Many Australians believe they eat very poorly and that they are likely to be deficient in vitamins etc. The truth is, our dietary problems are due to having too much food, especially fat and sugar. As stated above, vitamin and mineral deficiencies are rare in Australians.
- Some people believe that foods today are poorer in quality and have less nutritional value. There is no evidence that this is the case.
- People often feel their stress and tiredness are due to a nutrition deficiency of some kind. This is rarely the case, although people who are chronically tired should have their iron levels checked, especially women with heavy menstrual periods.
- Many people seem to believe vitamins have magical properties that will prevent a multitude of diseases. They often take the attitude, 'if some is good, more is better', and they feel that any increase in their vitamin intake is beneficial, or at least can't hurt. This is not true. There are some vitamins that are toxic to the body if taken in excess. This is especially the case with fat-soluble vitamins (vitamins A, D, E and K) which can be stored in the body in large quantities. Special care needs to be taken to avoid toxic doses of vitamin A (retinol) if taking supplements. (There is evidence that excessive intake has been associated with an increase of fractures.)

THE VITAMIN MESSAGE

Don't assume a vitamin deficiency is your problem. You will probably just be wasting your money and missing the real cause of your problem. If you are worried about your diet or have a problem, talk to your GP about your concerns. He or she can advise about proper nutrition and help find the cause of any underlying condition, should one be present. If you still feel you need to take supplements, do so for as little time as possible and take a supplement that has a wide range of vitamins etc. in concentrations that do not exceed your recommended daily allowance for each compound. Ensure that you purchase vitamins produced in Australia by reputable companies. Some less reputable products, usually from overseas, contain additives not mentioned on the label. These substances, which include compounds such as steroids, caffeine and ephedrine, are included because they give you more energy, at least temporarily. Athletes need to be especially careful as taking many of these substances may result in positive drug tests. (See the Australian Institute of Sport website www.ais.org.au/nutrition for more detailed information.)

Antioxidants

The oxidation of body tissues and compounds is a damaging process that is continually being fought by your body. It is principally caused by unstable compounds called free radicals. Free radicals are unstable because they lack an electron in their structure. In order to become stable, they steal electrons from other compounds they come in contact with. The loss of this electron is a process termed oxidation and the resultant changes in the structure of the oxidised compound often disrupt its ability to function properly.

Free radicals are produced by normal chemical reactions in the body, a process that can be increased in conditions such as diabetes and perhaps stress. Many different types of free radicals can be ingested, a principal culprit being tobacco smoke. Others include alcohol, animal fats, smoked and chargrilled foods, oils heated during deep-frying, pollutants, and many other chemicals in the environment. Oxidation by free radicals can affect blood lipids, the immune system, DNA (genes), enzymes, hormones, skin proteins etc. All this can lead to an increase in many diseases, including cardiovascular disease, cancers, and inflammatory diseases, such as arthritis.

As well as being fought by the body, oxidation reactions caused by free radicals can be prevented or reversed by the antioxidants consumed in the diet. These substances have an extra electron that they can give away. There are two main groups of antioxidants: nutrients, including vitamins C, E and betacarotene which play essential roles in processes in the body; and various other compounds found in foods, including carotenoids, polyphenols, flavenoids, catechins and theaflavins (found in tea). Hundreds of different antioxidants are present in vegetables, fruit, wholegrains, olive oil, nuts, tea, soy beans, dark grape juice and red wine, and many more are still being identified. Knowledge about which antioxidants are most beneficial is very limited at present and it is therefore advisable to have as wide a range of antioxidant-containing foods as possible. (See Appendix 13)

ANTIOXIDANT AND VITAMIN SUPPLEMENTS FOR HEART DISEASE AND CANCER PREVENTION

Antioxidants taken in your normal diet do help prevent coronary artery disease (heart disease). This fact has led to many people taking supplements of 'antioxidant' vitamins in the belief they will also help reduce heart disease. There is now good evidence that, unlike antioxidants in food, antioxidant supplements provide little or no benefit with respect to heart disease. Similarly, the protection against cancer that is provided so well by nutrients in vegetables and fruit cannot be replaced by supplements. In fact, taking large doses of only a few antioxidants has been shown to be harmful in some studies—they can even increase oxidation reactions.

The reason antioxidant supplements are unlikely to be of benefit is that there are hundreds of different antioxidants present in foods and we are likely to need a wide range of them for good protection. Also, as we don't know which are most beneficial or in what dose, it is not possible to know which antioxidants should be included in supplements. Antioxidant supplements just cannot match the hundreds of nutrients found in your normal foods and, unlike nutrients in food, they are not intimately mixed with this food. Until a great deal more is known about this topic, taking supplements for cancer or heart disease prevention is most likely a waste of your money and may even be causing you harm.

Selling nutritional supplements

You should be in no doubt that the priority of those selling you manufactured health foods and nutrient supplements, such as vitamins, is to do just that. Sell. Their message will always be that their product is good for you and you will rarely get an unbiased view. The producers of nutritional supplements (and herbal remedies) are not regulated by government organisations, such as Food Standards Australia New Zealand or the Therapeutic Drugs Administration. Thus, they are not required to give proof to these bodies that their claimed medicinal benefits are legitimate.

You should be sceptical of any information or advice provided at stores selling such products. They have a conflict of interest. Written opinions by so-called experts, often presented in the form of official looking articles, may be produced to support product claims. Remember, opinions are cheap and they mean nothing unless they are backed up by good research, something that is very difficult for you to determine in a shop.

Another often used sales method is to provide free in-shop advice by an expert about improving your health. Such advice is still only an opinion and, while it may have been given free, the products you are advised to purchase are not. This does not mean that their advice will necessarily be wrong or inappropriate. It will just be compromised.

Vegetarian diets

Vegetarian diets are generally a healthy option, especially if milk products and eggs are allowed in the diet. It is also an increasingly common option, especially amongst adolescent girls. About 25 per cent of girls choose to be vegetarian at some stage during their teenage years. Whilst some take this option for moral reasons, many do so to lose weight. Luckily, most remain quite well with the incidence of anorexia being about 1 per cent.

Animal products provide protein, energy and fat in your diet. As most Australians take excess fat and energy, the reduction of these from a vegetarian diet is often beneficial. However, some vegetarians have an energy-deficient diet and are underweight and unhealthy. As egg whites and milk products are rich in good protein, a vegetarian diet that includes these and a good variety of plant proteins is usually not protein deficient. Sources of plant proteins include cereals, nuts and legumes, such as soy beans, lentils, beans and peas.

Vegetarians who choose not to consume milk products and eggs need to be more careful to ensure their protein intake is adequate, both in the total amount and in the types of amino acids that are present in the protein. (Amino acids are the building blocks of all proteins. Some, called essential amino acids, cannot be made by your body and must be obtained from your diet.) Total protein intake needs to be at least 0.7 grams per kilogram of body weight each day in adults and 1 gram per kilogram of body weight per day in the elderly. A mix of 70 per cent from cereals and 30 per cent from legumes is ideal (Wahlqvist 2002). Nuts should also be included each day. These foods need to be a large part of the diet to ensure adequate protein and energy requirements. Vegetarians who do not consume milk products or calcium-enriched foods, such as calcium-enriched soy products, will need calcium supplements.

Vegetarian diets without milk products and eggs often provide inadequate levels of vitamin B12. (As body stores of vitamin B12 are large, a deficiency may not appear for several years after adoption of the diet.) Vitamin B12 deficiency also affects the unborn children of affected mothers, causing neurological problems, so women of child-bearing age on this diet should take supplements of vitamin B12. This issue should be discussed with your medical practitioner. Vegetarian diets without milk products and eggs are not suitable for children.

Iron can be deficient in some vegetarians and those requiring extra iron, especially teenage girls and pregnant women, may require iron supplements if they have been diagnosed to be iron deficient by a blood test.

Caffeine

Caffeine is an addictive drug and its intake needs to be regulated. In adults, intakes should be kept to a maximum of less than 200 to 250 mg per day, the equivalent of about two to three cups of coffee or four to five cups of tea. Coffee brands do vary somewhat in their caffeine content while all teas contain about 3 per cent caffeine (Stanton 2001). Decaffeinated coffee and tea contain only 0.3 per cent caffeine. New energy drinks also contain high levels of caffeine. This comes from guarana, a compound found in the seeds of a vine from the central Amazon.

Caffeine can cause increased stiffening of your arteries, which can increase your blood pressure. If you have high blood pressure, you may be well advised to restrict coffee intake to one or two cups per day or use decaffeinated coffee.

The commonest sources of caffeine

- fresh coffee (80–90 mg of caffeine)
- energy drinks (80 mg)
- instant coffee (60–90 mg)
- strong tea (50–60 mg)
- 375 ml can of cola drink (30–50 mg)
- weak tea (20–30 mg)
- chocolate products, including cocoa, hot chocolate and chocolate bars.

Source: Rosemary Stanton 2001

Some coffees, such as unfiltered Arabic or Robusta, can raise your cholesterol slightly. The responsible ingredient is not caffeine but a compound called cafestol. Filtered and instant coffees appear not to have this effect.

Caffeine causes anxiety-like symptoms, such as palpitations, tremors and sleep disturbances, especially when taken to excess by adults or when taken by children. As both cola drinks and energy drinks are high in caffeine and energy, children and adolescents should avoid them. The common use of these drinks in these age groups is an increasing problem, especially as obesity, mild anxiety and attention deficit hyperactivity disorders are some of the most common medical problems of childhood. (Some cola drinks are unsweetened and these do not cause the obesity problem.) All cola drinks are also quite acidic and this causes erosion of tooth enamel.

If you are cutting down on your caffeine, be aware that you are likely to suffer short-term withdrawal symptoms, such as headaches and difficulty concentrating, so you should do it slowly.

Organic foods, pesticides and food additives

Many people are concerned about the quality of the foods they are eating. Principal concerns centre on additives that may be harmful, pesticides, food allergies, and reduced nutritional quality in mass-produced foods. Most of these concerns are based on myths that have been propagated in the media. Such stories make good press and almost anything can be claimed by the selective use of evidence.

Most food allergies are caused by proteins in food, not food additives. While many people may think they have a food allergy, true food allergies, where people have a positive skin test to the food and symptoms after consuming it, are very uncommon. The main causes are eggs, peanuts, cow's milk, fish, shellfish, wheat, and soy. In Australia, only food additives that have been thoroughly tested by the Food Standards Australia New Zealand (FSANZ) and which have been found to be safe for general consumption are allowed to be used in foods. The FSANZ is a government body that has no commercial interest in the food industry. In allowing the use of an additive, FSANZ cannot guarantee that it will never cause adverse reactions. This is, however, an uncommon problem and very few additives have been associated with problems. (Tartrazine and monosodium glutamate are examples of additives that have caused illness in some people.) If you are worried about a reaction to a particular food, see your GP or dietitian. All food ingredients, including additives, are listed as numbers (or according to function) on food packaging and a list of these numbers is available on the FSANZ website (see page 127). Despite popular belief, there is good evidence that food additives are not responsible for behavioural problems, such as hyperactivity, in children (Wahlqvist 2002).

While pesticide levels in foods are not zero, they are very low and within accepted safety limits. Levels are regularly checked around the country by FSANZ.

Organic foods are those grown without pesticides and chemical fertilisers. Generally, organic products have few nutritional advantages over conventionally grown produce, although there is some evidence that their mineral content may be higher. Also, there should be no pesticide residues present and organic growers *may* choose more tasty varieties. Their main advantage is that they protect our environment and that is an important consideration for all Australians. However, if the extra cost of organically grown produce is likely to reduce your fruit and vegetable consumption, then conventionally grown produce is perhaps your best option. There is no evidence that the nutrient content of foods today, organic or not, is different from that of times past.

Poor food handling techniques that cause contamination are a far greater health concern than the concerns mentioned above. For more information on food additives etc., see the FSANZ website www.foodstandards.gov.au or the Dietitians Association of Australia website www.daa.asn.au.

Herbal and natural remedies

Many of the world's most useful drugs and lethal poisons are derived from plants and animals—that is, 'nature'. Natural, though, does not mean healthy. It is important that any medication recommended to you has been conclusively established as beneficial and free from unacceptable side effects. This book does not mention herbal medicines or natural therapies for the following good reasons.

The evidence for the effectiveness of herbal remedies is poor, with few properly controlled studies supporting any benefit from these medications. This is partly due to the fact that the companies promoting these products do not have exclusive rights to their use and thus they are not prepared to fund this often expensive research. Nevertheless, without such evidence, it is difficult to confidently recommend these medications.

There is little regulation regarding the preparation of these products. This causes two problems. Firstly, the ingredients in similar herbal remedies may vary significantly. Secondly, the products may be contaminated with potentially harmful ingredients. A recent study in the USA found that nearly 33 per cent of randomly selected Asian herbal remedies were contaminated with arsenic, lead or undeclared pharmaceutical drugs (Bellamy, 2001). Also, despite being 'natural' products, a significant number of people taking these preparations suffer side effects. (The same USA study showed 12 per cent of people using herbal remedies suffered side effects.) It goes without saying that prescription medications have many side effects too.

Another problem with natural remedies is that the person recommending and sometimes preparing the medication is often the person you are paying for the medication, so a conflict of interest exists. (Conflicts of interest also sometimes exist in traditional medicine.)

In making these comments, I am not saying that herbal remedies have no beneficial effects. It is just that very few have been scientifically proven and there is very little reliable information available about the side effects of these preparations. What is needed is proper government regulation of this industry. This would ensure good evidence is obtained to establish the benefits claimed for each medication and standards for the preparation of these medicines would be established and maintained.

Finally, it is important to mention that natural medications can interact with other drugs. You should mention all the substances you are taking when consulting your health professional.

Consumer food information

Almost all packaged foods in Australia have a nutrition label showing the ingredients and the presence of common food allergens. Labels also provide information about the nutritional contents, including energy, fat, protein, saturated fat, sugars and sodium. This is expressed as the amount in a usual serving of the product and in 100 grams of the product. By looking at the content of total fat, saturated fat, energy and sodium, you will be able to determine whether the food is a detrimental or beneficial addition to your diet. Hopefully, where appropriate, many packaged foods will also provide the fibre content and the glycaemic index on their labels to aid you in your purchasing decision. With regard to unlabelled foods, the food nutritional guides, together with the comments on the fat and energy content of foods in this book, should enable you to make an informed judgment regarding the nutritional value.

An example of a typical nutritional label appears in figure 8 and you will notice that the nutrients, such as saturated fat, are shown as two different amounts. When purchasing food items, the best way to compare the nutritional values of food alternatives, such as butter and margarine, is to look at the quantity of the nutrient, such as the saturated fat, in 100 grams of the product. This in effect tells you the percentage of the nutrient in each product and allows a meaningful comparison.

The amount in a typical serving is there to help you calculate how much of the ingredient you will consume when you eat a typical serving. The quantity of product in a typical serving is also stated. It is important to recognise that the typical servings quoted are only a guide, as your portion size may vary significantly from this level. (Some manufacturers suggest unrealistic portion sizes.) You need to weigh the portion on your plate to calculate its energy and fat contents accurately.

Nutritional information Servings per package: 3 Serving size: 150mg		
	Quantity per serving	*Quantity per 100g*
Energy	608kJ	405kJ
Protein	4.2g	2.8g
Fat, total	7.5g	4.9g
- saturated	4.5g	3.0g
Carbohydrate, total	18.6g	12.4g
- sugars	18.6g	12.4g
Sodium	90mg	60mg
Calcium	300mg	200mg
* percentage of recommended daily intake	(25%)*	
Ingredients: Whole milk, concentrated skim milk, sugar, strawberries (9%), gelatine, culture, thickener (1442).		
PRODUCT OF AUSTRALIA Bavarian Yoghurt Makers, 16 Allen Lane, Strahan, Tas.		
Best before 1 APR 03		

Figure 8 Sample of an Australian food label

Diet and cancer prevention

Environmental factors, a large percentage of which are dietary related, account for about 50 to 80 per cent of all cancers. It is not surprising therefore that dietary modifications can play an important part in cancer prevention. It is thought a reduction in cancer deaths of 30 to 40 per cent can be achieved in Australia (about 30 000 people each year) by dietary change alone. Well over half of this benefit originates from the consumption of at least 400 grams per day of vegetables and fruit.

Compounds in food can either increase or decrease the likelihood a cancer will develop, either by acting on the genes of potential cancer cells or by influencing other cancer-causing substances. A food compound may prevent cancer by protecting the cell from cancerous changes to genes, by inhibiting other chemicals that cause cancer, or by helping your immune system to help fight cancers, and vice versa. As well as influencing cancer initiation, food compounds may influence the rate of cancer growth.

Dietary recommendations to prevent cancer

The World Cancer Research Fund completed a three-year review in 1997 of over 4500 scientific studies relating to diet and cancer prevention (Potter 1997). The following dietary recommendations to reduce cancer were made from their findings.

- *Eat at least five (preferably seven) servings of a good variety of fruit and vegetables per day.* A serving of vegetables weighs 60 to 90 grams and a portion of fruit weighs 120 to 140 grams. Raw vegetables, salads, green vegetables, tomatoes, the onion family, carrots and citrus fruits are especially good, but a wide variety of all fruits and vegetables is vital.
- *Consume no more than 80 grams of red meat per day (about the size of a pack of playing cards).* One serve of meat per day is sufficient for a healthy diet. Alternatives include a variety of fish, poultry and red meat. All meats should be lean and have visible fat removed (or the skin removed in the case of poultry). Legumes or nuts can be substituted for meats occasionally as wished.
- *Charred foods and deep-fried foods should be avoided or reduced.* Fish or meat grilled on a direct flame should be eaten only occasionally. Low-heat cooking is best, such as steaming, microwaving, boiling and stewing. Limit the use of barbequing, grilling and pan-frying. Meat and fish juices should also not be burned.
- *Smoked or cured meat and pickled foods should be eaten only occasionally.*
- *Eat at least seven serves of cereals, rice, pasta, breads, legumes, roots and tubers per day.* One serve equals 90 grams of cooked rice or pasta, 30 grams of cereal, or one potato. Foods should be minimally processed and contain a minimum amount of refined sugar.
- *Limit the intake of fatty foods, especially those of animal origin.* Try to use low-fat dairy products.
- *Limit consumption of salted foods and limit the use of table and cooking salt.*
- *Do not drink alcohol or limit alcohol intake to two drinks per day for men and one for women.*
- *Maintain a healthy weight.* Especially avoid gaining more than 5 kilograms in your adult life. (Being underweight should also be avoided.)
- *Keep physically active.*

The effects of various types of foods on the incidence of cancers are shown in table 11. As can be seen, not all this evidence is conclusive. It is important to remember that most of the evidence relating to the benefit of foods in preventing cancer was gained by looking at consuming foods, not dietary supplements. The fact that a particular food helps reduce cancer does not imply that a supplement containing one or two of its constituent compounds will give the same benefit.

Vegetables and cancer reduction

Inadequate fruit and vegetable consumption is thought to cause about 2.5 to 3 per cent of the total burden of disease in Australia, and about 75 per cent of this disease burden is due to an increase in cancer. Most of this illness occurs relatively early in life, in the 55 to 74 year age group (and to a lesser extent in the 45 to 55 year age group).

Table 11 Nutritional risk factors for selected cancers—strength of evidence supporting relationship

	Convincing	*Probable*	*Possible*	*Insufficient*
Lung	• Vegetables, particularly green vegetables and carrots, and fruits decrease risk	• Carotenoids decrease risk	• Physical activity, vitamin C, vitamin E and selenium decrease risk • Retinol has no relationship • Total fat, saturated/animal fat, cholesterol and alcohol increase risk	
Stomach	• Vegetables and fruits decrease risk. In particular, raw vegetables, allium vegetables and citrus fruits • Refrigeration decreases risk by reducing the use of salt and risk of contamination	• Vitamin C decreases risk • Alcohol, coffee, black tea and nitrates (from vegetables) have no relationship • Salt and salting increases risk	• Carotenoids, allium compounds, wholegrain cereals and green tea decrease risk • Sugar, vitamin E and retinol have no relationship • Starch, grilled/charred/barbequed meat and fish increase risk	• Fibre, selenium, sesame oil, onion, garlic decrease risk • Cured/smoked meats, *N*-nitrosamines increase risk • Factors encouraging certain gastric microflora, like *Helicobacter pylori*, which may lead to atrophic gastritis
Bowel	• Physical activity decreases the risk of colon cancer • Vegetables decrease risk (not fruits)	• Non-starch polysaccharides decrease risk • Fibre, unless associated with low fat intake, increases risk • Alcohol, as beer, increases risk • Salicylates, aspirin, garlic and indoles decrease risk	• Starch, fish, carotenoids, decrease risk • High body mass increases the risk of colon cancer • Greater adult weight, frequent eating, sugar, total fat, saturated/animal fat, processed meat, eggs and heavily cooked/barbequed meat increase risk	• Resistant starch, vitamin C, vitamin D, calcium, whey proteins from dairy products, *Lactobacillus Bifidus* in fermented foods, vitamin E, folate, omega-3 fatty acids, methionine, wholegrain cereals and coffee decrease risk • Iron and omega-6 linoleic acid increase risk
Pancreas			• Energy intake, dietary cholesterol, trypsin inhibition, larger build and high protein/fat diet may increase risk	

	Convincing	Probable	Possible	Insufficient
Prostate		• Total fat, saturated/animal fat may increase risk • Lycopene (e.g. tomatoes), soy/phytoestrogens may decrease risk	• Vegetables (green leafy and yellow), soy decrease risk • High body mass, alcohol, vitamin C, coffee and tea have no relationship • Meat, milk and dairy products increase risk	• High energy intake, cadmium increases risk
Breast	• Coffee has no relationship • Rapid growth and greater adult weight increase risk	• Vegetables (green), legumes (soy), fruits decrease risk • Dietary cholesterol has no relationship • High body mass (postmenopausal), adult weight gain increase risk • Breastfeeding reduces risk with longer total duration • Alcohol (>5 g/day) increases risk	• Physical activity, non-starch polysaccharides/fibre and carotenoids decrease risk • Retinol, vitamin E, poultry and black tea have no relationship • Monounsaturated fats may decrease risk and omega-6 linoleic acid may increase risk • Total fat, saturated/animal fat, meat increase risk	• Vitamin C, Vitamin A from foods, isoflavones, lignans, fish decrease risk • Animal protein and DDT in tissues increase risk
Cervix/ ovaries			• Vegetables and fruits, carotenoids, vitamin C and vitamin E decrease risk • Folate and retinol have no relationship • Galactose (milk) may increase risk of ovarian cancer	

Source: Food and Nutrition, Mark L. Wahlqvist, 2002; adapted from World Cancer Research Fund/American Institute for Cancer Research 1997.

As can be seen from table 11, vegetables and fruit are protective against many types of cancer, including lung, bowel, stomach, breast and prostate cancers (and possibly, cervical and ovarian cancers). The study of many individual compounds in vegetables, including nutrients such as vitamins and other phytochemicals (i.e. chemicals in plants), has produced no conclusive evidence that any one compound has anti-cancer properties on its own. The study of these compounds individually is very difficult due to interactions between the many different compounds present that may be of benefit, including salicylates, tannins, phytoestrogens, isoflavones, flavenoids, polyphenols, isothiocyanates etc. It is very likely that we need the full range of compounds available from a wide variety of vegetables to receive a beneficial effect and that no single chemical will be shown to be particularly beneficial.

It is also likely that taking supplements of vitamins, antioxidants etc. is not beneficial in reducing cancer. This is because we do not yet know which nutrients/chemicals are beneficial, let alone in what quantity, and because supplements do not provide the diversity of nutrients/chemicals required. Also, more is not necessarily better when consuming natural compounds, and in some cases, taking quantities significantly in excess of normal dietary requirements can increase the risk of disease, including cancers. With our present level of knowledge, supplements are not recommended and your money will be much better spent at the greengrocer.

Hints for preserving protective nutrients in vegetables

- Start with fresh vegetables and herbs whenever possible.
- Store fresh foods in a cool, dark place.
- Do not store fresh foods for long periods (a week at most).
- Keep pieces of fresh food as large as possible when chopping/slicing.
- When cooking vegetables, minimise both cooking time and cooking water to reduce vitamin losses. The preferred cooking method should be microwaving, followed by steaming, stir-frying and, lastly, boiling. If boiling, add food only when the water is boiling and boil in the smallest amount of water possible. Do not soak vegetables before cooking.
- Do not use copper pots or utensils as they can increase losses of some vitamins, particularly vitamin C.
- Use cooking water and liquid from canned foods in sauces, gravies etc.
- Do not use baking powder to preserve vegetable colour during cooking as it increases vitamin losses.

Water soluble vitamins are the ones destroyed by cooking as they dissolve in water. Maximum losses during cooking vary from 10 per cent for vitamin B12 to 100 per cent for more unstable vitamins, such as folate and vitamin C. Fat soluble vitamins are more hardy and don't dissolve in cooking water.

Food and bowel cancer

There is overwhelming evidence that the majority of bowel cancers occur due to environment factors and these factors are mostly dietary in origin. A better diet and healthier lifestyle can reduce the risk of colon cancer by 65 to 75 per cent. Bowel (colorectal) cancer is the second most common cancer in both men and women and reducing its incidence by such a huge amount would be a tremendous health benefit.

The National Health and Medical Research Council advises that the most important factors in reducing bowel cancer are:

- Eat at least five portions of vegetables per day. A portion of vegetables weighs 60 to 90 grams.
- Eat a high-fibre diet.
- Reduce dietary fat intake to 25 per cent of total energy (calorie) intake and avoid large amounts of animal fat.
- Maintain a normal weight—obesity increases the risk of bowel cancer. This can be achieved by restricting fat intake and consuming an appropriate energy intake for your level of physical activity.
- Avoid smoking.
- Partake in regular physical activity. There is convincing evidence that regular physical exercise, especially if done throughout life, protects against bowel cancer.

Other important measures include avoiding excess alcohol consumption, and charred foods, increasing resistant starch in the diet and avoiding large amounts of red meat. The evidence linking bowel cancer and red meat is controversial at present. However, meats with a high content of fat, such as processed meats, are probably a greater risk. (Stanton 2002). The cause of any increased risk remains uncertain and may be due to the meat, the fat or additives.

Vegetables, fruit and bowel cancer

Eating at least five portions of vegetables and fruit per day is the most important dietary measure in preventing bowel cancer. A wide variety of vegetables and fruit is essential.

Vegetables offer especially strong protection against bowel cancer with the most effective vegetables being the cruciferous varieties, which include bok choy, broccoli, Brussels sprouts, cabbage, cauliflower, Chinese cabbage, collards, kohlrabi, mustard greens, swedes and turnips. Their cancer-reducing effect is due to the sulphur-containing compounds, such as indoles and isothiocynates, they contain. All these vegetables are also high in fibre and antioxidants.

Salicylate-containing foods are also of probable benefit in reduced gut tumours, including stomach and oesophageal cancer as well as colorectal cancer. Salicylate-containing foods include fruit (dried fruit, cherries, pineapples, oranges, rockmelons, strawberries, apples), vegetables (gherkins, mushrooms, capsicums, zucchini, eggplant and green beans), condiments (thyme and oregano) and some beverages. Some people are sensitive to salicylates.

Charred foods and bowel cancer

Charred foods, including meat, toast and vegetables, can create chemicals that increase the risk of cancer, particularly bowel cancer. These chemicals include polynuclear aromatic hydrocarbons and heterocyclic amines. Polynuclear aromatic hydrocarbons are absorbed by foods when they are smoked (especially fatty meats) or are produced by charring foods. High-temperature cooking (frying, grilling and barbequing) of meats and fish turns some protein compounds into heterocyclic hydrocarbons, which are weakly carcinogenic.

Wherever possible, try to cook using low-heat methods such as steaming, microwaving or stewing. When barbequing, the production of these chemicals can be reduced by cooking over the hotplate rather than over coals. Also, microwaving the meat briefly first reduces the creatine content that gives rise to heterocyclic amines. Try using marinades to add extra flavour rather than charring food. (Avoid too much soy sauce as it has a very high salt content, even in the low-salt variety.)

Other food constituents and bowel cancer

High-fat intakes generally increase the incidence of bowel cancer, particularly saturated fats. The exception is omega-3 fatty acids, which actually offer some protection against bowel cancer. These are mainly present in fish and fish oils.

It appears likely that dietary resistant starch is of benefit in reducing bowel cancer. Starches are carbohydrates found mostly in grains, vegetables and fruit. Most starch is broken down in the small intestine. Resistant starch is starch that is not broken down in the small intestine and therefore reaches the large bowel, where it is broken down by bacteria. As it breaks down, it generates beneficial substances, especially butyrate, that help keep bowel cells healthy. They also reduce the chances of cancer-causing chemicals (carcinogens) affecting cells. Resistant starch also acts to increase faecal bulk, which dilutes carcinogens, encourages the growth of healthy bacteria, and reduces the growth of unhealthy bacteria. To be beneficial, at least 20 grams a day is needed. Hi-maize contributes a small amount of resistant starch to the diet and is found in some breads (e.g. the 'Wonder White' brand), breakfast cereals and muffins. Wholegrain cereals, rice, pasta (when eaten firm, i.e. not over-cooked), legumes, slightly unripe bananas and potato also contribute.

There is some evidence that the excessive consumption of alcohol may contribute to bowel cancer, with beer perhaps being a more important contributor.

Maintaining your recommended calcium intake may be protective against bowel cancer. Calcium's effect in reducing bowel cancer is thought to be due to a reduction in bile acids and fatty acids in the colon. There is no evidence that achieving a greater calcium intake through calcium supplements is of any benefit.

Folate may reduce cancers, including bowel cancers, by helping to repair damaged DNA (genes) in cells that may otherwise become cancerous. It is provided in leaf vegetables, spinach, asparagus, baked beans, citrus fruits and folate-enriched breakfast cereals and breads.

Selenium is an essential trace element that we must have in our diet, but require only in very small quantities. It acts to reduce colon cancer by reducing oxidative damage to the DNA (genes) of cells that may otherwise become cancerous. It also helps improve immune function in the body. Selenium is found in grains, vegetables, brazil nuts, fish and meat. The amount of selenium in grains depends on the soil content of selenium in which they were grown. Australian soils are generally adequate in selenium.

Food and prostate cancer reduction

As the early diagnosis and treatment of prostate cancer is of questionable benefit, trying to prevent this common cancer in the first place is an important goal. Several foods have been shown to influence the rate of prostate cancer.

Lycopene, found in tomatoes, has been shown to probably reduce prostate cancer incidence. Likewise, there is evidence that soy products/phytoestrogens may decrease prostate cancer risk.

Increased total fat intake, especially the saturated/animal fat component, is likely to increase prostate cancer risk. There is, however, some evidence that the consumption of fatty fish, such as salmon, herring and mackerel, reduces the risk of prostate cancer (Terry 2001). This may indicate that the omega-3 fatty acids contained in these fish are protective against prostate cancer. These fatty acids also offer significant protection against vascular disease, including coronary artery disease.

There is possible evidence that vegetables also decrease the prostate cancer risk.

Other dietary influences on cancer

Cancers of the colon, breast, kidney and digestive tract are associated with obesity. The most important event is actually gaining the weight. Adults should be encouraged (unless underweight) not to gain any weight, and definitely not more than 5 kilograms in their adult lives.

Alcohol increases liver cancer, breast cancer, most gastrointestinal cancers and pancreatic cancer. (See alcohol section in Part 2.)

Smoked/salt-cured foods contain nitrites, which can form nitrosamides in the stomach. These compounds may increase the incidence of stomach cancer. Such foods include smoked fish, hot dogs, corned beef, bacon and ham.

Further information

Nutrition Australia
A non-government, community-based organisation with offices in all states and territories. It is an independent body that aims to promote the health and well-being of all Australians. Its website is: www.nutritionaustralia.org

Food Standards Australia New Zealand (FSANZ)
Provides current recommendations regarding food standards in Australia. Lots of good information. Ph: (02) 6271 2222; Website: www.anzfa.gov.au

Dietitians Association of Australia
Website: www.daa.asm.au

Recipe Books
These wonderful recipe books will ensure that you don't make homemade dishes that drive the family from home.

Great Food for Men by Rosemary Stanton, Allen & Unwin, Sydney, 2001.
A great book for healthy, easy and delicious recipes for everyone. It also has total fat, fibre and energy content calculated for each meal.

Simply Healthy by Sally James, JB Fairfax Press, 1999.
Great, low-fat recipes.

Fresh & Healthy by Sally James, JB Fairfax Press, 2000.
This is the National Heart Foundation's new cookbook. It also has fat, fibre, and energy contents calculated for each recipe.

Healthy Vegetarian Eating by Rosemary Stanton, Allen & Unwin, Sydney, 1998.
Looks at the potential advantages and disadvantages of vegetarian eating.

Vegetables by Rosemary Stanton, Allen & Unwin, Sydney, 2000.
An A to Z of vegetables, with information and recipes to help you eat more veggies.

Books giving information about specific nutritional topics

Rosemary Stanton's Fat & Fibre Counter (revised), Information Australia, 1999.
Lists fat and fibre for 15 000 foods and notes which contain 'bad' fats.

Good Fats, Bad Fats by Rosemary Stanton, Allen & Unwin, Sydney, 1998.
A small book with detail about fats, LDL and HDL cholesterol, trans fats and triglycerides.

Vitamins by Rosemary Stanton, Allen & Unwin, Sydney, 1999.
A concise but thorough look at each of the 13 vitamins.

Part 4

Obesity and physical inactivity

Obesity

What is it and how does it affect us?

Obesity is an increasing problem in developed societies due to an increasingly sedentary lifestyle and the ready availability of foods high in fat and sugar. In Australia, the incidence of obesity has reached epidemic proportions. It directly causes about 4.4 per cent of the total burden of disease in Australia. The combination of obesity and physical inactivity is Australia's greatest health problem.

Figure 9 shows that excess weight increases with age. This is partially explained by the increase in fat stores that accompanies increasing age. Fat comprises 20 and 30 per cent of body weight in lean young men and women respectively and 25 and 35 per cent in lean older men and women. Ageing is, however, only a minor factor in causing obesity when compared with poor diet and lack of exercise.

Australia is fast becoming a 'takeaway food society'. Of the money spent on food, 33 per cent is used to purchase foods prepared and eaten outside the home. Most of these foods have both a high-fat content and a high saturated fat content. They are also usually high in energy (calories/kilojoules). Even so-called 'low-fat' foods, such as low-fat biscuits, muffins etc., are sometimes still relatively high in fat and they usually still have the same high-energy content. A change towards healthier low-fat/low-energy foods is needed to ward off the diseases that are associated with obesity.

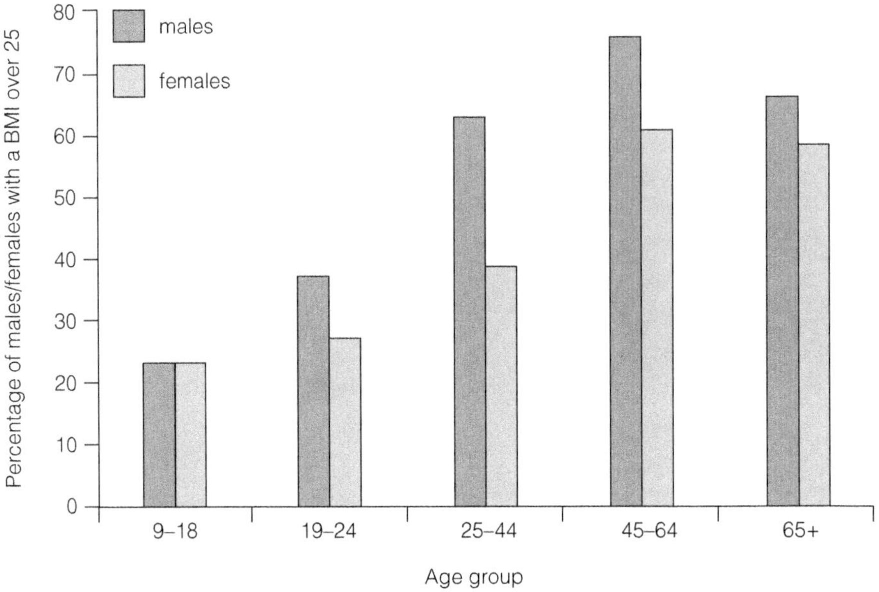

Source: Australian Institute of Health and Welfare, 2000.

Figure 9 Prevalence of excess weight in Australians

Defining excess weight

The traditional way of defining weight categories is by using the Body Mass Index (BMI), which can be calculated with the formula on page 145 or from the graph shown in Appendix 7. Table 12 shows the generally accepted weight categories for BMI readings. Anyone with a BMI of 25 or above is classified as having an excess weight problem.

Table 12 BMI levels for adult weight categories

BMI	*Weight category*
Less than 18	Very underweight
18–19.9	Underweight
20–24.9	Normal
25–29.9	Overweight
30–39.9	Obese
Greater than 40	Morbidly obese

$$\text{BMI} = \frac{}{\text{Height (in m)}^2}$$

For example, if you weighed 75 kg and were 1.70 m tall your BMI equals:

75 divided by 1.7 squared = 75 / 2.89 = 26

Excess weight and disease

To minimise your risk of illness from being overweight, you need to keep within a normal weight range and not increase your weight during adult life. After the age of 25, your risk of developing diabetes or coronary artery disease is increased with any weight gain over 5 kilograms if you are female, and with any weight gain at all if you are male.

If you are obese or have increased your weight in adult life, do not despair. Losing weight does help. For example, a 9-kilogram weight loss in an otherwise well, obese woman aged between 40 and 65 can give a 25 per cent reduction in overall mortality.

The numerous consequences of obesity are detailed below and figure 10 shows their contribution to total burden of disease caused by obesity. The burden of disease due to obesity is at its maximum in the 45 to 65 year age group in men and in the 55 to 75 year age group in women.

The distribution of fat in your body also has a profound influence on your health, with abdominal obesity being a major problem. Abdominal fat is composed of fat under the skin (two thirds) and fat surrounding the organs in your abdominal cavity (one third). It is the fat around your abdominal organs that is the main culprit as it is thought to be the major cause of insulin resistance in obese people. (See Appendix 15 for a fuller explanation.) This insulin resistance results in numerous serious health problems that together are called 'the

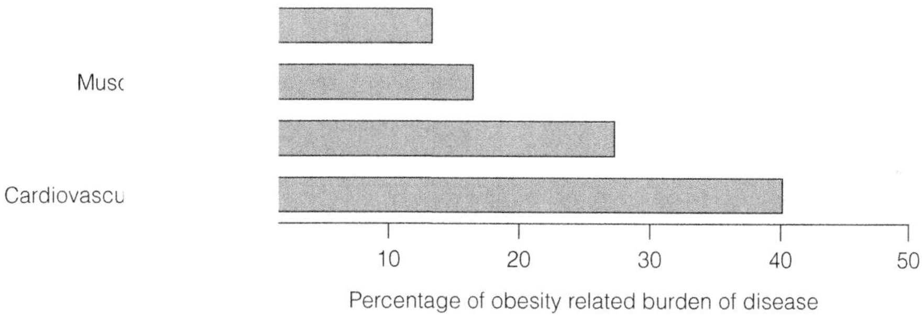

Source: Adapt | Institute of Health and Welfare, Mathers, 1999.

Figure 1 on of burden of disease caused by obesity

Table 13 Waist measurements in relation to health risk

	Ideal waist measurement	*Moderately increased waist measurement*	*Seriously increased waist measurement*
Vascular disease and diabetes risk	*Normal*	*Moderately increased*	*High*
Men	Less than 94 cm	94 to 102 cm	Greater than 102 cm
Women	Less than 80 cm	80 to 88 cm	Greater than 88 cm

Notes:
1. The waist should be measured at the level of the navel.
2. Waist measurements should be about 10 cm lower for Indian and Asian people.
3. Waist measurements are a better predictor of vascular disease risk than BMI levels.

metabolic syndrome' or syndrome X' (see below). Excess amounts of this harmful intra-abdominal fat increase your waist measurement and this explains why having a large waist measurement is so dangerous. Safe waist measurements for men and women are shown in table 13. Excess fat located around the hips ('pear shaped' people) is associated with far fewer medical problems.

If your reading is above the maximum safe level, your mortality level is increased. Many authorities now consider waist circumference may actually be a better indicator of the risk of heart disease from obesity than BMI measurement. For this reason, weight loss programs should focus particularly on abdominally obese people—males with a waist circumference over 100 centimetres and females with a waist circumference over 90 centimetres.

Also of concern is the fact that 20 per cent of young women in Australia are classified as underweight. This causes health problems, such as osteoporosis or weak bones, and very underweight people also have an increased general mortality rate. This is discussed further in the section on childhood obesity.

METABOLIC SYNDROME (OR SYNDROME X) AND OBESITY

This serious condition is becoming more common in Australians, especially males. The syndrome occurs when obesity is central or abdominal, giving a large waist measurement. The syndrome is associated with a marked increase in some or all of the following conditions:

- Deleterious changes in blood lipids, including a reduction in high-density lipoprotein (good cholesterol) and an increase in triglycerides. Both are bad for vascular disease and need to be treated aggressively in people with this condition.
- Atherosclerosis (vascular disease), including coronary artery disease and stroke.
- High blood pressure (hypertension).

- Diabetes or insulin resistance, a 'pre-diabetes' condition.
- Protein in the urine.
- Gout.
- Sleep apnoea.
- Fatty liver disease.

While this syndrome may be partly genetic in origin, there is also a large environmental component. It is imperative these environmental components, namely poor diet and lack of exercise, are treated aggressively to reduce the increased risk of coronary artery disease and death.

Success in treating this condition relies primarily on weight loss. The medical treatment of the consequences of this syndrome, such as drug therapy for hypertension, diabetes and high blood lipids, will only have limited success unless it is accompanied by a reduction in abdominal obesity.

CORONARY ARTERY DISEASE (AND RESULTANT SUDDEN DEATH)

Obesity is associated with several factors that increase the risk of coronary artery disease, including an increased workload on your heart, increased blood pressure, and increased vascular disease due to deleterious changes in blood lipids, such as reduced HDL and increased LDL (bad cholesterol). This situation is worse in 'Syndrome X' individuals.

DIABETES TYPE 2 (NON-INSULIN DEPENDENT DIABETES)

This type of diabetes, which occurs mostly in adults, is responsible for 90 per cent of diabetes in Australia and is closely related to obesity levels. If you have a BMI of say 22, you are very unlikely to get diabetes. However, if you are overweight with a BMI of 25 to 30, your risk of developing diabetes increases ninefold. Very overweight people with a BMI greater than 35 have a diabetes incidence about 20 times that of a person with normal weight. Obesity is one of the causes of increased resistance to the hormone insulin, and it is this insulin resistance that is responsible for type 2 diabetes in overweight people.

CANCER

Obesity will increase your risk of developing a variety of cancers, with about 14 per cent of the disease burden caused by obesity due to an increased incidence of cancer. In obese women, the extra fat tissue causes increased production of the hormone oestrogen. This extra oestrogen increases the risk of developing post-menopausal breast cancers and endometrial cancer (cancer of the uterus or womb). They occur to a greater extent if you have abdominal rather than hip obesity. Other cancers increased by obesity include colon, kidney and digestive tract cancers.

GALL BLADDER DISEASE AND LIVER DISEASE

Cholesterol is excreted from the liver into the intestine via the bile ducts and the gall bladder. This cholesterol is a major component of most gallstones. Increased gall bladder disease in obese people is probably due to increased secretion of cholesterol from the liver into the gall bladder.

Fatty liver disease is common in Australia, affecting up to 20 per cent of the population. It is caused by fat deposits damaging the liver tissue and is more common in obese people. Weight loss has been shown to reduce the incidence of this problem. It also occurs in people with diabetes or high blood triglycerides. Generally, fatty liver disease produces few symptoms and it is usually found when tests of liver function are performed for other reasons. It can occasionally go on to cause significant liver damage in severe cases. Weight loss and abstinence from alcohol have been shown to reduce liver damage associated with this problem.

ARTHRITIS—OSTEOARTHRITIS AND GOUT

Obesity is associated with increased osteoarthritis in both weight-bearing joints, such as the hips, and non-weight-bearing joints, such as those in the hands. The incidence of gout also increases in obesity. This is due to impaired uric acid clearance via the kidney. (Uric acid is the compound that causes gout.)

HORMONE (ENDOCRINE) PROBLEMS

In females, abdominal obesity is associated with increased levels of androgens (male hormones). This can cause masculine features such as facial hair growth. Obesity can also cause infertility. (Weight loss can reverse this in a significant number of cases.) Extremely obese men have decreased testosterone (a male hormone) levels and this causes feminine-like features, such as breast enlargement.

DEPRESSION, SLEEP APNOEA AND OTHER PROBLEMS

There is evidence that obese people with a BMI greater than 30 are more likely to suffer from depression (Roberts 2000). Whether the depression or the obesity comes first is uncertain.

Significant obesity is a common cause of sleep apnoea. This can be helped with continuous positive airways pressure machines, hopefully while weight loss is being achieved. Reflux, stress incontinence, skin problems, back pain, fatigue and shortness of breath with exercise, social isolation, and psychological problems may also occur when someone is obese.

Heart failure is also more common in overweight individuals and there is recent evidence that obese people may have an increased risk of stroke.

Prevention of obesity

Danger times for developing obesity

By far the best way to avoid obesity and its associated problems is to avoid becoming overweight in the first place through a healthy diet and adequate exercise. However, there are specific times during your life where weight gain is more likely. These need to be anticipated and managed appropriately through increased exercise or decreased energy intake. (See the section on 'Causes and principles of treatment' pages 150–165.)

CHILDHOOD

The cornerstone of healthy weight management throughout life is having a healthy home environment during childhood, where good food and physical activity are encouraged. It is vital you provide this sort of environment for your children. The older children are when obese, the more likely they are to become obese adults. Families where obesity is a chronic problem that appears in several generations need to be particularly vigilant to ensure their home environment is a healthy one. Their children may have a significant genetic predisposition to developing obesity.

ADOLESCENCE

Inactivity during the teen years, especially in girls, predisposes adolescents to obesity. Weight gained after growth in height is complete is more difficult to remove. Males are usually active and grow quickly during their adolescence and they eat appropriately. Unfortunately, they often stop playing sport late in their adolescence, just when their growth is also finishing. This double reduction in energy expenditure makes weight gain a particular problem.

PREGNANCY

Pregnancy itself does not usually cause abnormal weight gain. However, stress levels are often high during this time and post delivery and this can lead to weight gain, especially if depression is a significant problem. Other factors that increase the likelihood that a net gain in weight will be present several months after delivery include a large weight gain with the pregnancy, a greater number of pregnancies, a later return to work after the pregnancy, and not breastfeeding. (The additional energy needed for breastfeeding can lead to some weight loss.)

MENOPAUSE

A slight weight gain is common around this time in most women, mainly due to lifestyle changes, such as reducing levels of physical activity and more time for socialising, and a decrease in the body's metabolic rate. Fat is also redistributed from the hips to the abdomen (a bad change). There is no evidence that hormone replacement therapy increases this slight 'natural' weight gain.

LIFE EVENTS

Any major life event has the potential to cause weight gain, either because of the stress involved or because the event causes changes to your lifestyle, such as less time for exercise. Such events might include the death of a parent or spouse, retirement, marriage, or a new relationship.

QUITTING SMOKING

Weight gain is common with 'quitting' and occurs due to a decreased metabolic rate, improvements in taste, and increased appetite. Before quitting, it is essential to get dietary advice as weight gain is a common cause of 'quit' failure.

Causes and principles of treatment

An increase in body fat can be due to an increase in the size of fat cells, which occurs in almost all obese people, and/or an increase in fat cell number, which is common in most forms of severe childhood obesity. Obesity has numerous and varied causes and there are usually several factors operating. Most cases are due to environmental factors with genetic susceptibility also playing a role.

Environmental factors

Poor diet and lack of exercise are by far the most important causes of obesity. If you are overweight, they are extremely likely to be the cause of your problem. Excessive alcohol intake is another important cause in many people. These factors are influenced by habits learned throughout life and by the quality of the coping skills you have developed. Good skills enable a positive long-term approach to weight control.

In general, men tend to care less about becoming overweight and health issues in general than women, thus they tend to disregard these important environmental factors.

Genetic susceptibility

Genetic factors are complex in nature and involve multiple genes that ultimately act by enhancing the storage of fat. They accomplish this by altering factors such as appetite and satiety levels and by controlling the proportion of energy from the diet that is stored rather than expended (i.e. altering your metabolic rate). For example, appetite has been shown to be altered by a hormone called leptin, which is produced in fat cells. In this way, leptin acts to control long-term body energy reserves (i.e. body fat). Its production is at least partially genetically determined. Overall, genetic susceptibility is an important factor in about 40 per cent of obese patients.

A few rare genetic abnormalities, such as Prader-Willi, Ahlstrom's, Cohen's and Carpenter's syndromes, are associated with obesity.

Other factors

Hormonal (or endocrine) diseases causing obesity include injury to the hypothalamus (the part of the brain that produces hormones), Cushing's disease, polycystic ovarian disease, hypothyroidism, hyperinsulinaemia, acromegaly and hyperprolactinaemia.

The principal drugs that can cause obesity are phenothiazines, tricyclics, sodium valporate, carbamazepine and steroids. Oral contraceptives (the pill) can also slightly increase weight. Hormone replacement therapy for menopausal women has also been implicated but there is good evidence it does not contribute to obesity.

Drugs and hormonal diseases cause only a small fraction of the obesity problem and these should be dealt with through consultation with your GP. The environmental factors of poor diet and lack of physical activity are by far the most important causes.

The energy equation

For body weight to remain unchanged, energy intake in the diet must equal energy expended by the body. If the energy intake is greater than the energy expended, then you store the excess energy, mostly as fat. If energy intake is less, then you use stored energy to make up the difference. Most of the body's energy stores are in the form of fat (triglycerides), although glucose is also an important form of stored energy. (It is stored as glycogen in the liver and muscles.) The body uses energy in three different ways:

To keep the body functioning normally: Approximately 70 per cent of the energy expended by the body is used to keep the body functioning in its resting state; that is when not exercising or eating. The amount of energy used when resting during the day is termed your resting metabolic rate (RMR). (It is very similar to your basal metabolic rate, which is measured at night while sleeping.) RMR levels vary from person to person and thus, while resting, some people will burn up more energy than others. While resting, muscle consumes only 20 per cent of the energy you use. (The liver, brain and heart use 29, 19 and 10 per cent respectively.) During exercise, muscle energy use can rise by 50 times or more. Most of the factors that affect your RMR you cannot change. These include your genetic make up, your height, your age, illness, and the level of some hormones.

Some factors, however, you can change. The most important of these is your lean body mass—your body weight without any excess fat. People with more muscle have a greater lean body mass and a higher RMR, and therefore they use up more energy. Increasing physical activity can increase your body muscle mass so that your RMR increases up to 10 per cent. This results in a large increase in the body's energy consumption and can result in significant weight loss. On the other hand, very low energy diets can reduce muscle mass and thus reduce RMR. This lessens the achieved weight loss from the diet. Drugs such as caffeine and nicotine increase your RMR slightly, which is one reason why you gain weight when reducing their intake.

Physical activity: Physical activity usually accounts for about 20 per cent of energy expenditure. However, there is considerable individual variability in energy used in physical activity and it is the major way you can increase your body's energy use.

Digestion: About 10 per cent of your energy intake goes into digestion.

What foods increase body fat?

Most food groups provide energy to the body, however, the energy content and the way it is used by the body differ greatly with each group. Table 8 (on page 106) showed the energy content of each major nutrient group and how it is used by the body. This is very important when considering fat storage and thus obesity.

There are two main dietary causes of fat deposition in the body: excess energy (calories/kilojoules) and excess fat. The main cause of excess fat storage in the body is excess energy in the diet. By weight, fat and alcohol provide significantly more energy than carbohydrates and protein, therefore, they are very important sources of excess dietary energy. Reducing your fat and alcohol intake is imperative if you are to restrict dietary energy intake to levels that will maintain a healthy weight and not cause obesity.

Fat plays largely an energy storage role, and it is this storage system that gives us our body shape. A large proportion of the fat eaten in Western diets is stored as body fat and used later for energy, if required. At present it is uncertain whether the type of fat consumed makes any difference to the way it is stored. However, the type of fat consumed does make a big difference to cardiovascular disease risk and saturated fats should be avoided.

Fat stores can originate from dietary fat or from dietary carbohydrates that are converted to fat. However, the body prefers to store fat as fat. The main reason for this is that the process of storing carbohydrates as fat is an inefficient use of dietary energy. Storing carbohydrate as fat consumes about 25 per cent of its energy content whereas fat only loses about 3 per cent of its energy content when being stored as fat. For this reason, carbohydrates are stored as fat only if dietary energy intake from carbohydrates is considerably excessive. (The amount of carbohydrate used for energy can be increased by the body by increasing its metabolic rate.)

In an energy-balanced diet, all the fat eaten is eventually consumed to produce energy. It may be used as soon as it is eaten or may be stored as fat and then used later. A diet that has more than 15 to 20 per cent of the body's energy needs provided by fat is adequate to maintain body function and provide the few fatty aids your body can't produce (the 'essential' fatty acids). Western diets often have about twice this amount of fat and such diets will always have surplus dietary fat ready to be kept in storage should your diet contain energy greater than your body's requirements.

Problems with common attitudes to weight loss

For a long period, society has had simplistic and often misguided attitudes towards obesity and weight loss. It has centred on blaming obesity on laziness or gluttony and assumed everyone could be slim with a disciplined approach to diet and exercise. It also assumed that being thin optimises health and happiness. The problems with these attitudes are they do not give a real understanding of the complex nature of the causes of obesity and its treatment, and do not distinguish between weight and health.

Your focus should be on attainable and sustainable solutions that will deliver you a comfortable weight and improved health. Your solutions will need to encompass behavioural change in both diet and exercise.

CONCENTRATE ON ACHIEVABLE BEHAVIOURAL CHANGE NOT WEIGHT LOSS

Concentrating on changing your eating and exercise behaviour is a more successful approach than concentrating on short-term weight loss and these behavioural changes should be your main long-term priorities.

The behavioural goals in your weight-loss strategy should be focused on what you can realistically achieve and sustain. Almost all obese people have tried to lose weight on numerous occasions and failed. The prime reasons for this are that they impose dietary restrictions they will never be able to maintain in the long term and have unrealistic weight-loss goals. This starts the 'weight-loss cycle', seen in figure 11, and leads to repeated failure, making future success very unlikely. Repeated weight loss followed by weight gain has also been associated with generally poorer health and can cause a reduction in lean body mass (i.e. muscle), thus making future weight gain more likely.

It is probably best not to have any definite weight-loss goal at all and just concentrate on strategies that improve your health.

THE PROBLEM OF TAKING A SHORT-TERM VIEW

Healthy weight loss is usually slow—about 0.5 to 1 kilogram per month (or waist size losses of 1 to 2 centimetres per month). A weight loss of 5 to 10 per cent over six to 12 months

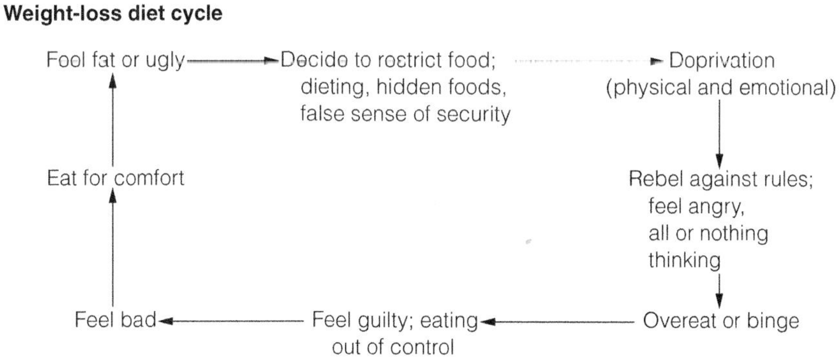

Source: Kausman, 'A New Perspective to Long Term Weight Management', *Australian Family Physician*, 2000; 29(4): 303–306, The Royal Australian College of General Practitioners.

Figure 11 Unhealthy diet cycle

is good progress and will give significant health benefits. (Women often lose weight slower than men.) Remember, by keeping to your long-term weight-loss strategy, you are losing actual body fat permanently. One kilogram of fat lost is equivalent to two 500-gram tubs of margarine.

An example demonstrating why fat loss is slow

Let us assume that your weight is stable on a diet containing 8000 kilojoules and you initially plan to decrease your dietary energy intake to 7000 kilojoules per day, a reduction of 1000 kilojoules or 12.5 per cent of your energy intake. As you still weigh the same, you will still need to use 8000 kilojoules and the extra 1000 kilojoules of energy would need to come from burning body fat. If we assume that 1g of fat produces 37 kilojoules of energy, you would burn up about an extra 27 grams of fat per day. At this rate, it would take about 37 days to lose one kilogram of body fat. As your body gradually loses weight, its energy requirements also gradually reduce and this already slow rate of fat loss will gradually become even slower. Eventually a new equilibrium will be set up where your 7000 kilojoules energy intake is the correct amount to maintain a new lower weight and no further weight loss will occur. This means that your diet change will continue giving weight (fat) loss benefits for months. This is a very simplistic calculation and your weight loss may be quicker than this. However, it does give an idea of why fat loss is a slow process. This slow change does have one benefit; it means an *occasional* 'night out' will not suddenly increase your body fat stores.

Early weight loss in 'quick fix' diets is usually due to changes in body water content rather than loss of body fat. Also, muscle weighs more than fat and the increased body muscle mass that occurs with increased exercise may actually increase body weight while decreasing body volume (i.e. you will still appear thinner). A better guide to progress is change in body shape. This can be measured by noting changes in waist measurement.

POSITIVE ATTITUDE TOWARDS YOUR DIET AND YOUR BODY

Foods should not be categorised as 'bad' or 'good', as this can increase your feelings of guilt and failure. It is better to categorise foods as being 'everyday' or 'sometimes' foods.

You should also not focus exclusively on the negative side of your body image. You should accept your body while you are trying to change it. A good method is to write down positive things about your body, for example having good eyesight or musical ability.

Poor eating behaviours

NON-HUNGRY EATING

Identifying why you eat will help find solutions to your weight problems. Normally, you will feel hungry three to five times per day. This occurs because your blood sugar (glucose) level decreases when you have not eaten for some time. Non-hungry eating occurs in most people and is an important factor in obesity. Many obese people have lost the ability to tell when they are hungry. A hunger scale (from 0 to 10) is useful for assessing your hunger levels. To assess the extent of your non-hungry eating problem, your 'degree of hunger' needs to be written down each time you eat.

Once your level of non-hungry eating is established, the reasons can be determined. They may include eating when you are supposed to eat, for example when the clock says it's lunchtime; the feeling that everything on the plate must be finished; tiredness or boredom; emotional problems; and the association of eating with another activity, such as watching TV or playing cards. Many young adults retain the eating behaviours they learned while growing up. When they stop growing, this food intake is too large and they become obese young adults.

Some people will find they are not hungry at meal times. This can be due to snacking or because their previous meal was too large. If large meals are your problem, try cutting down the quantity of food you eat by reducing portion size or not eating dessert. Or you can try not eating all that is provided on your plate and see how you feel. If you're not hungry, don't finish it. Some people are not even hungry at breakfast. Breakfast, however, should never be missed as it gets your body going for the day. People who skip breakfast also tend to snack more during the morning and are often obese.

If snacking is your problem, you should stop it, especially if your snacks comprise foods high in fat or sugar, as most commercial snack foods are. A helpful way to reduce eating between meals is to brush your teeth after each meal. This signifies the end of the eating period and the fresh mouth feel is a reminder that your eating time has now finished. It is also good for your teeth and gums. As well as reducing total food intake, a reduction in non-hungry snacking will allow you a more varied and interesting diet at meal times.

DELAYING HUNGRY EATING

If you are hungry between meals, you should delay the feeling of hunger by ensuring each meal contains foods that take a long time to digest. This means your blood sugar level following a meal stays elevated longer, which delays the onset of hunger. The glycaemic index (GI) used by people with diabetes categorises each food according to the speed that it raises blood sugars once it is eaten. Foods with a high GI, for example white bread, potato chips and biscuits, cause an early and high rise in blood sugar after eating. The body then initiates an early release of insulin to reduce this elevated blood sugar level and as this occurs hunger starts to return.

Foods with a low GI, such as apples, pasta or a bowl of muesli, are digested over a longer period. Thus, the rise in blood sugar occurs more slowly, is not as high and lasts longer. The subsequent fall in blood sugar also occurs later, delaying the onset of hunger. Thus, low GI foods should be incorporated into each meal (see pages 117–119 and Appendix 6).

BINGE EATING

Binge eating is a significant contributor to weight gain; in women the incidence is as high as 40 per cent. It is part of the unhealthy diet cycle that occurs with weight-loss programs imposing unsustainable dietary restrictions. The resultant dietary failure is accompanied by subsequent feelings of guilt and loss of self-esteem and these feelings make future attempts at weight loss even less likely to succeed. Binge eating often occurs with stress, after exercise (as a reward), when eating with others, at festive occasions, and with alcohol consumption. The answer is to make more modest dietary modifications that are sustainable in the long term and to be aware of the problem.

QUICK FIX DIETS THAT EXCESSIVELY RESTRICT ENERGY INTAKE

Most commonly used diets work by severely restricting energy (calorie/kilojoule) intake to the extent that the energy consumed is considerably less than the energy used by the body. This results in a relatively quick weight loss as large amounts of the body's glycogen stores (the storage form of glucose in our bodies) are used to supplement the reduced energy provided in the diet. As these glycogen stores are used up, water needed for storing the glycogen is also lost. While this initial loss of glycogen and water can result in a weight loss of 2 kilograms, it is replaced by the body as soon as energy intake increases again.

Diets that significantly restrict energy intake are unpleasant and difficult to maintain. Also, it is obviously not possible to continue with severe energy-restricting diets; you can't continue to use more energy than you consume. These diets are therefore usually associated with large fluctuations in weight but little overall weight loss in the long term.

Another problem with such diets is that, as a protective mechanism, your body reduces its energy needs (i.e. its resting metabolic rate [RMR]) when dietary energy supply is significantly reduced. (This strategy is also used by the body in times of famine.) This reduces the effect of the energy-restricting diet. Also, such diets result in a loss of muscle mass (lean body mass) and this reduces RMR further.

Diets that excessively restrict energy intake are also associated with numerous side effects, including impaired concentration, which affects work and study; poor nutritional balance; and decreased self-esteem associated with diet failure. This decrease in self-esteem can in turn affect many aspects of your life and lead to, or worsen, depression. Finally, these diets also increase the likelihood of developing eating disorders, such as anorexia, as they discourage normal eating patterns and give the message that good foods, such as bread and pasta, are bad for you.

In contrast, the dietary advice given in this book revolves around reducing fat intake (especially saturated fat) and using predominantly carbohydrates to provide an energy intake that equates to the energy your body would use if you were a healthy weight. The aim is to improve health and attain sustainable weight losses through long-term dietary change.

Diets—do they work and which is best?

Firstly, it needs to be stressed that 'diet' is being discussed in the context of long-term changes in eating behaviours, not short term attempts at weight loss. It also needs to be stressed that the principal aim in attempting such changes should be improved health. For many people, an integral part of this will be fat (weight) loss. However, there are other issues to be considered, such as lowering blood cholesterol, cancer prevention, lowering high blood pressure and providing enjoyable food alternatives that increase life enjoyment.

There has been considerable discussion in the media about which type of diet is best at achieving long-term fat loss. This debate has been hindered by the limited amount of good research on the topic. Unfortunately, it has to be said very few people (about 5 to 15 per cent) are successful in their attempts at long-term fat loss, no matter which diet they adopt. General advice, such as that provided in health promotion programs, is rarely successful unless it is accompanied by dietary counselling, or better still, supervised dietary therapy (Wahlqvist 2002). However, do not despair. Fat loss can be achieved if you take the approach described in this book.

All diets which appropriately restrict energy intake will result in fat loss. The problem is that people find keeping to them very difficult. Over recent years, Australians have experienced an increasingly sedentary lifestyle, increasingly larger meal sizes, and a dramatic increase in the availability of convenient pre-prepared foods that have a high energy content. These three factors have all contributed to making dietary energy restriction even more difficult and have resulted in the obesity epidemic that Australia is now facing. Recently, low-fat diets have been accused by some as being the cause of this epidemic. This criticism is unfair as a reduction in dietary fat content was never going to be enough to compensate for the changes in eating habits and physical activity. Buying supposedly 'healthy' low-fat foods such as muffins and icecream that are packed full of energy is a dietary disaster.

There are four things that a healthy fat loss diet must do to be successful. These are:

1. Restrict energy intake.
2. Maintain a lowish to medium fat intake (about 25 to 30 per cent is good). A higher fat intake makes body fat (weight) loss difficult.
3. Minimise saturated fats.
4. Provide a wide variety of nutritious food options that are enjoyable to eat.

The energy contained in food comes from the fat, carbohydrates and protein that it contains. Alcohol also contributes significantly in some people. These components are quantified in terms of the energy they supply. For example, saying a diet contains 30 per cent fat means that fat contributes 30 per cent of the total energy contained in the diet.

Having established the optimum fat level in our diet, the remaining energy consideration is the balance between the levels of carbohydrates and protein.

The overall health benefits provided by the wide variety of nutritious foods available in low fat/high carbohydrate diets mean that these diets are still the clear preference of most dietitians in Australia and are the diets advised in this book. Fat levels should be between 25 and 30 per cent of energy intake and carbohydrate levels can vary from about 50 to 60 per cent. Protein provides the remainder, about 15 to 25 per cent. It needs to be emphasised that these levels are approximate; you are eating, not studying maths.

High protein diets have been around for a long time and are certainly becoming more popular at the moment. There is a wide variety of such diets and the protein and fat they contain can vary significantly. Diets with very high protein levels have been shown in the past to be difficult to keep to and are not a healthy choice because their fat content also tends to be high and because they can cause calcium loss and thus osteoporosis. Diets containing a moderate amount of protein that are also low in fat are a much better dietary option and, in fact, are not greatly dissimilar to low fat/high carbohydrate diets. They just have a bit more protein and a bit less carbohydrate. These diets are being intensively investigated at present and may, in the end, prove to be another dietary option for fat loss.

It should be noted that for those people who are not overweight, a diet may contain a slightly higher level of fat (up to 35 per cent) as long as the fat is mostly healthy unsaturated fats (the Mediterranean-type diet). Losing weight is more difficult with this level of fat intake.

Thus, loss of body fat is best achieved by a low fat/high carbohydrate diet, the cornerstones of which are reducing your fat intake, maintaining a sustainable energy intake appropriate for your activity levels, and ensuring that the dietary restrictions you undertake to achieve these two goals are sustainable in the long term.

As this dietary change keeps energy levels within the range for maintaining a healthy weight, it does not allow for an unlimited intake of carbohydrates or protein. If you are overweight, you are likely to have an excess energy intake and you will find that, as well as restricting fat and alcohol intake, this diet requires you to eat smaller quantities of food.

Ways to reduce meal sizes

- Only make enough for one serving for each household member.
- Don't go back for seconds.
- Eat your food slowly.

- Use smaller plates.
- Drink lots of water with the meal.

While weight loss is usually slow, it is permanent. Continued monitoring of your weight control program during and after weight loss needs to be an integral part of your program if it is to be successful.

Regulating energy intake

Energy is stored mostly as fat (with some as glycogen). To maintain the body's energy (fat) stores, the energy provided by the food we eat must be equal to the energy we use each day; that is, an energy balanced diet.

In order to lose weight, dietary energy intake needs to be reduced to the level that a person within a healthy weight range (a BMI of 20 to 25) would use during their daily activities. This level is less than the amount an obese person would be consuming to maintain his/her weight and thus fat will be slowly 'burnt off' until a healthy weight is achieved. As stated above, reducing your fat and alcohol consumption is unlikely to produce a sufficient reduction in energy consumption, so the volume consumed will probably need to be reduced also. The best way to do this is to reduce the size of the portions you consume while maintaining a large variety of everyday foods, including fruit and vegetables, salads, wholegrain breads and cereals, pasta and fish. Try to choose foods with a low glycaemic index and a high-fibre content. Soft drinks are a source of large amounts of energy and should be avoided. (They are especially a problem in children.)

If weight loss is very slow on this balanced energy intake, the consumption of energy in the diet can be reduced further. However, as explained previously, too great a restriction in energy intake leads to a diet that is hard for you to keep to, thus resulting in failure.

Tables 14 and 15 assist in determining the appropriate energy intake for people wishing to maintain their weight in the healthy weight range. Weight is measured in kilograms. Table 14 is the simplest to use.

Table 15 gives you the adjustment factors (for age and activity level) to substitute into the following energy calculating equations and is a slightly more accurate estimate, although all these figures should be used as guides only.

Male energy expenditure (in calories per day) = (716 + [15 × weight]) × adjustment factor
Female energy expenditure (in calories per day) = (716 + [12 × weight]) × adjustment factor

(To convert the answer to kilojoules, multiply the answer in calories by 4.2.) By substituting into the equation the weight you would need to give you a BMI of 25, these equations allow you to calculate the energy intake you would require to maintain a BMI

Table 14 Energy intake needed to maintain a healthy weight

	Energy intake in kilojoules (calories)	*Fat intake with 25% of energy intake as fat (g per day)*
Women		
Moderately active	8 400 (2 000)	54
Sedentary	6 300 (1 500)	40
Men		
Moderately active	0 500 (2 500)	70
Sedentary	8 400 (2 000)	54

Note: When attempting to lose body fat, try to keep your total fat intake to about 40 g a day (30 g if you are small and inactive). Do not reduce levels below these as your body requires an intake of some fat and very low-fat diets are hard to maintain.

of 25. (Those having initial difficulty with weight loss may benefit from further energy restriction and thus need to use a slightly lower weight.)

For example, if a 65-year-old inactive man had a height of 179 centimetres, he would need to weigh 80 kilograms to have a BMI of 25 (see page 145 for the formula to calculate BMI). By substituting 80 kilograms and the appropriate adjustment factor from the table of 1.06 into the male equation, he could calculate the dietary energy content that would eventually bring him down to this weight, as follows:

$$\text{Energy level} = (716 + [15 \times 80]) \times 1.06 = (716 + 1200) \times 1.06 = 1916 \times 1.06 = 2031 \text{ calories}$$

In kilojoules, this would = 2031 × 4.2 = 8530 kilojoules.

Reducing energy intake to normal levels requires you to calculate your daily energy intake from the foods you eat. This can be done with the aid of information provided on packaging and food calorie charts. (Rosemary Stanton's *Fat & Fibre Counter* is a good guide.)

Table 15 Adjustment factors (for age and activity level)

	Activity level		
Age	*Inactive*	*Active*	*Very active*
18–30	1.25	1.70	2.25
30–35	1.19	1.61	2.14
36–49	1.13	1.53	2.03
50–69	1.06	1.45	1.91
70+	1.00	1.36	1.80

Source: Adapted from Eggar, 2002.

An even easier option is to use recipes where the energy content has been calculated for you. Many modern recipe books (including those mentioned at the end of this chapter) have such information. These calculations will initially take some time. However, you have to do the calculation once only for each meal. Planning the energy content of diets is an area where an experienced health professional can be of great benefit. Please remember that such calculations are useful only when you keep to the suggested serving sizes!

Reducing fat intake

Fat is eaten in excess by most Australians. The reasons so many fatty foods are consumed is that they can be eaten quickly, they taste good, they are readily available, they are conveniently packaged (ready-to-eat), and they are profitable and well marketed. To reduce your fat intake to optimum levels, you need to know the amount of fat you are allowed in your diet and the amount of fat in the food you wish to consume. From a cardiovascular disease viewpoint, you also need to know the type of fat present in each food.

Dietary fat intakes for most people should be between 25 and 30 per cent of total energy intake. (One gram of fat equates to about 9 calories or 38 kilojoules.) For example, to detemine the fat content in a 8000 kilojoule diet that obtains 25 per cent of its energy from fat you would calculate:

Energy content in 25 per cent of a 8000 kJ diet = 8000 kJ × 0.25 = 2000 kJ
Number of grams of fat needed to give 2000 kJ = 2000 kJ divided by 38 kJ/g = 53 g

Thus, a 8000 kJ diet obtaining 25 per cent of its energy from fat should contain 53 g of fat.

Dietary fat intakes that are equivalent to 25 per cent of total energy intake are shown in Table 14.

A fat intake of 25 per cent of total energy intake will probably be a significant reduction from your present intake as, on average, Australian men consume (at least) 100 grams of fat per day and women 68 grams per day. As mentioned, if you are trying to lose weight you can reduce your intake below these levels but 30 to 40 grams of fat per day should be a minimum as you do need some fat in your diet.

Working out the fat content of your meal can be done by working out the fat content of the individual ingredients you use if your recipe doesn't show a fat content as previously mentioned. This need only be done for the products that contain significant amounts of fat. The amount of fat in all packaged foods, such as breakfast cereals, is displayed in the nutritional information panel provided. The fat content of unpackaged foods, such as meats, can be calculated from figures given in fat guides that are available in most book stores. To calculate the amount of fat in a serving, you will also need to know the weight of your serving.

$$\text{Weight of fat per serve} = \frac{\text{fat content (in g of fat/100 g of food)} \times \text{weight of food (in g)}}{100}$$

For example, the fat content of 80 grams of avocado (22.6 grams of fat in 100 grams of avocado) would be determined as follows:

$$\text{Fat content} = 22.6\text{ g} \times \frac{\text{weight of avocado}}{100} = 22.6 \times \frac{80\text{ g}}{100} = 18.1\text{ g}$$

Remember that these figures are accurate only if you keep to recommended serving sizes.

This process may take a little time at first, but, as with energy content, you will only have to do it once for each recipe. You will soon get a rough feel for the amount of fat in the foods that you like to eat and can adjust your diet accordingly. (A list of foods that are major contributors to fat in Australian diets is included in Appendix 3.)

Remember also, the type of fat in each food is important (tables 9 and 10 give a guide to the type of fats present in many foods). As stated previously in this book, omega-3s and monounsaturated fats are preferred. All foods containing fat will have a combination of several types of fat, including saturated fat. For example, olive oil contains 75 per cent monounsaturated, 13 per cent polyunsaturated and 12 per cent saturated fat. It is saturated fat that you need to watch and you should try to keep this as low as possible and no more than 30 per cent of your total fat intake.

Some practical advice on ways to reduce your fat intake

- Reduce the use of spreads on bread etc. If you need a spread, try using some avocado.
- Use low-fat dairy products; for example, skim milk, reduced-fat cheese.
- Reduce red meat intake and use only lean cuts of meat. All visible fat should be removed from the meat. Restrict using red meat to two to three times a week and increase the amount of fish eaten. Red meat is still useful in the diet as it is an important source of proteins, iron and other nutrients. A piece the size of a pack of cards is a good indication of an appropriate serving size for red meat (about 80 grams).
- When using chicken, use lean cuts such as the breast and remove the skin.
- Grill, stir-fry or steam your foods; and avoid fried foods.
- Don't skip meals as this increases snacking.
- Don't snack. Make sure you have nutritious morning and afternoon tea foods available.
- Use some foods with a low glycaemic index in each meal to delay the onset of hunger.
- Avoid the purchase of fatty foods when shopping. Remember that commercially prepared foods labelled as low-fat often have a high energy content and are thus still bad for you. Check the label or prepare your own low-fat, low energy meals.

- Plan your meals! Much of the fat consumed is contained in food prepared outside the home, either purchased as a takeaway or eaten in restaurants. This can be avoided by ensuring you always have adequate appropriate food at home to prepare quick nutritious meals when needed.
- Take low-fat food to work.
- Frequent restaurants you know have low-fat meal options.
- Put a reminder on the fridge or in the pantry to help you avoid fatty foods.

Remember that recipes in cookbooks are not cast in stone. They can often be significantly altered to reduce fat content without detrimentally affecting taste. Some easy changes include reducing the quantity of meat (substitute a vegetable instead); using cuts of meat with a minimal fat content; reducing the use of cooking oils; and substituting low-fat alternative ingredients where available. Recipes that require large amounts of full-fat dairy products, coconut products or other foods high in saturated fats should be avoided.

Recommended food intake for a low-fat diet

Bread, pasta, potatoes (prepared without fat), grains

Six serves a day. One serve equals one cup of mashed potato or cooked pasta or cooked rice, three-quarters of a cup of breakfast cereal, or one slice of bread or fruit loaf or a small roll.

Meat, fish, chicken, eggs, legumes

One serve a day. One serve equals 80 grams of red meat, 100 grams of cooked chicken or fish, one to two eggs, or ⅔ of a cup of cooked legumes. Foods should be prepared in as little fat as possible. Avoid frying/roasting. Meat must be lean with all visible fat removed and chicken should be skinless.

Vegetables

Eat as much as you like, but not less than four serves per day. One serve equals about half a cup or about 60 to 90 grams. Try to make vegetables the central part of at least some of your main meals (for example, vegetarian lasagna or ratatouille). Use a wide variety of vegetables and add a variety of herbs and spices (preferably fresh) to vegetarian dishes to improve flavour (they should be an integral part of vegetarian recipes). Fresh herbs and spices are also nutritionally very beneficial.

Fruit

Eat two to three serves a day. One serve is about 120 to 140 grams and equals one medium or three small (e.g. apricot) pieces of fruit, about 20 grapes, a cup of berries, or half a cup of canned/stewed fruit; Fruit is great after a meal or as a filler during the day.

Nuts

A small handful several times a week (unsalted). Nuts, especially peanuts, should not be given to young children due to the risk of inhalation.

Milk products

Two serves a day. One serve equals one cup of low-fat milk or skim milk, 30 grams of low-fat cheese, or 200 grams of fat-reduced yoghurt. Keep to low-fat dairy products wherever possible. Avoid butter and cream.

Fats and oils

A maximum of two serves per day. One serve equals one teaspoon of oil for cooking, one teaspoon of margarine or a quarter of an avocado (50 grams). Monounsaturated oils are best. If using spreads, those containing plant sterols can help reduce cholesterol; or try using avocado.

Indulgences

Enjoy a maximum of one to two serves each day. One serve equals two standard alcoholic drinks, a tablespoon of jam or honey, or one cup of homemade popcorn. Try to avoid high-fat foods, such as potato or corn chips, sausage rolls and meat pies, chocolate, sweet biscuits and pastries.

Fluids

- Water is best. You should try to drink at least two litres a day. A jug of iced water at the lunch or dinner table should be a household ritual.
- Low-fat milk (as allowed above) is an equally good choice. A good way of ensuring an adequate calcium intake is to have two cups of calcium enriched low-fat milk per day.
- Alcohol needs to be restricted to two standard drinks per day and alcohol intake should be part of your indulgence allowances. You should also have at least two alcohol-free days a week.
- Non-sweetened fruit juices should be restricted to one serve per day, about 150 millilitres.
- Soft drinks need to be avoided.

In what order should dietary changes be made?

More often than not, numerous dietary issues need to be addressed. It is often unrealistic for you to attempt to change all dietary problems at once as this may lead to too drastic a change, one that you (and other members of the household) cannot tolerate. The changes you need to make vary in importance but should be addressed in the following order.

1. Reduce fat intake.
2. Reduce alcohol consumption.
3. Further reduce energy content by reducing food volume.

Physical activity and obesity

The other major cause of obesity in Australia is lack of exercise. It has been shown that 30 per cent of adult Australians engage in no exercise at all, and 54 per cent do not do enough to gain any benefit. Exercise is an integral part of any weight-loss program. This topic is dealt with in detail in the section on 'Physical activity'.

Other weight loss options

SPECIAL VERY LOW-CALORIE DIETS

These diets are an option for people who have properly tried a low-fat diet and been unsuccessful, for people requiring rapid weight loss prior to essential surgery, and for those who are so obese they are unable to exercise. They should be attempted only under proper medical supervision. Side effects include constipation, gallstones, hunger, hypotension, gout and low blood potassium.

SURGERY

This option is used only in the morbidly obese (BMI greater than 40) and where all else has failed. It can be permanent (gastric stapling) or temporary (a removable gastric band) and has a success rate of 30 to 50 per cent. Complications include surgical problems as well as long-term nausea, vitamin deficiencies, constipation, and the possibility of obstruction. Surgical complications can be reduced by performing the procedure by laparoscopy.

DRUGS

Generally drugs have no role as they are addictive, have numerous side effects, and are ineffective in the long term. Appetite suppressants are especially bad as they are addictive and cause agitation and insomnia. Other drugs that can cause weight loss are thyroxine, diuretics and laxatives. None of these drugs should be used for achieving weight loss.

Orlistat, one of the newer drugs in the market, inhibits the lipase enzymes in the gastrointestinal tract that help break down dietary triglycerides to fat acids, resulting in about 30 per cent of consumed triglycerides remaining unchanged in the bowel. These triglycerides cannot be absorbed and are lost as fat in the bowel motion. Overall Orlistat has been shown to achieve a slightly higher weight loss than with diet alone. Weight loss is usually slow with losses of less than 1 kilogram a month. Trials have shown that diet plus Orlistat can provide a 5 to 10 per cent weight loss after one year (Marks 2001). This degree of weight loss helps in reducing cardiovascular risk factors, such as hypertension and diabetes, and Orlistat can reduce LDL cholesterol by about 8 per cent.

It is prescribed for those with a BMI greater than 30 or a BMI greater than 27 plus other risk factors for vascular disease such as hypertension, diabetes etc. Side effects are usually mild, but do occur in many patients. They are mostly due to unabsorbed fat being passed in the bowel motions. This causes oily spotting, flatus with discharge, faecal urgency and faecal incontinence. The best way to minimise these side effects is to keep to a low-fat diet (less than 50 grams of fat per day). Two-year studies have shown the drug also causes a reduction in the absorption of fat soluble vitamins, including vitamins A, D, E and K. The blood levels of these vitamins did not, however, fall below normal ranges. Whether longer-term therapy causes a greater problem needs further investigation. People with nutritional vitamin deficiencies may need vitamin supplements which should be taken at least two hours after their Orlistat dose. Interactions with other drugs do occur. These need to be discussed with a medical practitioner. Ninety-seven per cent of the drug is not absorbed; it is excreted in the faeces.

Sibutramine is a new drug that acts to modify hunger and reduce the decline in energy expenditure that occurs during weight loss. It can achieve a weight loss of 5 to 10 per cent. It can also give improvements in blood lipids. It is used in people with a BMI of over 30 or over 27 if they have other vascular disease risk factors. Its side effects include a slight rise in blood pressure, dry mouth, insomnia and constipation.

Some problem diets

High protein/low carbohydrate diets (for example, the Atkins diet): These diets have been fashionable on and off for years and are being promoted actively at present. They tend to restrict foods such as fruit, grains, and some vegetables. They therefore tend to lack fibre and some nutrients, which is bad for the bowel, the heart and cancer protection.

They also often have no fat restrictions, allowing the consumption of saturated fat which can raise LDL cholesterol and increase vascular disease. Their high-protein content can lead to several other medical problems including high uric acid levels, which may cause gout; dehydration due to the need to excrete larger quantities of water to dispose of the extra urea and uric acid; and osteoporosis, due to excess calcium loss. On diets such as these, you initially lose a few kilograms due to water loss, but in the long term few people can maintain the dietary restrictions and the diet fails. Finally, protein deficiency is very rare in Western diets, so consuming more does not make a lot of sense.

Liver-cleansing diet: This diet is not factually well founded. The diet does not cleanse the liver—the liver does not need to be cleansed as it does this by itself. The diet, however, is low in fat and follows many accepted dietary principles. (It also recommends 'natural' liver-proactive remedies that are unnecessary.)

Pritiken diet: This diet is very low in fat and very high in high-fibre vegetables. It suits some people but many find it too strict to follow.

Fit for life diet: This diet has many rules about which foods can be mixed together and when certain foods can be eaten. None of these rules has any basis in fact and the diet is best avoided.

Programs offering prepared diet foods: While many of these programs are well planned nutritionally, they suffer from two problems. Firstly, the food offered is usually relatively expensive. Secondly, they do not teach the overweight person how to choose and prepare a well-balanced diet for themselves. Thus, when they stop using the prepared foods, they usually revert to their old eating habits and fail in the long term.

Achieving change in eating habits

The previous sections have described what you need to do to lose weight and become healthier. Implementing these changes is not easy, especially if you need to make numerous changes. This section provides a practical approach to changing your eating habits.

It is very beneficial to involve other household members, especially your partner, in the process. They will know your dietary problems and be in a position to help you. They will also be at least partly responsible for the purchasing and preparation of food and intimately involved in its consumption. Sharing meal planning will help keep everybody happy and all will benefit from better eating habits.

Food diary—identifying dietary problems

Before commencing any dietary change program, your present dietary habits need to be assessed so that problem areas can be identified. Hopefully many aspects of your eating patterns will not require change and, obviously, the less that needs to be changed the easier the task will be.

This task is best accomplished with a three-day food diary in which all the foods you eat are documented. The days should include two weekdays and one weekend day. It is also useful to note the degree of hunger by recording hunger level, on a scale of one to eight as outlined below, each time you eat. Once again, this process is often best done in consultation with a dietician or medical practitioner.

Hunger scale (Egger 2001)

1. Ravenous
2. Hungry
3. *Slightly hungry* } *Preferred levels of hunger*
4. *No hunger*
5. *Feeling satisfied*
6. Slightly full
7. Very full
8. Beyond full

From this assessment, areas requiring change can be identified and your dietary strategy worked out. This food diary needs to be fairly detailed, so please allocate sufficient time to do it properly and be accurate. Do not underestimate the amount of food you consume. Your medical practitioner or dietitian is there to help, not judge you.

A good way to identify dietary problems is to look at each day of the week and, as much as possible, group them into days that are similar. For example, many people have working day routines that are fairly similar. Once you have done this, you can use your food diary

Table 16 Sample of food diary

Day..............................

Meal	*Time*	*Food eaten*	*Amount (weight in g)*	*Total fat (in g)*	*Hunger scale*	*Other comments*

to look at your eating habits throughout the day. This can be done by dividing the day into six eating time zones: breakfast, between breakfast and lunch, lunch, between lunch and dinner, dinner and after dinner.

In each eating period, look at what you eat and see how your diet fits in with your objectives. This will require purchasing a book detailing the energy (calories/kilojoules) and fat contained in each food you eat. You should also look at regular changes you know will occur in your routines and do not appear in your food diary. For example, do you go out for lunch once a week? Eating habits at dinner time and after dinner do vary during the working week. However, these evening activities are often patterned on a weekly cycle, such as regular sporting commitments, meetings or social drinking on a Friday.

Eating habits during time off (often the weekend) do tend to be more varied and again, you should note any significant patterns that aren't represented in your food diary, especially if they are detrimental to a healthy lifestyle. There is not much use moderating your food and alcohol intake during the week if you then binge on food and drink on the weekend.

Dietary planning initiatives

Having identified your problem areas through your food diary, it is now time to plan strategies to overcome them. Here are some important initiatives that should be incorporated into your plan.

PLAN MEALS AHEAD

Family members should make an extensive list of suitable evening meals that everyone enjoys and then plan the week's meals a week ahead from this list. You will need to allow adequate time for food shopping. Planning the meals a week ahead will allow you to minimise the number of trips to the shops that need to be done. Your planning should also include a few easy options for those 'I couldn't be bothered' nights. You can do this by ensuring you always have the ingredients for a couple of easy nutritious meals in the fridge and making healthy meals ahead that can be stored frozen. Freezing sandwiches ahead for work is also a good idea. All this planning will reduce the need to revert to takeaway meals during the week. As well as being bad for you, takeaways are usually more expensive.

PLAN FOR FAMILY MEALS

Make sure there are at least several days during the week when the whole family sits down to eat together. These times are especially important if families are to keep in touch with how members are getting on and they can be used to help in planning family activities. Ensure you allow enough time to enjoy family meals.

REMINDERS

Reminders in the kitchen (and at work) are a great help. A 'healthy heart' reminder (you or your child could draw a 'red heart') stuck on the fridge or the pantry door can assist greatly in reducing non-hungry eating and snacking temptations.

AVOID NON-HUNGRY EATING

Non-hungry eating occurs in most people and it is very important to be aware of this problem. Remember, reducing this type of eating allows a more varied and interesting diet at meal times.

MAKE MEALS MORE EQUAL

In Australia, the evening meal is usually the largest. This is unfortunate as it is usually followed by your period of least activity. If possible, try to change this practice by reducing the size of your evening meal and making the three main meals of the day more equal. Family lunches on the weekends are a great start. Larger breakfasts and lunches will also help reduce snacking during the day.

Planning your dietary day

At this stage you should have assessed the information contained in your three-day food diary to detect your dietary problems. It is now time to go over your days again and correct your problem areas. This section looks at each part of the day and suggests ways to help reduce common dietary problems areas.

BREAKFAST

> 'The critical period in marriage is breakfast time.'
>
> A.P. Herbert

It is important to have a substantial breakfast because you have been fasting overnight and need energy to commence the day. Skipping breakfast is commonly associated with obesity, mostly because it leads to increased snacking and larger, fattier lunches. It also interferes with cognition or thinking, reducing morning work performance. Unfortunately, about a third of adults miss at least one breakfast during the week. Make time for breakfast. Get up early enough to avoid running late. It just makes you, and all those around you, irritable and is a bad start to the day. Breakfast is a great time to find out what is happening with your family during the day. (This will help you in the evening when you are trying to determine why your daughter/son/spouse is out of sorts and vice versa.)

Cereals high in fibre with low-fat milk and low-fat yoghurt, perhaps with a few nuts added, are a great start to the day. So is fruit and wholegrain bread. Try to ensure your food selections have a low glycaemic index. (Breads or cereals with linseeds are a good choice as they add omega-3s to your diet.)

If you are running late, have an alternative breakfast plan. This may mean taking breakfast with you. (A piece of fruit with perhaps some nuts and a small tub of low-fat yoghurt would do the trick.) You can eat this on the way to or when you get to work. Remember, if you do not have time for breakfast at home, you certainly do not have time to drop into fast-food chains or the local muffin and coffee outlet for breakfast. Also avoid muesli-type bars as they often have lots of added sugar and sometimes added saturated fat.

If you are unlucky enough to have a boss who feels 7 a.m. breakfast meetings are beneficial to your working life, please remember you have the right to ask for healthy breakfast foods to be offered. The same goes for those who have regular 'in house' lunch meetings where the employer provides the food.

BETWEEN BREAKFAST AND LUNCH

There is often a considerable period between breakfast and lunch and hunger may occur during this time. On working days this is not a time when you can buy food easily and you will need to rely on food in your workplace. For this reason you need to provide your own nutritious food or ensure the food provided by your employer is of good nutritional value and does not continually run out. Unfortunately, this is often difficult as others working with you may not share your enthusiasm for healthy food and healthy food is sometimes a more expensive option for the employer—a packet of biscuits is cheaper than fresh fruit. When choosing food, again look for options with a low glycaemic index so their hunger-reducing effect lasts longer.

LUNCH

People usually have more time to eat at lunch than at morning tea, therefore there are more options available. Try to make lunch a reasonably substantial meal. Bringing your own lunch has several advantages; it is almost always cheaper and it is always available. If work commitments are such that you do not have time to go out to get your lunch, it is there for you. (Such commitments are not always known ahead of time.) Try to use foods that keep well and store them in a fridge if you have one. If you don't, talk to the boss.

The local food bar is a popular alternative and has the advantage of providing a greater variety of fresher foods. If it doesn't, change food bars. Choose your foods carefully as almost all food bars will have plenty of high-fat, high-sugar options available, especially as little extras. This is a great time to purchase some fresh fruit for afternoon tea.

Work will not always allow you to leave the premises at lunch time or there may not be any food outlets close to your workplace, so your lunch may need to be delivered. Providing the food quality is satisfactory, this option is fine. If the options or quality provided by your regular supplier are not good enough, complain. The prospect of losing business will often dramatically change the food choices offered. Try to have a regular 'standby' lunch that can be ordered when you haven't got the time to think about food alternatives.

If in-house lunch meetings are common in your workplace, you will need to look at the type of food provided. Remember, you have the right to ask for healthy foods to be offered. For those fortunate enough to have restaurant lunches reasonably regularly, it is important that the restaurant offers healthy food choices. If you go to a steak house, that is probably what you will get. So spend some time looking at the restaurant choices in your work area.

When making meal choices, healthy options include salads, dishes based on rice or pasta with plenty of vegetables, dishes that are steamed, grilled, stir-fried or baked and perhaps fruit or sorbets for dessert. Avoid fried foods, foods coated with batter, and creamy sauces. Eat breads with a little margarine or olive oil and avoid butter wherever possible. Limit alcohol to one glass (if any) and ensure you have plenty of water on the table. Avoid soft drinks.

BETWEEN LUNCH AND DINNER

The same comments that were made for mid-morning also apply here.

DINNER

Dinner will often be your main meal of the day and it deserves some forward planning. This planning will avoid having to take the easy takeaway option. It is always worth having some prepared meals in the freezer for those days when you don't feel like cooking. As stated previously, dinner is usually preparing us for a low-activity period, therefore, try to reduce the size of portions. Dinner can still be a place of lively conversation without the huge servings. When dining out, the same rules apply as for lunch.

SOCIALISING AFTER WORK, ON WEEKENDS AND FOR CELEBRATIONS

Socialising after work or on the weekend is the time we like to enjoy ourselves. In moderation, it does not significantly influence the benefits of healthy lifestyle practices. However, as in most things, moderation is the key. If your socialising involves excessive food and alcohol, it should probably be restricted to once a week. If your occupation requires more than this, then stricter controls on your food and alcohol intake will be necessary.

Excessive alcohol consumption has historically been a problem in Australia and remains so today. When you relax with friends or celebrate, ensure you don't significantly depart from the maximum levels of alcohol consumption for good health. Exceeding six standard drinks in one day for males and four for females puts you at increased risk. This practice of binge drinking is especially prevalent in young adults. Its associated problems go well beyond putting on a few extra kilos and waking up feeling less than perfect.

Excess consumption of high-calorie fatty food goes hand in hand with relaxation time, and is exacerbated by alcohol. If moderation is not practised, all your good work during the rest of the week will be undone. This will hurt your self-esteem and put you back on an unhealthy diet cycle. If this type of socialising is a common feature of your lifestyle, you may need to change the environment in which you socialise. An example might be playing sport with friends—Saturday afternoon tennis for example—instead of a round in the pub.

Dietary change—doing it!

Before commencing your dietary modification, you need to have decided you want to change. You will not succeed if you are not sufficiently motivated. There are several stages that you need to progress through to be ready.

Stage 1—Not interested.
Stage 2—You've given the matter some thought, but are not committed and have made no plans to proceed.
Stage 3—You have made the decision to change and have taken active steps towards this goal, such as assessing your dietary problems. You are much more likely to succeed if you take an active role in planning rather than just being told what you should do; although good advice is obviously a great help.

Hopefully reading the earlier chapters has helped you progress through these stages. If you are still undecided, see your doctor to discuss the issue further. Do not start unless you are ready.

PREPARATIONS FOR CHANGE

It is important to emphasise that dietary change is usually best accomplished in several small steps. Changing lifetime eating habits is not easy and attempting to change everything at once is, for most people, an unrealistic expectation and a recipe for failure. With the help of your GP or dietitian, pick a few problem eating habits you think you can modify and address these first. Once you have incorporated these permanently into your routine, a process that will probably take several months (at least), you can move on to the next group of changes.

You should have a definite starting date. Try to choose a day that is usually not too stressful and have your strategies worked out well before this time. Ensure you have suitable meals ready to choose from and have some prepared meals already in the freezer. Try to reduce your alcohol intake for the first few weeks as it tends to reduce your resolve. (This may be one of your goals anyway.)

Remind yourself regularly why you have changed your eating behaviours and the advantages for you. Have them displayed at work and at home. Reward yourself during the period of change and after. Remember, avoiding fatty food and takeaways often leaves you with more money to spend on other treats.

Don't be afraid to get help. Hopefully your GP or dietitian has already been involved in formulating your plans. Regular visits to monitor your progress will help with any problems you are facing and provide positive feedback when things are going well. If you are having problems, seek help early on—don't leave it until you have substantially broken away from your plan as this will reduce your self-esteem and your resolve to succeed. Other professional help can be gained from exercise specialists—make sure they are accredited. Quality shared-care programs, such as Weight Watchers, can also be useful. For those with psychological problems, such as stress at home or anxiety disorders, referral to a psychologist may be in order.

Your family should already be well aware you are trying to change your eating habits and hopefully they are participating in the changes. It is much easier to change as a family. Likewise, your friends should also be aware you are trying to improve your eating behaviours so they can be supportive and hopefully join in. If this doesn't happen, it may be time to change the way you socialise with your friends. The odd drink while playing an afternoon's tennis is much better than sitting down watching the football on TV.

Maintaining your dietary change

Hopefully, good planning will have made your initial dietary change relatively easy. Now your program needs to be monitored for progress. There are several issues you will need to consider.

Weight loss from a diet you can maintain in the long term will be slow, especially for women. Losses of 1 to 2 kilograms per month or waist measurement reductions of 1 to 2 centimetres per month are common and are a good result.

People who have used low-energy (calories/kilojoules) diets previously are used to a quick, initial weight loss due to water and glycogen loss that reverses as soon as energy intake is increased. This quick weight loss will not occur in a diet that has a well-balanced supply of energy. However, unlike quick-fix low-calorie diets, the weight you lose with long-term changes is actual fat tissue that will stay lost.

Monitoring your fat loss is often best done by measuring your waist circumference rather than your actual weight loss, especially early on in your weight-control program. (In pre-menopausal women, fat loss can occur from sites other than the waist first, so a better assessment of initial fat loss may be gained from the arms, thighs, buttocks or bust measurements.)

PLATEAUING

After a period of three to six months, you will usually notice that your weight stops reducing; you will have reached a plateau. Maintaining this plateau is one of the most important tasks in your weight-loss program. It is a sign that your initial dietary changes have succeeded in achieving this initial weight loss, not a sign of failure. You may even have reached an acceptable weight for you.

For most people, however, reaching their first plateau will not coincide with reaching a healthy weight. After maintaining your plateau for two to three months, further changes to diet or exercise routines can be planned in order to stimulate further weight loss. These more challenging changes will be easier to embrace as you will be more confident following your initial success and fitter following your increased exercise. Also, as discussed previously, change usually needs to be done in a step-by-step fashion, and part of your initial weight-loss program should have encompassed this approach to planning. Good ways of breaking through a plateau include trying new foods, reducing the amount of food eaten, changing eating times, changing eating patterns, such as being a vegetarian for a few days a week, or changing your exercise regimen.

Your overall weight reduction should be a pattern of weight loss and plateau. You will find your rate of weight loss becomes slower as your weight diminishes and that plateau periods become progressively longer. This is normal. This overall pattern will be slower for women and people who have been obese for a long time. However, please remember, weight loss is a long-term goal and it is getting there that is important, not how fast you do it. Slow weight loss is not a sign of failure.

RELAPSE AND LONG-TERM WEIGHT LOSS MAINTENANCE

Relapses are not failures. They are temporary set-backs. Some can be anticipated and avoided with good planning. The others should be viewed as part of your weight-loss program, just as plateau periods are. Having said this, you need to address the cause of your relapse very quickly so that minimal damage is done. There are numerous factors that can lead to relapse including:

- Failure to attain results—this may be due to unrealistic expectations or a weight-loss program that was incorrectly planned with respect to reducing energy intake. More commonly, it is due to non-compliance with the diet.
- A history of failure—if you have a past history of failure, you need to be very carefully monitored, especially during the initial stages of weight loss.
- Food cravings—these last about three weeks after changing your diet and can be overcome by eating low-fat, low-energy snacks, such as fruit.
- Excess alcohol or other drug intake.
- Increased stress levels.
- Other psychological problems including depression.
- Physical problems such as injury—some of these may be caused by increasing activity levels too quickly.
- An exercise schedule that has been interrupted by bad weather.
- Lack of support at home from your partner.
- Changing circumstances, such as reduced time available for exercise.
- Hours of TV watched—the amount of weight regained after weight loss increases with the number of hours of TV watched.

When relapse occurs, your initial response should be to check your plan with your doctor or dietitian. If the plan provided an insufficient reduction in energy consumption or an insufficient increase in energy expenditure, then adjustments need to be made. If you are not keeping to your plan, then you need to sort out why.

A quick perusal of the above list shows that many problems occur due to change in circumstances, such as reduced time, increased stress, or injury. Your life is continually evolving and it is important you have a plan that is flexible. Some circumstances, such as short illnesses or injury, can be allowed for as part of your plan. Other problems, such as decreased support from your partner or a long-term injury, are not under your control and modifying your program to account for them will need the help of your doctor or dietitian.

Life is never stress free and times of increased stress act to reduce your resolve. Some actions that may help include: avoiding alcohol as it further reduces your resolve; giving yourself an extra reward, such as going to the pictures; avoiding situations where you are likely to eat or drink too much; and trying to reduce your stress load by getting help from family and friends. If you have chronic problems with stress, part of your weight management program should be a course in stress management as the ability to manage stress is an important component in successful weight control.

Some physical problems, such as sore feet or joints or chafing between the upper legs, may be directly attributable to increased physical activity levels. They can be prevented or treated by proper attention to footwear, an increase in the amount of non-weight-bearing exercise such as swimming, and the use of lycra bicycle shorts. Problems such as excess alcohol are best addressed before weight reduction programs are commenced.

Most importantly, do not give up. There is always a solution to your problem! There is always someone there to help you.

RELAPSE OF FELLOW DIETERS

Family and friends who diet with you will often lose weight. However, as they are not the primary subjects of the program, they are usually not given individual advice, support or follow-up. Thus, while they may initially lose weight, they may not be able to maintain this weight loss. The message in this situation is to encourage others joining in your weight-loss program to have their own program worked out at the same time and to ensure they are also continually monitored during their program. Otherwise, their failure may affect their involvement in and support of your weight-management program.

Further information

Nutrition Australia

For those wishing to know more about diets and their relative merits, a wealth of information can be found on the Nutrition Australia website.

Website: www.nutritionaustralia.org (see Frequently Asked Questions—Weight Loss and Exercise, in particular)

Weight Watchers
Website: www.weightwatchers.com.au

Recipe books
These wonderful recipe books will ensure you don't make homemade dishes that drive the family from home.

Great Food for Men by Rosemary Stanton, Allen & Unwin, Sydney, 2001.
A great book for healthy, easy and delicious recipes for everyone. It also has total fat, fibre and energy content calculated for each meal.

Simply Healthy by Sally James, JB Fairfax Press, Sydney, 1999.
Great, low-fat recipes.

Fresh and Healthy by Sally James, JB Fairfax Press, Sydney, 2000
More low-fat recipes. This is the National Heart Foundation's new cookbook. It also has fat, fibre and energy contents calculated for each recipe.

Healthy Vegetarian Eating by Rosemary Stanton, Allen & Unwin, Sydney, 1998
Looks at the potential advantages and disadvantages of vegetarian eating.

Vegetables by Rosemary Stanton, Allen & Unwin, Sydney, 2000
An A to Z of vegetables, with information and recipes to help you eat more veggies.

The following books deal specifically with nutrition.

Rosemary Stanton's Fat and Fibre Counter (revised), Information Australia, 1999
This lists fat and fibre for 15 000 foods and notes which contain 'bad' fats.

Good Fats, Bad Fats by Rosemary Stanton, Allen & Unwin, Sydney, 1998
A small book with details about fats, LDL and HDL cholesterol, trans fatty acids and triglycerides.

Vitamins by Rosemary Stanton, Allen & Unwin, Sydney, 1999
A concise but thorough look at each of the thirteen vitamins.

Childhood Obesity

Obesity in Australian children and adolescents has been an increasing problem over the past 30 years. At present, more than 20 per cent of children are either overweight or obese. This is twice the incidence of ten years ago! The maximum incidence in girls is just prior to puberty. In boys, however, the incidence continues to increase throughout adolescence, with about one-third of 16 to 18 year old boys being affected. This presents a major problem as many obese children will go on to become obese adults.

The likelihood of childhood obesity persisting into adult life increases with the severity of the problem, the presence of at least one obese parent and the older the age of the obese child (after age three years). Fifty per cent of obese six year olds and 75 per cent of obese adolescents become obese adults. Preventing or successfully treating obesity in children is the best method of preventing obesity in adults.

At present there is no universally accepted classification of childhood obesity. Most classifications are based on an interpretation of the child's body mass index (BMI).

$$\text{Body Mass Index} = \frac{\text{Weight (in kg)}}{\text{Height (in m)}^2}$$

The method most commonly adopted in Australia is to use percentile charts that relate a child's BMI to their age. Those above the 85th percentile are classified as overweight. Those above the 95th percentile are classified as obese. There are different charts for boys and girls. The charts can be downloaded from the internet at: www.cdc.gov/nccdphp/dnpa/bmi/bmi-for-age.htm

Another good method for determining obesity levels in children is to use the BMI readings in table 17.

Table 17 BMI classification for overweight and obese children and adolescents according to age

	BMI			
	Overweight		*Obese*	
Age (years)	*Males*	*Females*	*Males*	*Females*
5	17.4–19.2	17.1–19.1	19.3 +	19.2 +
6	17.6–19.7	17.3–19.6	19.8 +	19.7 +
7	17.9–20.5	17.8–20.4	20.6 +	20.5 +
8	18.4–21.5	18.3–21.5	21.6 +	21.6 +
9	19.1–22.7	19.1–22.7	22.8 +	22.8 +
10	19.8–23.9	19.9–24.0	24.0 +	24.1 +
11	20.6–25.0	20.7–25.3	25.0 +	25.4 +
12	21.2–25.9	21.7–26.6	26.0 +	26.7 +
13	21.9–26.7	22.6–27.7	26.8 +	27.8 +
14	22.6–27.5	23.3–28.5	27.6 +	28.6 +
15	23.3–28.2	23.9–29.0	28.3 +	29.1 +
16	23.9–28.8	24.4–29.3	28.9 +	29.4 +
17	24.5–29.3	24.7–29.6	29.4 +	29.7 +
18	25.0–29.9	25.0–29.9	30.0 +	30.0 +

Source: T.J. Cole et al., 'Establishing a standard definition for child overweight and obesity worldwide: International survey', *British Medical Journal* 2000; 320: 1240–3. Reproduced with permission from the BMJ Publishing Group.

Causes of childhood obesity

An increasingly sedentary lifestyle with a great deal of time spent watching television or in front of the computer is a major cause of the increase in childhhood obesity. A recent study in the USA showed that childhood obesity levels are directly related to the amount of television watched (Crespo 2001). Families with two active parents are six times more likely to have active children than families with inactive parents.

Also of significance is the increasing intake of soft drinks, fatty foods and takeaway/fast foods. As stated before, one-third of food expenditure in Australia is on foods not produced or consumed in the home. Parental preferences significantly influence child food preferences, so try to set a good example.

Some children have a genetic predisposition to becoming obese. However, obesity develops only in an environment conducive to weight gain (i.e. low exercise and poor diet).

Older teenagers are at significant risk of developing obesity for two reasons. Firstly, they are finishing their growth, which reduces their energy requirements. Secondly, physical activity levels are often reducing at this time, due to either school emphasis moving more towards study or the child leaving the school and its environment, which encourages sport.

Childhood obesity is only very occasionally due to a specific medical cause. Short stature for age, developmental delay, and the early onset of obesity are warning signs that there may be an underlying medical cause that needs to be investigated by your medical practitioner.

Problems caused by obesity in children

Obesity causes impaired glucose tolerance, which increases the risk of developing diabetes in adolescence or later life. At present, there is an increasing incidence of type 2 diabetes in adolescents. The presence of obesity and impaired glucose tolerance, defined as 'the metabolic syndrome', increases the risk of coronary artery disease (heart attacks) in later life.

Those children most likely to suffer from impaired glucose tolerance or even diabetes are those with a BMI above the 95th percentile (i.e. obese children) who also have either a family history of type 2 diabetes, come from an ethnic group predisposed to diabetes, or suffer from hypertension or obstructive airways disease. (A purplish-brown pigmentation between the legs or on the neck, called acanthosis nigrans, is another warning sign.) Some experts are at present suggesting that screening for diabetes should be considered in these children.

Obesity also causes adverse changes in blood fats including high levels of total cholesterol, LDL and triglycerides and low HDL which further increases the risk of developing vascular disease. Obese children also have a higher incidence of gallstones, fractures and, rarely, sleep apnoea.

Psychological problems are also more prevalent in obese children. These include poor body image and decreased self-worth, partly as a result of peer teasing, which in turn may lead to depression. Overweight children are often taller for their age. This makes them look older but they cannot perform to the level expected for their older appearance. Thus they appear to under-perform. Thirty per cent of very obese girls have an underlying eating disorder, although preoccupation with weight is a problem with almost all young women. Obesity in adolescence may reflect family discord, boredom or depression.

A family problem, not a problem with the child

In dealing with childhood obesity, adopting a family approach is likely to lead to greater success. As is the case with nearly all aspects of life, parents can often help their children most by being good role models and, by sharing healthy meals, all family members will benefit. Making childhood obesity a family problem rather than a problem with the child can also prevent the child developing feelings of guilt regarding their size. Such guilt can initiate body–image problems, which can lead to other serious problems, such as anorexia in adolescents and young adults.

As with adult obesity, it is important to concentrate on long-term changes in behaviour rather than a particular weight goal. Again, this will help avoid guilt. Usually all that is needed is to aim to maintain weight and, as the child grows taller, the obesity problem will gradually disappear.

Parental (carer) attitudes

When dealing with an obese child, parents need to recognise their child's obesity is an issue of concern. Many parents see their child's obesity as 'normal'. Be observant of their behaviours and reward desired behaviours. You should direct praise at good behaviour rather than towards any reduction in weight.

As a parent, you also need to be consistent with eating habits in the home and model desired eating and exercise habits yourself. Limits can be set for eating behaviours if necessary. However, do not allow food or diet to become an obsession and avoid causing guilt by being too judgmental. You should also include your children in meal planning and take this opportunity to educate them in making healthy food choices. Providing a caring and loving environment for your children where communication is encouraged helps them know they are loved irrespective of any problems they have.

Control of the child's eating environment

As a parent, you need to assist your children's behaviour modification through control of their environment. Improving the quality of food available at home is an important start. Provide a wide range of good foods, including plenty of breads, healthy cereals, vegetables and fruit. Fruit and vegetables are especially important and are often lacking in children's diets.

Reduce the use of takeaway food and especially avoid having unhealthy snack foods in the home as they encourage eating when your child is not hungry. You should reduce the use of foods containing large amounts of sugar and salt. Soft drinks are a very important source of excess sugar in children of all ages, even two to three year olds, and they should be avoided. Water (without cordial) is a much healthier and cheaper option and should be your child's preferred drink. Do not provide different foods for each child. It is not fair to expect your overweight child to choose an apple while the others have chocolate biscuits.

Breakfast is a particularly important meal for all members of the family. Missing breakfast or having a less nutritious breakfast is often associated with being overweight.

Missing breakfast increases the likelihood of snacking during the morning, often on high-energy, high-fat foods. It has also been shown to decrease cognitive (thinking) functioning.

Any goals should be directed at eating habits, not specific weight targets. Encouraging your children to monitor their own food intake and activity levels will enable them to learn how to successfully manage their weight and fitness throughout their adult lives.

As stated above, good (and bad) eating habits are learned from parents and the family meal is a great place for children to start learning. As well as benefiting from more family interaction, children who regularly eat family meals have a 50 per cent increase in the likelihood of consuming the recommended five daily servings of fruit and vegetables, have significantly higher intakes of calcium, iron and vitamins, consume more fibre, and have lower intakes of saturated fats. They are also 30 per cent less likely to consume soft drinks and fried foods away from home (Gillman 2000).

Finally, you should also be able to have a say regarding the foods offered at your child's school canteen. You should lobby your school to remove fatty foods, such as chocolates, and high energy, low-nutrient foods, such as soft drinks, from the shelves and encourage the canteen to offer a range of healthy foods including fruit.

Nutritious snacks for children

- Bread-based snacks such as sandwiches, fruit loaf, fruit buns
- Breakfast cereals
- Fruit—fresh, dried or canned (unsweetened)
- Vegetables
- Dairy products—milk, yoghurt, cheese, fruit smoothies
- Home-made popcorn
- Fruit sticks.

Snacks, when not used for afternoon or morning tea, should be consumed only occasionally, not every day. They should occur at specific times during the day and be low in fat, especially saturated fat.

Reduced fat diets and children

Low cholesterol and low total fat diets (25 per cent of total energy intake) are quite safe for children over the age of five years (Obarzanek 2001). As stated in the section on obesity, they are the best method for reducing weight and can have the added advantage of being low in saturated fats. Such diets can be used by the whole family and can help with adult obesity and lipid problems. The aim is to establish healthy long-term eating habits for the whole family.

Under the age of five years, fat should make up about 35 per cent of total energy intake to ensure total energy intake is adequate for this rapid growth period. A strict low-fat diet is not appropriate in this group; children of this age require some good quality foods that contain fat. One really good source is whole milk and this should be used in preference to low-fat varieties in this age group. Others are cheese, lean meats, peanut butter, yoghurt and eggs. (Nuts, especially peanuts, should not be given as they can cause choking.) Saturated fat intake should be limited wherever possible and poor quality fatty foods, such as crisps, chocolate and takeaways, should still be omitted or used as occasional (not daily) treats. Otherwise, the dietary advice in the preceding two sections is suitable for children as well as adults.

Control of the child's activity

As a parent, you also need to increase your child's physical activity options. Promoting family physical activities, such as walking and bike riding, and encouraging participation in sports they enjoy or have shown interest in is a good start. Make sure you participate too by helping with their practice, being the team coach etc. Most children prefer participating in team sports and they are very important for socialisation as well as physical activity. However, many team sports are stopped when the child leaves school. It is therefore important to encourage sports and other physical activities that will be easy to continue throughout adult life. Such activities include walking, cycling, golf, tennis or swimming. The golden rule is the activity should be fun and any sport or activity your children are interested in should be encouraged! If they enjoy it, they are more likely to continue participating.

In order to increase time for physical activity, you need to restrict access to passive activities, such as TV and computer games. A maximum of 30 minutes per day in front of the TV or computer is usually more than adequate. Watching less TV also reduces the consumption of snack foods and reduces exposure to advertisements for poor quality foods, which in turn helps to improve food preferences. Such advertisements are very commonly shown in child viewing times. Intervention programs that reduce sedentary behaviour have been shown to be as effective at inducing weight loss as those that aim solely at increasing physical activity.

Obtaining professional help

A weight-control program can be a difficult and frustrating task for both parents and children. Thus, it is often beneficial to enlist the help of the family's GP or a dietitian. They can also help recognise any underlying medical cause, if present. When the overweight person is an adolescent, an outsider's point of view can be invaluable. In addition, more serious eating disorders, such as bulimia, are a problem in this age group and health professionals will be needed to help with treatment in these cases.

As a team, the family and health professional can assess the family's dietary problems, initiate an appropriate weight-loss strategy for all members of the family, and help with monitoring the family's progress through regular follow-up visits. These consultations may be done without your child if he or she is under the age of 11 years, as repeated visits can cause feelings of guilt about body shape, resulting in body-image problems in adolescence.

When weight loss goes too far—anorexia and bulimia

Eating disorders are important psychological illnesses. In Australia, about 25 per cent of girls aged 13 to 17 eat to control weight and about 47 per cent exercise to control weight. However, only about two per cent of girls suffer from bulimia and 0.5 per cent suffer from anorexia. Males are occasionally affected, mostly in association with substance abuse.

Characteristics associated with anorexia include low body weight, food avoidance, excessive concern about being fat, distorted body-size image, the use of purging, and excessive exercise. Medical problems are related to low body weight and include weakness, osteoporosis, growth retardation, depression, and hormonal problems, such as periods ceasing, impaired fertility and the appearance of fine body hair. Death from weight loss and suicide also, rarely, occurs.

In bulimia, the person is usually overweight but has tried or is trying to lose weight by food restriction. A period of food restriction is followed by binge eating and induced vomiting and the use of laxatives is common. This cycle continues with the person having haphazard eating patterns. The anxiety related to food and weight lead to relationship problems and often depression. Other side effects include weakness and teeth problems.

Anyone suspected of having an eating disorder should see their GP.

Diagnosis of eating disorders

A positive response to two or more of the following five questions indicates an eating disorder is present (Morgan et al. 1999).

1. Do you make yourself sick because you feel uncomfortably full?
2. Do you worry that you have lost control over what you eat?
3. Have you recently lost over 6 kilograms in weight in a three-month period?

4. Do you believe yourself to be fat when others say you are too thin?
5. Would you say that food dominates your life?

It is important to note that this is a screening test to help identify people with eating disorders. You do not need to wait for these symptoms to appear to seek help if you are worried that you or a friend has a problem with eating.

Weight criteria suggested for anorexia

- At 13 years—a BMI of 15.5 or less
- At 14 years—a BMI of 16 or less
- At 16 years—a BMI of 16.5 or less
- 17 years and over—a BMI of 17.5 or less.

(RACGP 2002)

Physical inactivity

A major cause of both vascular disease and obesity in Australia is insufficient physical activity. Thirty per cent of Australian adults engage in no exercise at all and 54 per cent do not do enough to gain any benefit. This has a huge influence on illness in Australia, with 7.5 per cent of all male burden of disease and 6.0 per cent of all female burden of disease directly attributable to physical inactivity.

With respect to reducing coronary artery disease, all physical activity is good, including mild exercise such as walking. As well as being beneficial itself, physical activity helps by reducing other risk factors such as obesity and diabetes.

A recent study involving 72 000 women (Manson 1999) showed that any exercise is significantly beneficial, with the benefit increasing with the amount of exercise. Just walking one to three hours per week reduced the risk of a heart attack or death by about 30 per cent. Recent evidence (Myers 2002) from a study of 6000 males over an average of six years in the USA showed that, in both healthy men and those with cardiovascular disease, being fit halved the risk of dying from any cause. The degree of benefit was directly related to the level of fitness and the greatest benefit occurred by moving from the least-fit 20 per cent to the next least-fit 20 per cent—indicating that even small amounts of exercise are beneficial. The level of fitness was also found to be a better predictor of risk of death than other cardiovascular risk factor.

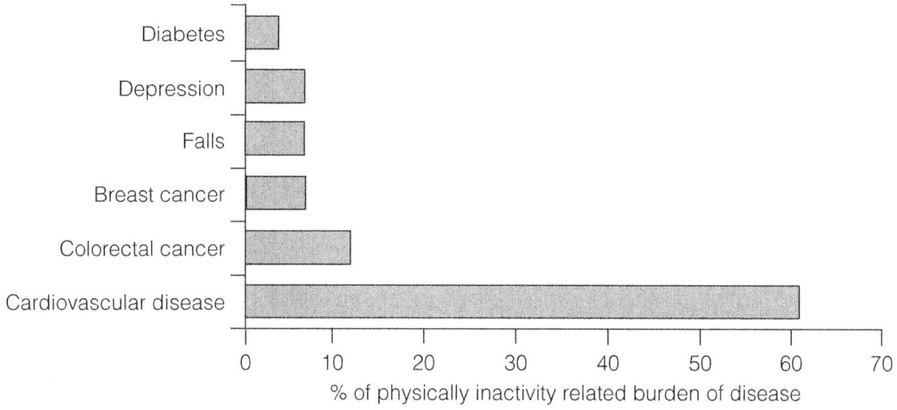

Source: Adapted from Australian Institute of Health and Welfare: Mathers, 1999.

Figure 12 Distribution of burden of disease caused by pyhsical inactivity

Research by Blair (1989) showed that people whose sole risk factor for cardiovascular disease was a low fitness level had a higher death rate from vascular disease than fit people with three other risk factors.

Whilst the main benefits from increasing physical activity relate to reduced cardiovascular disease, figure 12 shows that important benefits are also gained from the prevention of colorectal and breast cancers, depression and falls.

Benefits of physical activity

A REDUCTION OF BODY FAT

Physical activity increases the body's energy requirements by the actual energy needed to do the activity and by increasing the body's basal metabolic rate through an increase in lean body mass (i.e. muscle mass). This overall increased energy requirement results in the breakdown of some body fat. Exercise also decreases body fat by reducing your appetite. A reduction in body fat decreases your weight and helps improve your body shape.

A REDUCTION IN CARDIOVASCULAR DISEASE RISK

Exercise reduces cardiovascular disease risk (and thus decreases mortality) by a reduction in blood pressure, an improvement in blood fats (reduced total cholesterol and increased HDL)

and an increase in heart muscle fitness, which acts to decrease the overall workload of the heart.

IMPROVED PSYCHOLOGICAL WELL-BEING

Exercise has many psychological benefits including an enhanced body image, enhanced self-esteem and well-being, providing a feeling of vitality, and improved mood. Mild anxiety or depression can be helped by exercise. These psychological benefits occur with as little as ten minutes of simple exercise (e.g. walking) a day.

CANCER REDUCTION

Physical activity significantly reduces the risk of several different cancers, including colon, uterine or womb, and breast cancers (Stanton 2002).

OTHER PHYSICAL BENEFITS

These include improved sleep, improved balance that can reduce the incidence of falls, and reduced likelihood of osteoporosis. Exercise also reduces the loss of cognitive function (thinking ability) that occurs with increasing age and improves your health overall.

Preventing injury from exercise

Physical injuries are more common in older people, especially when they exercise irregularly. These can be minimised by a five-minute warm up and cool down with each activity, the use of correct equipment and technique (an exercise trainer or coach can be helpful here), and adequate nutrition and fluids. A resistance and strength-training program before or with training for cardiovascular fitness is also of benefit.

Everyone has heard stories about people dropping dead while exercising. In those under 30 years of age, this is mostly due to an underlying unknown heart abnormality, such as a congenital heart valve problem. In those over 30 years, it is most likely due to coronary artery disease. While the risk of sudden death is increased during vigorous exercise, this risk is still very, very small and its significance is easily outweighed by the reduction in cardiovascular deaths associated with a physically active lifestyle (i.e. you are at much less overall risk if you exercise). Also people who exercise regularly have a reduced risk of sudden death while exercising.

Proper medical assessment prior to commencing an exercise program and increasing exercise levels gradually can help minimise any risk. If you are an inactive person, you should take at least eight to 12 weeks to build up your general level of fitness.

Get assessed first

Professional assessment before you commence your exercise program is essential. All people are different and assessment allows the selection of the most appropriate exercise program for you. Remember, this is a lifestyle change, not a once in a lifetime event, and your exercise program therefore warrants careful planning.

Also, if you are to avoid injury, the risks involved in partaking in a particular exercise program need to be discussed with a qualified health professional before commencing that program. This especially applies if you are over 35 years of age, have any heart-disease risk factors, or have other significant medical problems. It is good to minimise cardiovascular risk factors, such as blood pressure, before exercise is undertaken. This is also a good time to assess and treat other health issues that are concerning you.

Planning your exercise modification program

The first thing that needs to be done is to look at your lifestyle. As with dietary assessment, this will take some time and you need to look at each day of the week separately, dividing each day into several components, including working time, time spent travelling to and from work and recreational time. Look at non-physical recreation activities and work out how these can be changed to physical ones.

When examining your daily schedule, consider the exercise you already do and the opportunities available to increase this exercise. Remember to look for similarities and differences in each day. It is often helpful to put all this information in a table, such as table 18. This can be used to assist in planning modifications to your present physical activity. Include in the table the type of activity, its duration, and when it occurs during the day.

Hopefully, assessing your daily activities will show where time for extra physical activity can be fitted in. This may involve filling in gaps present in the day, such as opportunities to do exercise to and from work (and at work), or using alternatives to present-day activities that will allow increased exercise. For example, when driving to work, use a parking station further away and do some extra walking.

Changing your lifestyle priorities/choices so more time can be found for exercise will also be of benefit. Non-physical activities, such as watching TV, can be swapped for physical activities—you can even do both at the same time. Try having an exercise bike for use while you are watching TV.

Concentrate on changing behaviours, not outcomes, such as cycling 10 kilometres in a certain time. Don't have unrealistic expectations. Rather, aim for achievable changes initially, increase goals gradually, and don't aim to achieve all your dietary and exercise goals at the same time.

Table 18 Exercise assessment table

Day	*Physical activity as part of normal daily activities*	*Planned physical activities (include type of exercise, time done and duration)*	*Total time per day (duration and time of activity)*	*Opportunities for extra physical activity (include type of exercise and time period)*
Monday				
Tuesday				
Wednesday				
Thursday				
Friday				
Saturday				
Sunday				

Changing circumstances may necessitate a change in your program. Ensure your exercise routine is flexible as performing some activities will depend on factors beyond your control, such as the weather, changes in your schedule and your health. Plan a structured exercise regime with the help of a qualified exercise consultant if needed.

How much and what type?

There are two main types of physical activities: those that are part of your normal daily routine, such as walking to the bus stop, and those you do for their own sake, such as tennis or jogging. Both are effective at improving health. The national physical activity guidelines for Australians, shown in figure 13, indicate how you should allocate your weekly physical activity. You should note that most of your energy should be (and usually is) expended in day-to-day activities, not doing specific exercise programs.

In becoming more active, you should increase your normal daily activity. You need to think of movement as an opportunity, not an inconvenience! This may include walking instead of driving, walking at work rather than telephoning, using stairs rather than lifts or escalators, or getting off the bus/train a stop earlier than needed and walking the rest of the way. Increasing this type of activity is very beneficial if you are very overweight as strenuous exercise can be more difficult for this group. Your everyday activity can be measured by a pedometer, which measures the number of steps you take. You should aim for about 7500 to 10 000 steps per day. This will burn up about 1000

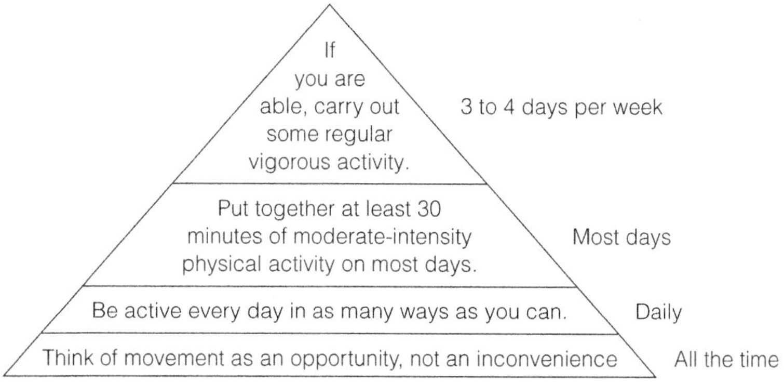

Source: Eggar et al., 2001.

Figure 13 National physical activity guidelines

kilojoules of energy. Small amounts done often are just as effective as fewer longer periods.

Your structured exercise program should be composed of lifestyle activities, such as gardening, and leisure-type sports as well as more formal exercise programs. It should also ideally be based around increasing contact with family and friends.

You should initially aim to build up to 20 minutes of structured physical activity per day and every opportunity to move should be encouraged. Your structured physical activity should then be gradually increased to and then maintained at a level of at least 30 minutes of medium intensity activity per day for most days of the week. Medium intensity exercise is the best level for 'burning off' fat, although lower levels are also very beneficial. With walking or running to achieve weight loss, it is the distance covered that matters most, not how fast you do it. A good indicator of medium exercise is getting slightly puffed and returning with a 'glow'. Fitness levels can be assessed by measuring heart rates during exercise.

Optimum (moderate) exercise levels can be achieved by exercising at 65 per cent of your maximum heart rate. Your maximum heart rate equals 220 beats per minute minus your age in years. As an example, the maximum heart rate for a 50 year old would be:

220 – 50 (beats per minute) = 170 (beats per minute).

Sixty-five per cent of this figure would be 111 beats per minute. Heart rates for moderate exercise according to age are shown in table 19. This level needs to be gradually worked up to, especially if you have not been regularly exercising—50 per cent would be more appropriate for a beginner.

Table 19 Optimum heart rates during exercise

Age (years)	*Heart rate at moderate exercise level in beats per minute (equivalent to 65% of max. heart rate)*
20	130
30	124
40	117
50	111
60	104
70	98

Remember, with respect to burning up excess fat, the length of time spent exercising is more important than the intensity of the exercise. If desired, you can attempt more strenuous exercise later on to improve your cardiovascular fitness. Vigorous exercise equates to exercising at about 75 per cent of your maximum heart rate (or getting reasonably puffed). Excessive exercise that is beyond your fitness level should be avoided as it is more likely to cause injury.

To improve weight loss, try exercising prior to eating, especially before breakfast. Blood glucose levels are lower at these times and a greater proportion of the energy used comes from the breakdown of body fat. Cooling down slowly rather than quickly and not eating too soon after exercise will also help body fat use.

Energy expenditure with exercise

The amount of weight you lose will depend on the energy you expend while exercising.

Low energy exercise

Includes slow walking or swimming, and bowls.
Expends less than 17 kilojoules per minute (or about 500 kilojoules in 30 minutes)

Moderate exercise

Includes brisk walking, cycling for pleasure, golf (when walking), social tennis, water activities, low impact aerobics or dancing.
Expends about 17 to 30 kilojoules per minute (or about 500 to 900 kilojoules in 30 minutes).

Vigorous exercise

Includes jogging, running and active cycling, tennis (singles), swimming, aerobics or dancing.

Expends over 30 kilojoules per minute (or over 900 kilojoules in 30 minutes). Very vigorous exercise can expend considerably more energy than this.

Walking and weight loss

Weight loss with walking varies depending on the number of steps you take each day. One kilojoule of energy is expended in taking 5 to 6 steps (for a 75 kilogram person). You should work out how many steps you are taking at present using a pedometer. (They are relatively cheap and can be purchased from most electronics or fitness stores.) Record your number of steps over a week and determine your current steps per day. You can increase this gradually in increments of 500 to 1000 steps per day. Taking more than 8000 steps per day is likely to result in fat loss in most people but you may need to reach this level slowly, especially if you are very overweight. (This would expend about 1600 kilojoules of energy per day.)

(Kron 1999)

Which planned physical activities are right for you?

Activities that can be successfully incorporated into a long-term physical activity program need to be ones you enjoy and should fit into your lifestyle easily. A variety of physical activities is best. They should involve both upper and lower limbs and include some weight bearing exercise to help prevent osteoporosis. Good choices are walking, jogging, cycling, weight training, rowing, tennis, golf, aerobics and swimming. Your activities should also aim to increase social contact with friends and family. Join a club associated with a physical activity, such as a sports club or a bushwalking club, or try walking with your partner or another family member or friend. This will provide some of the much needed communication time that often goes missing when work life becomes increasingly demanding. Also, the concern of 'letting friends down' by not participating will help prevent you missing regular activities.

Your activities should include indoor and outdoor activities so that bad weather doesn't cause too much disruption. Also, as your goal should be aimed at long-term change, you should introduce some activities that you will be able to perform for many years to come and enjoy doing. Often you can resurrect activities you enjoyed when younger but gave up.

Occasionally there are barriers to regular activity that need to be addressed. Concerns about appearance can deter people from exercising and any exercise program should be done in a non-threatening environment. Also, do not feel that any present lack of fitness means you will not be able to gain benefit from starting an exercise program. All exercise is beneficial and exercise levels can be gradually increased from initial modest levels. The 'no pain, no gain' slogan is neither helpful nor truthful. A lack of time should not stop you from exercising. There are many ways of incorporating activity into your daily routine.

Commencing and maintaining a new physical activity program

Once you have planned your physical activity program, decide on a definite starting date. As with dietary change, try to choose a day that is usually not too stressful and ensure you have the equipment you need to carry out your activities.

Remind yourself regularly why you have changed your activity behaviours and the advantages they will bring to you. These reminders can be displayed at work and at home. Family pictures displayed at work could perhaps show you engaging in physical activities together. Reward yourself during the period of change and after.

Don't be afraid to get help at any time. Hopefully your GP has already been involved in formulating your plans. Regular visits to your GP to monitor your progress will help with any problems you are facing and act as positive feedback when things are going well. If you are having problems, seek help early on. Don't leave it until you have substantially broken away from your plan as this will reduce your self-esteem and your resolve to succeed. Your family and friends should already be well aware you are trying to change your exercise habits. Hopefully they are participating in the changes as well.

Good planning will have made your changes in physical activity relatively easy. However, weight loss from exercise is often slow. Do not be discouraged and remember there are many other benefits to be gained from exercise.

While a good exercise program will help avoid most injuries, there will still be the occasional strain, and there are always coughs and colds to knock you about. These interruptions have to be accepted and not seen as failures in the program. Note that after a period without exercise, it is necessary to build up to your previous level gradually to avoid injury.

Life is never stress free and times of increased stress act to reduce your resolve. You need to be especially focused at these times and try to give yourself an extra reward as encouragement.

Physical activity for children and the elderly

Physical activity and children is covered in the section on 'Childhood obesity'. However, several points are worth emphasising here.

Exercise is important for all children and, as Australian children are becoming more sedentary, they should be encouraged to be physically active. It is important to remember that your good example is their best education! If you are active, they will be too. Remember, families with two active parents are six times more likely to have active children than families with inactive parents.

Any sport/activity that children enjoy should be encouraged. However, it is worthwhile encouraging at least one physical activity they will be able to continue into their adult life, such as walking, cycling, running, golf, tennis and swimming. Many team sports are great to do when young and help develop socialising skills. However, they are often ceased after leaving school.

From a peak at age 20, exercise levels fall steadily with increasing age. By the age of 70 they have dramatically reduced in most people, with 40 per cent of people over this age doing no exercise at all. This is unfortunate as exercise has numerous benefits for the elderly. It is impossible here to recommend specific exercises as all elderly people have different levels of fitness and different medical conditions that need to be taken into account when advising on an exercise program. However, there are exercises for almost everyone.

The numerous advantages of exercise for the elderly include prolonged independence and a reduction in the incidence of falls due to better muscle tone and balance, maintaining heart and lung fitness, a reduced risk of osteoporosis, reduced pain from arthritis, and an increased number of years without disability. Exercise also offers increased socialisation if performed with others, improves thinking, and generally enhances your feeling of well-being.

See your doctor and physiotherapist and then start up!

Part 5

Preventing heart attacks and strokes

Vascular disease—an overview

Vascular disease accounts for 38 per cent of all male deaths and 40 per cent of all female deaths in Australia. Coronary artery disease and stroke are the two most important contributors and together they cause about 18 per cent of the total burden of disease. Coronary artery disease is the disease that is most likely to cause you to die prematurely, irrespective of whether you are male or female and even in people with no (known) risk factors, vascular disease is still the most likely cause of death. This section needs to be read by everyone.

An outline of the vascular system

The vascular system is basically a system of tubes, known as blood vessels, for transporting the blood. Those tubes taking blood from the heart to the various organs of the body, such as the muscles, brain and heart muscle itself, are called the arteries. Those returning blood from these organs to the heart are called the veins. The power to move the blood through these vessels is supplied by the heart, which is really just a pump. The blood in the arteries takes essential nutrients, including the oxygen needed to produce energy in the body's cells, to the organs. Without an adequate supply of oxygen, body cells soon die. The time it takes cells deprived of oxygen to die varies. Brain cells can last for only a few minutes. Heart muscle cells can last for up to several hours.

Table 20 Incidence of vascular disease in Australia

Disease	*Incidence in Australians %*
Coronary artery disease	
Men over 40	50
Women over 40	33
Stroke	
Men over 45	25
Women over 45	20
Male deaths from vascular disease	38
Male deaths from coronary artery disease	22
Female deaths from vascular disease	40
Female deaths from coronary artery disease	20

Source: Australian Institute of Health and Welfare, 2000.

What is vascular disease?

It is your arteries that are involved in vascular disease. Vascular disease acts to block these arterial vessels and, in doing this, blocks the supply of oxygen and nutrients to the tissue the artery supplies. These blockages occur in the inner section of the artery, adjacent to the lumen. They occur as multiple discrete small lesions rather than as a generalised blockage along the whole length of the artery. They occur in most people in Western society as they age.

Each individual lesion arises from the thickening of the vessel wall that occurs when cholesterol accumulation forms a fatty deposit in the wall. This process depends on the events outlined below. Before commencing this discussion, it is important to review the information on cholesterol in the nutrition and exercise section of this book, especially that relating to lipoproteins (pages 114–115).

Vascular disease initiation

The initial event in vascular disease is an injury to the inner part of the artery wall that lines the vessel lumen. There are numerous possible causes for this injury, including forces associated with high blood pressure, chemical injury from compounds originating outside the body (such as chemicals from cigarette smoke), raised blood levels of normal body compounds, and perhaps even infection. This injury makes the cells lining the inner artery wall leakier, allowing the entry into the vessel wall of extra LDL (bad cholesterol) from the blood. (A high blood level of LDL obviously makes this situation worse.)

Normal LDL in the vessel wall supplies the cholesterol needed for the construction of cell components, such as cell membranes. This is a normal body process and does no harm.

However, LDL in the vessel wall can be oxidised by numerous chemicals called oxidants or free radicals, especially when excessive levels of LDL are present. The cholesterol contained in this oxidised LDL is not used for normal body processes and accumulates in the artery wall. This abnormal accumulation of oxidised cholesterol is irritating to the tissues, causing further injury and inflammation to occur, thus perpetuating the whole process.

As these cholesterol deposits gradually enlarge, they become harder due to the deposition of calcium and fibrous tissue into the fatty deposit and the whole process causes the artery lumen to become increasingly blocked. Also, part of the artery wall forms a distinct layer (a fibrous cap) between the cholesterol deposit and the lumen of the artery.

The development of such lesions is termed atherosclerosis. Each lesion takes at least 10 to 20 years to form and new lesions are continually starting up, so lowering your total cholesterol and LDL cholesterol and reducing other risk factors needs to be a life-long project.This process is described more fully in figure 15 and appendix 8.

All is not lost, however, as three mechanisms can be used to slow down or partially reverse this process. Firstly, it is thought that consuming lots of antioxidants in your diet may help neutralise the effects of the oxidants/free radicals and reduce the oxidisation of LDL. Secondly, diet or drugs can influence cholesterol deposition and removal. (Decreasing your blood LDL and total cholesterol levels reduces cholesterol deposition in the vessel wall and increasing HDL helps with cholesterol removal.) Finally, reversing factors causing the initial injury, such as high blood pressure, can reduce further injury to the artery wall.

What happens to vascular atherosclerosis lesions?

The fate of your vascular lesions (and yourself!) depends on how well you look after your vascular disease risk factors. People with fewer, less severe risk factors will develop far fewer lesions and they will appear significantly later in life. Thus, they are unlikely to be troubled by vascular disease until very late in their life if at all. If you have numerous risk factors, you can expect trouble a lot earlier.

LESIONS CAN DECREASE IN SIZE

If you take care of your arteries by minimising your risk factors for vascular disease, these lesions actually get smaller by reducing the amount of cholesterol in the lesion. This acts to reduce the pressure and inflammation that the fatty lesion exerts on and causes in the artery wall, thus making it less likely to rupture. It's a bit like letting air out of an overfilled balloon that is likely to burst.

LESIONS CAN INCREASE IN SIZE—STABLE AND UNSTABLE LESIONS

If you disregard vascular disease risk factors, the vascular lesions will get larger. The way this occurs depends on whether the inner artery wall over the lesion is thin or thick.

If the inner wall is thick and the lesion just continues to gradually increase in size, there will be a corresponding decrease in the size of the lumen vessel (a stable lesion). The body

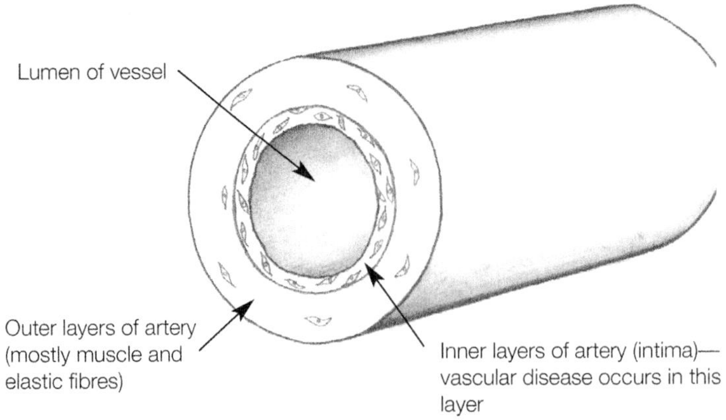

1. Normal artery (at birth)

This is a simplified view of a normal artery wall with no vascular disease present. The inner layer (or intima) is where the vascular disease occurs. In Western society, vascular disease gradually increases from early in life. Even at the age of 10, many children would have signs of the early stages of vascular disease.

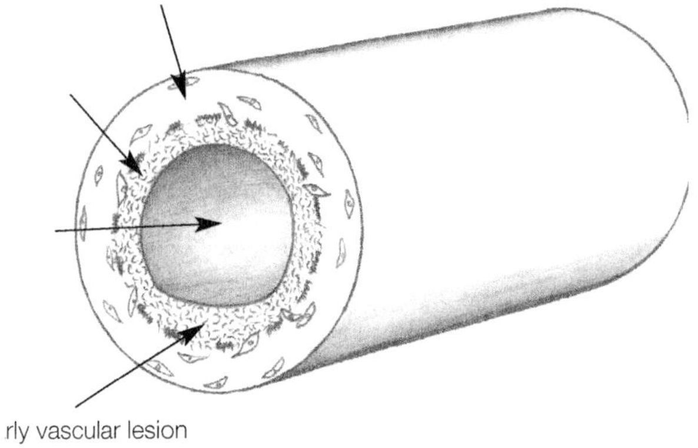

2. Early vascular disease (called a 'fatty streak')

A small deposit of cholesterol containing cells ('foam cells') and cholesterol itself has formed in the intima section of the artery. This process occurs adjacent to a site where there has been damage to cells lining the inner artery wall (the endothelial cells). The lesion shown has thickened the intima layer slightly and consequently reduced the size of the lumen (and thus the blood flow).

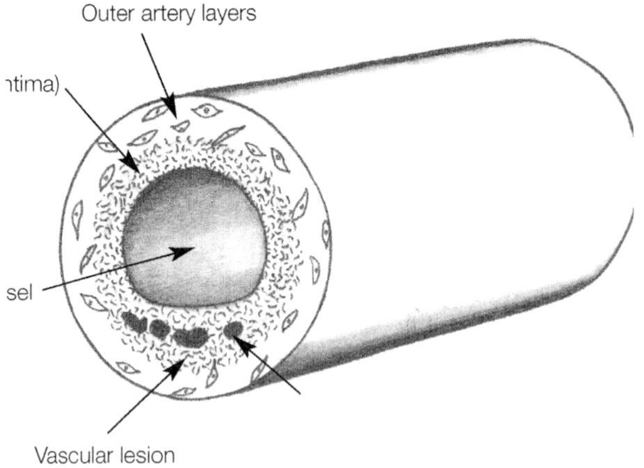

3. Futher progression of vascular disease

(Occurs from the third decade of life onwards)

Further enlargement of the lesion has occurred and distinct cholesterol deposits have developed. As well as containing cholesterol, the lesion will be starting to accumulate some connective tissue and calcium, a process that hardens the lesion. The rate of this enlargement process depends on the number of risk factors for vascular disease you possess and their severity.

Figure 15 Artery

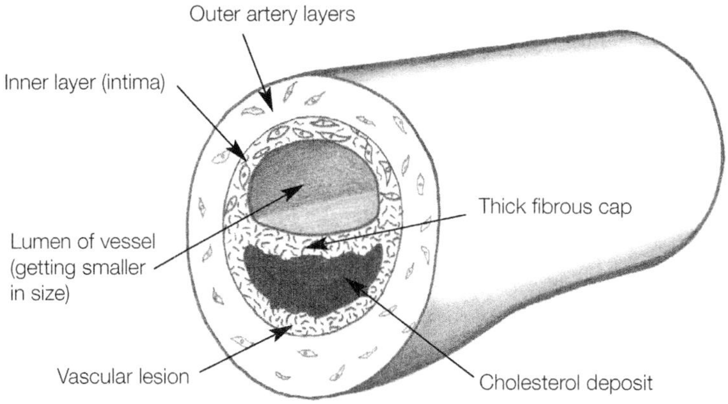

4. Established lesion with a thick capsule—a stable lesion

(Occurs from the fourth decade of life onwards)

With further enlargement, the vessel becomes more blocked and a distinct layer (a fibrous cap) develops between the lesion and the artery lumen. In this diagram, the fibrous cap is farily thick. This is important as it means the fibrous cap is relatively strong and decreases the likelihood that it will rupture or tear. These types of lesions are more common in people with more favourable vascular disease risk factors and these people are also more likely to develop such lesions later in life.

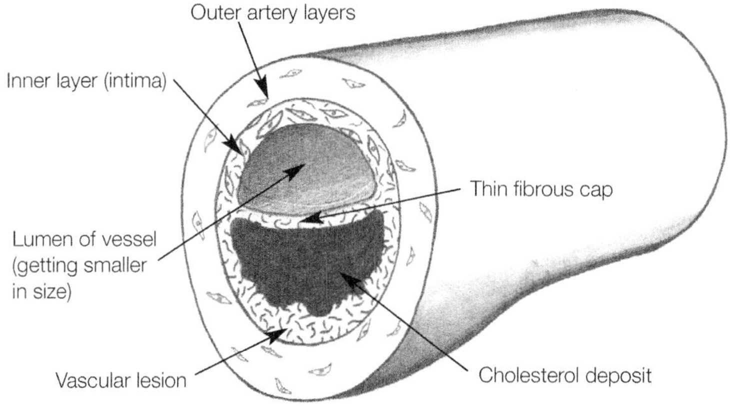

5. Established lesion with a thin capsule—an unstable lesion

(Occurs from the fourth decade of life onwards)

In this diagram the lesion has progressed further. Importantly, the vascular lesion is covered by a thin fibrous cap that is weaker and more likely to tear or rupture. Thin fibrous caps from over lesions for several reasons, including increasing pressure on the fibrous cap from the enlarging underlying lesion and further injury (and inflammation) to the inner lining of the vessel or the cap itself. These lesions are more likely to occur in people with more severe risk factors.

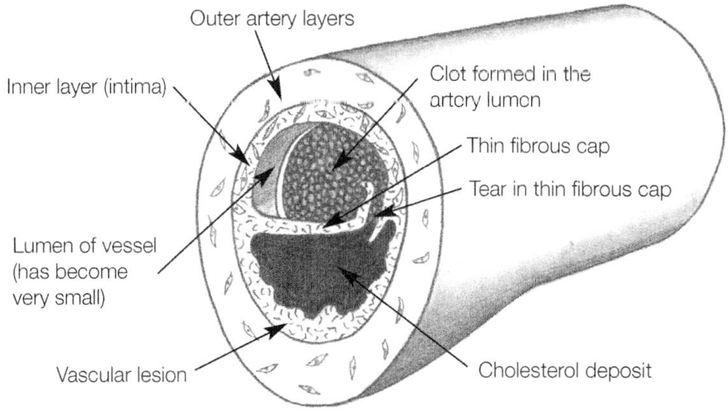

6. Rupture of a vascular lesion

(Occurs from the fourth decade of life onwards)

When this weakening process is severe enough, the thin cap will tear or rupture. This brings the underlying lesion into direct contact with blood in the artery lumen. The natural response of the body is to repair this break and it starts this process by establishing a blood clot over the rupture site. This clot will vary in size depending on the size of the tear. However, the clot can often be quite large and when this is the case, it can cause a sudden severe reduction in blood flow through the already significantly blocked artery. This deprives the tissues the artery supplies with oxygen and this tissue may die as a result. This is the process that causes almost all heart attacks and many strokes.

Removal of clots

With respect to the heart, removing this clot quickly (by drugs or surgery) can avoid or significantly reduce permanent damage to heart muscle. This is one reason why anyone with symptoms suggestive of a heart attack needs to go to hospital as quickly as possible. Every minute counts! Similarly, people with a suspected stroke need to be assessed in hospital quickly to minimise brain damage.

can compensate for this to a degree by making new smaller vessels to bypass the increasingly blocked vessel. However, the blockage will eventually become great enough to cause problems due to inadequate supply of oxygen (via the blood) to the tissue the artery supplies. Initially this gives symptoms only when the person is exercising as tissues require more oxygen during exercise. Angina heart pain that occurs with exercise is an example of this process. Eventually the blockage may be large enough to cause symptoms even when you are resting.

Lesions in people with multiple severe risk factors tend to increase in size more quickly and have inner vessel walls that are thin. They are termed unstable lesions. As the fatty deposits increase in size, they stretch the inner vessel wall that lies over them. The inflammation that occurs causes further weakening of these already thin walls, making them more likely to rupture. Any factor exacerbating this inflammation, such as an infection derived from the blood, can make this process occur more quickly. This may explain why people who have gum infections tend to have more heart attacks.

Eventually the thinned wall becomes too weak and a rupture occurs. A clot forms over the break in the inner surface of the vessel wall to try to seal it off and allow the break to mend. This clot formation occurs over a few minutes and causes the blockage to suddenly increase in size and the blood flow through the vessel to suddenly decrease. There is no time for new vessels to grow to compensate for the sudden blockage.

The consequence of this rupture and clot formation depends on the degree of blockage it causes. A large blockage will cause a dramatic reduction in blood flow (and thus oxygen) provided by the artery to the tissues it supplies and results in the death of this tissue. This is how almost all heart attacks and many strokes occur. If the rupture is not this large, it may just cause symptoms to occur with exercise, like the angina heart pain mentioned in association with stable lesions. Smaller ruptures may give no symptoms but do act to further weaken the inner vessel wall and make future ruptures much more likely.

An integral part of treating heart attacks is to try to dissolve newly formed clots. A single aspirin tablet can help this process and should be taken as soon as a heart attack is suspected.

Heart attacks and angina

Coronary Artery Disease is vascular disease in the arteries that supply the heart muscle. These are called the coronary arteries and are shown in figure 16. Even though the heart is full of blood, a system of small arteries is still required to supply the heart muscle with the blood it needs to function.

If the blockage associated with this vascular disease is severe enough, it deprives the heart muscle of sufficient oxygen for the heart to function normally. It is this lack of oxygen that causes the chest pain associated with this disease, termed angina pain.

Episodes of angina usually occur when the heart needs more oxygen than normal, such as during exercise. In this situation, the blocked vessel can supply adequate oxygen while

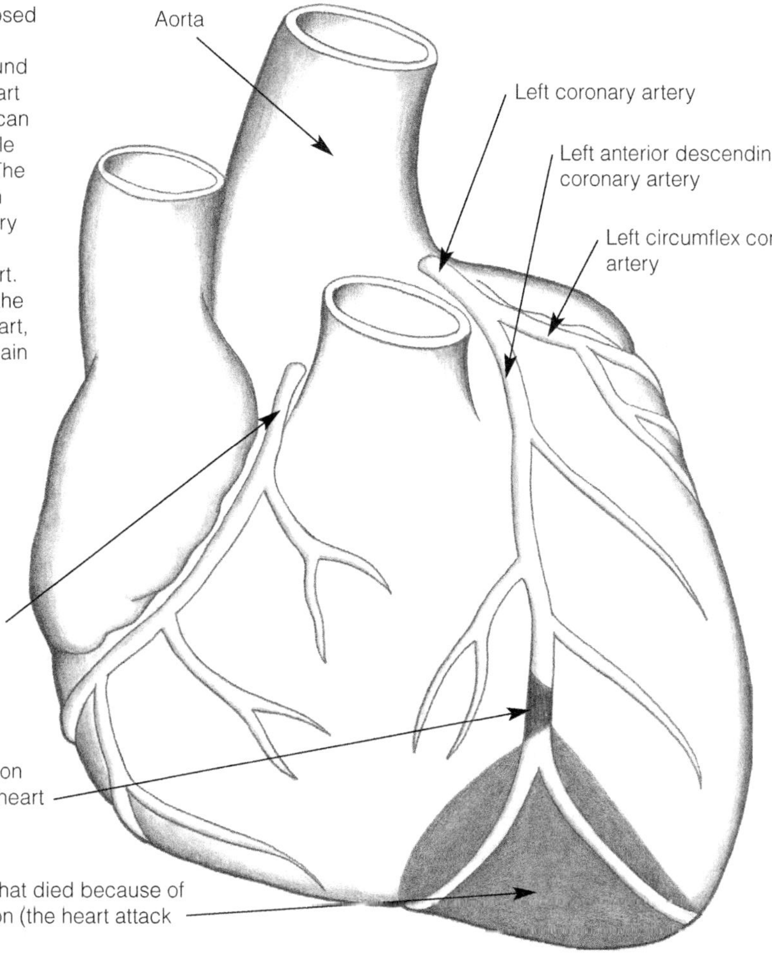

Figure 16 The heart showing the coronary arteries

you are resting, but inadequate oxygen to allow your heart to work harder during exercise. The angina episode and the associated pain are only temporary (less than 20 minutes) and there is no permanent damage done to the heart muscle.

Myocardial infarct or heart attack

Sometimes a sudden large increase in the degree of artery blockage can occur. When this happens, the reduction in blood flow causes the heart muscle to suffer a prolonged period of inadequate oxygen supply and this kills the heart muscle and, not uncommonly, the person! The death of heart muscle is called a myocardial infarct or heart attack. This dead tissue cannot be replaced.

The actual death of heart muscle cells starts after about one hour. After several hours, irreversible damage is being done to the heart muscle. This is why any anti-clotting therapies, such as taking aspirin, or procedures to open up your suddenly blocked artery, such as stenting, must be done very soon after the blockage occurs. To take advantage of such surgical treatments, you must go to a hospital as soon as possible after your chest pain symptoms start. Do not delay!

What is heart chest pain like and what should you do if you have it?

All chest pain needs to be taken seriously and any pain that might be angina needs to be assessed in hospital. While it is reasonable to speak with a local doctor on the phone regarding an episode of chest pain, this should be done after the ambulance has been rung. Do not go to a doctor's surgery as this will only delay treatment in hospital and this delay may prove fatal. The correct procedure is to ring for an ambulance to take you to hospital if they are close by or get another person to drive you to hospital if there is no ambulance available. You should not drive if you have chest pain.

It needs to be emphasised that, for some people, angina pain can be very unusual and therefore difficult to diagnose. Thus, help should be sought even if the pain being suffered is not 'typical' angina pain. Typically, angina pain is felt centrally in the chest. However, it can also be felt in the neck, jaw, left arm, back or in the upper abdomen where it can be confused with dyspepsia-like symptoms. The pain is usually described as a crushing, vice-like pain. However, it can mimic other types of pain, especially stomach pains. It is usually not related to breathing. The pain is also usually (but not always) significant and stops any activity the person is doing at the time. It usually comes on gradually and lasts for a few minutes at least. During this time it is fairly constant and does not tend to come and go. It will often come on with exercise although this is not always the case, especially when it is associated with a heart attack rather than a short angina attack.

Surgical treatments for coronary artery disease

Coronary artery disease can be treated by bypassing the blockages in the arteries. This procedure, called coronary artery bypass grafting, is done using a vessel from another part of your body, often veins from your legs. Over 19 000 were done in Australia in 1998. Angioplasty uses an inflatable balloon to expand the blocked coronary artery. The artery is then usually kept open by placing an expanding metal mesh tube, called a stent, at the blockage site. Newer stents are impregnated with chemicals that reduce the risk of them becoming blocked in the future by clots. Over 19 000 angioplasties were done in 1999.

Table 21 Risk factor incidence in adult Australians

Risk factor for vascular disease	*Incidence in adults* Males %	Females %	*Degree risk factor increases death rate*
Diabetes	8	7	2 times in men 4 times in women
High cholesterol	51	51	3 times (4 times at a total cholesterol of 8 or greater)
Lack of physical activity	34	35	2 times
Smoking	27	20	At least 2 times
High blood pressure	31	28	2 times 4 times if the heart is affected by blood pressure on testing
Overweight (BMI > 25) Obese (BMI > 30)	68 19	53 22	2 times
Family history of coronary artery disease before age 60			2 times
Early menopause			2 times
Personal history of vascular disease			5 to 7 times

Risk factors for vascular disease

The risk factors for vascular disease are the same for all arteries, whether they supply blood to the heart, brain, legs, kidneys etc. However, risk factors have been studied most extensively in relation to the heart and, as heart disease is by far the most important type of vascular disease in Australia, the discussion of risk factors will be in the context of how they affect coronary artery disease.

For people with no symptoms of heart disease, evidence to date shows that an assessment of the risk factors for coronary artery disease is by far the best way of predicting those most likely to suffer from coronary artery disease symptoms in the future. The more risk factors you have, the greater your chance of developing symptoms of coronary artery disease and the greater your chance of having an unstable lesion that might lead to a heart attack. Tests such as ECGs (cardiographs) and exercise ECGs (stress tests) are not good at predicting future sufferers of heart disease symptoms and they certainly cannot predict those more likely to have the unstable lesions that lead to heart attacks. The newer CT scans that detect the amount of calcium present in arteries are being used to predict those that require investigation for heart disease. However, there is no good evidence to date that they are as helpful as

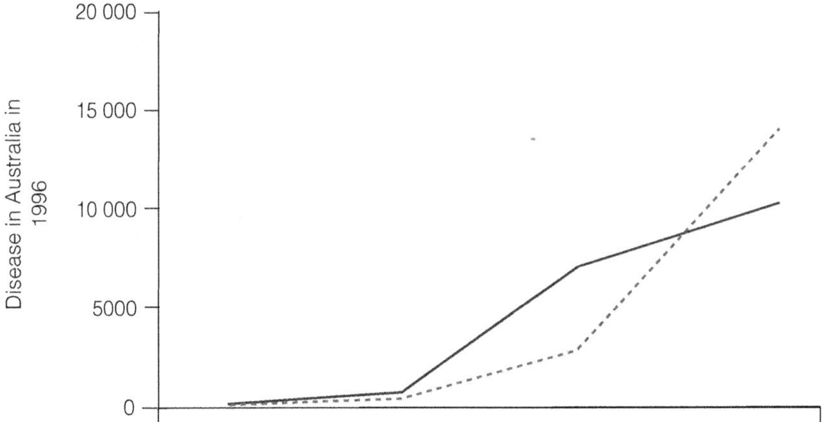

	15–34	35–54	55–74	75+
—— Males	66	1168	6524	9505
---- Females	20	233	2738	12 427

Age group

Figure 17 Age-related death rates from coronary artery disease in Australia in 1996

Source: Australian Institute of Health and Welfare, Mathers 1999.

assessing risk factors. These tests are discussed in greater detail later. The above is only the case in people with no heart symptoms. Medical investigations are essential for people with heart disease symptoms.

The established risk factors for coronary artery disease are listed, with their prevalence, in table 21. These risk factors, together with age and gender, are responsible for much of the increased risk of coronary artery disease that is present in the community and reducing these risk factors will help reduce the overall incidence of vascular disease. Having said this, there is still a lot that is not known about the causes of vascular disease and this explains why many of cases of coronary artery disease occur in people without known risk factors for the disease. (Remember that the commonest cause of death in people with no known risk factors for vascular disease is still vascular disease.) For this reason, it is not possible to guarantee that you will definitely benefit by reducing your personal risk factors. (However, until the whole story is known, it is still by far your best option!)

RISK FACTOR INCIDENCE

The large mortality associated with cardiovascular disease is not surprising when the prevalence of cardiovascular risk factors is examined, as follows.

- 80 per cent of the adult population has at least one major risk factor for coronary artery disease.
- 10 per cent of adults have at least three major risk factors.
- In both males and females at age 60, the prevalence of hypertension and physical inactivity is at least 35 per cent and the incidence of high cholesterol and obesity levels is over 60 per cent.
- High cholesterol levels occur in 51 per cent of the adult population overall and this figure reaches 70 per cent in 70 year old women.
- Over 66 per cent of adult males and 50 per cent of adult females are overweight. Interestingly, society often has the view that it is women who have the higher levels of obesity, probably because many overweight men are unaware of their problem.

The incidence of death due to heart attack is shown in figure 17. It indicates that coronary artery disease increases with age and that females develop significant levels of coronary artery disease soon after menopause.

ASSESSING RISK FACTORS

As stated previously, the more risk factors you possess, the greater is your likelihood of having a heart attack. Quantifying the individual effect of each risk factor is difficult. However, as a rough guide, each lifestyle risk factor (i.e. smoking, hypertension, diabetes, physical inactivity, obesity and high cholesterol) has the effect of at least doubling a person's risk of a heart attack in the next ten years, while a past history of vascular disease increases your risk by at least five times.

Attempts have been made to 'add' risk factors together to obtain an overall 'risk factor level'. The New Zealand cardiovascular disease risk calculator is an example of such an attempt and is the one most commonly used in Australia. (See Appendix 11.) Adding risk factors is quite a difficult process as risk factor severity varies greatly in each individual. To make identifying at risk people easier, the National Heart Foundation of Australia and the Cardiac Society of Australia and New Zealand have produced a list of the groups that are at significantly increased risk from coronary artery disease. They appear in the boxed section below. Are you included?

National Heart Foundation classification of groups at increased risk of coronary artery disease

- People with known coronary artery disease.
- People with other vascular disease, such as peripheral vascular disease.
- People with diabetes.
- People with chronic renal failure (or a kidney transplant).

- Aborigines or Torres Strait Islanders.
- People with raised cholesterol that runs in the family (i.e. familial hypercholesterolaemia).
- People with raised cholesterol and triglycerides that runs in the family (i.e. familial combined hyperlipidaemia).
- An absolute risk of 10 to 15 per cent or greater in the next five years according to the New Zealand cardiovascular disease risk calculator (see Appendix 11).
- People with an LDL cholesterol over 4.4 mmol/L or a total cholesterol over 6.0 mmol/L with any two of the following:
  —HDL less than 1.0mmol/L
  —significant family history of cardiovascular disease
  —obesity
  —smoking
  —glucose intolerance or impaired fasting glucose (but have not yet got diabetes)
  —microalbuminaemia (small amounts of protein in the urine) or renal impairment
  —age over 45 years.

If you are in one of the groups listed, you need to make every effort to reduce your risk factors for coronary artery disease. With respect to lowering cholesterol, the National Heart Foundation feels that most people in the groups listed should be treated with lipid-lowering drugs if diet alone does not give sufficient improvement in blood cholesterol levels. Unfortunately, due to cost considerations, the Australian Government's pharmaceutical benefits scheme does not include all of the above groups in their criteria for subsidised lipid-lowering drug treatment.

Over the past 40 years, the combination of reducing risk factors and better medical care has reduced death rates from coronary artery disease by 60 per cent. However, the high overall incidence of risk factors and vascular disease in the community indicates there is still a long way to go. Remember, not only are diseases such as coronary artery disease still very prevalent, they can affect people at a relative young age.

The main preventable risk factors (in order of importance) are high cholesterol, hypertension (high blood pressure) and smoking. However, the dramatic rise in the levels of diabetes, physical inactivity and obesity occurring in Australia at present will increase their relative importance in the not too distant future! They may even start to reverse the continuing reduction in the incidence of coronary artery disease.

How to approach the important non-modifiable risk factor of a family history of heart disease is dealt with below.

EVERYONE NEEDS TO REDUCE THEIR RISK FACTORS, EVEN THE YOUNG

Everyone needs to worry! Vascular disease is the major killer of Australians and all adults need to be assessed for risk factors on a regular basis from the age of 45 years or earlier if they are at increased risk from a strong family history. Even people without risk factors for vascular disease should be fully informed about the disease as it is also the most common cause of death amongst this group; although the rate is obviously much less than for those with risk factors and it also usually occurs later in life if at all.

A recent study (Grundy 2000) involving 80 000 men found that there was a direct relationship between raised cholesterol levels in the 18 to 39 year age group and later incidence of coronary artery disease. Deaths from coronary artery disease were three times as common in those with cholesterol levels over 6.2 mmol/L. Men with normal total cholesterol lived on average four to nine years longer.

Another study (McGill 2000) looked at the coronary arteries of young people aged 15 to 34 years who died as a result of trauma. Twenty per cent of men and 8 per cent of women had significant atheroma lesions in their arteries, with such lesions being 2.5 times more common in those who were obese or had a high total cholesterol.

MODIFYING RISK FACTORS—HOW MUCH DOES IT HELP?

Many studies have shown that reducing major risk factors does make a huge difference in preventing vascular disease. One worth examining is an ongoing study of 80 000 female nurses in the USA (Stampfer 2000). This study has identified five key lifestyle modifications that assist in lowering coronary artery disease. These were not smoking, exercising at least 30 minutes per day, good weight control (BMI less than 25), consuming over 5 grams of alcohol per day (but with a maximum of 20 grams per day) and a healthy diet (including an intake of more unsaturated fat, especially omega-3 fatty acids, less saturated fat, a low glycaemic load, and a high intake of folate and cereal fibre).

Adopting all five of these lifestyle factors produced a reduction in coronary artery disease in the order of 80 per cent! Women who achieved less than the optimal levels stated above still gained significant benefit. (For example, the risk of coronary artery disease was reduced by 64 per cent in those women who had a BMI less than 28, exercised for 15 minutes per day and drank over 2 grams of alcohol.) Refraining from smoking was found to be the most beneficial factor.

FAMILY HISTORY—A RISK FACTOR YOU CAN'T CHANGE

Many people inherit an increased risk of vascular disease. This is defined as having a first-degree relative (parent or sibling) who developed coronary artery disease (angina or heart attack) before the age of 60 years. A family history of coronary artery disease is an important risk factor and if you have such a history, it is imperative you take all measures possible to reduce any other risk factors you have.

It is also important to look for the cause of your relative's coronary artery disease. If your relative had risk factors that you can prevent, such as smoking, high blood pressure, obesity or lack of exercise, you may be partially off the hook; as long as they do not affect you too. If diabetes or high cholesterol were problems, then you should be regularly tested for these conditions as they are to some extent inherited.

If your relative who developed coronary artery disease did not have any obvious risk factors and the family history is relatively strong, then you should consider being tested for a raised homocysteine level in the blood as this can be associated with increased vascular disease and is usually an inherited condition. Homocysteine is dealt with later in the section 'Other influences on vascular disease'.

NEW RISK FACTORS—IDENTIFYING INFLAMMATION IN VASCULAR LESIONS

Recently, there has been considerable investigation of compounds present in the blood that indicate the presence of inflammation in the body. While such inflammatory disease markers are raised in many types of inflammatory disease, such as arthritis, it is hoped some will assist in predicting which people have high levels of inflammation resulting from significant vascular disease and thus be useful additions to the present list of risk factors in at least some people.

The most studied marker for vascular inflammation is a compound called C-reactive protein. There is evidence that the level of this compound in the blood is a good predictor of future vascular events, such as heart attacks. Unfortunately, as there are many causes of inflammation in the body, there is considerable individual variability in results and there is also a problem with test variability between laboratories. While these problems may make C-reactive protein difficult to use as a future risk factor, it may turn out to be useful in identifying which people are not at risk—a helpful thing to know. Recent study has shown that a particular form of this compound, called highly sensitive C-reactive protein, provides a more accurate indication of coronary artery disease risk. Further study still needs to be done to confirm the usefulness of these tests.

Medical tests—investigating coronary artery disease

There are numerous tests available for determining the presence and extent of coronary artery disease. Testing for coronary artery disease needs to be discussed in terms of whether the person has symptoms of the disease or not. Tests to determine the presence of coronary artery disease are essential in people who have symptoms suspicious of coronary artery disease. They are also very useful in determining the extent of the disease. If you have had episodes of chest pain suggestive of angina heart pain, you should see a doctor immediately.

Medical tests are much less accurate and can be difficult to interpret in people without symptoms of heart disease, with numerous false positive and false negative tests occurring (see below). Tests that patients without symptoms of coronary artery disease might encounter will be discussed briefly here because they are commonly done and are currently the topic of considerable public debate. Investigations done on patients with established disease such as coronary angiography are beyond the scope of this preventatively oriented publication.

ECGS (CARDIOGRAPHS)

As a general principle, ECGs tell you what has happened to your heart muscle rather than what will happen. Thus, with respect to coronary artery disease, they can really only show damage that has already occurred to the heart. While this is still very useful information, it unfortunately misses many individuals who are at risk of having a heart attack. A normal ECG just means nothing has happened to your heart yet. It should be stressed that ECGs provide much useful information in addition to that related to coronary artery disease, and they are necessary and relevant in many clinical situations.

EXERCISE ECGS (STRESS TESTS)

As well as showing heart muscle that has died, ECGs can become abnormal in appearance when there is an oxygen supply to the heart muscle that is only just adequate. An exercise ECG is a cardiograph done while you are exercising. It will pick up more people with coronary artery disease because, during exercise, the heart muscle requires more oxygen, and thus blood supply, than it does at rest. A normal resting ECG may become abnormal in appearance during exercise because an artery supplying adequate blood/oxygen at rest may be too diseased to be able to supply the exercising heart's increased blood/oxygen demand.

This test is useful in helping diagnose patients who already have symptoms such as chest pain. Unfortunately it is often inaccurate in those who do not, giving both false positive and false negative results. False positive tests can result in these people undergoing additional unnecessary and potentially hazardous testing, such as coronary angiography, while a false negative test misses the individual who has a small artery blockage that still might suddenly rupture, causing a heart attack.

In about half the patients with coronary artery disease, the first symptom is a heart attack, and for many of these individuals an ECG and, probably, a stress test prior to the event would not have been much help in predicting this event.

DETECTION OF CALCIUM IN ARTERIES BY ELECTRON BEAM COMPUTED TOMOGRAPHY

This is a relatively new and controversial method of determining the extent of disease in coronary arteries. It does this by measuring the amount of calcium in the walls of the coronary arteries, the assumption being that this relates to the degree of disease. The investigation is non-invasive but quite expensive (and you pay for all of it as Medicare does not cover any of the cost).

The controversy surrounding this procedure relates to whether the information gained from the test improves the ability to predict your likelihood of developing symptomatic coronary artery disease (i.e. angina or heart attacks). At present, there is little evidence the information gained gives additional benefit to that provided by risk factor assessment.

Following on from this, it is difficult to know what advice is appropriate regarding further management and investigation if you have an abnormal test result. However, it is early days in the assessment of this test and further evidence may show the test does have a significant place in assessing asymptomatic individuals. Time will tell.

CORONARY ANGIOGRAPHY

Coronary angiography is a specific test to determine the extent of coronary artery disease in individuals with symptoms suggestive of this disease. It is not a screening test for individuals without symptoms.

Strokes

The death of brain tissue due to a problem with its blood supply is termed a stroke. There are two quite different mechanisms by which strokes occur. The least common (15 per cent) is caused by a haemorrhage (bleeding) into the brain tissue from a break in the wall of a small artery. These breaks usually occur at weak points in the artery called aneurysms. As most of these weak spots are present from birth, they are difficult to avoid. However, they are much more likely to rupture when a person has high blood pressure. Avoiding this risk factor is the best way to minimise your risk from this type of stroke.

The more common type of stroke (85 per cent) is called an ischaemic (i.e. due to lack of blood) stroke. A result of vascular disease, as described previously, it involves the arteries supplying the brain. As with heart attacks, these arterial blockages deprive the brain tissue of blood and thus oxygen. Brain tissue is much more sensitive to lack of oxygen than heart muscle and tissue death commences after only three to four minutes of oxygen deprivation.

Blockages causing ischaemic strokes can be due to either of the following: an obstruction at the vessel wall lesion itself, similar to the process that causes heart attacks; or a piece of clot that forms over the vessel lesion breaking off and causing a blockage further down the vessel. This piece of clot is called an embolus and it usually arises from lesions in the major arteries of the neck, the carotid arteries. Once the embolus breaks off, it travels down the progressively narrowing artery until it is the same diameter as the artery lumen it is travelling through and cannot pass further. The artery becomes blocked at this point.

Sometimes, if the embolus is brittle, it can break up into smaller pieces and the artery can become unblocked. This is more common with small emboli and the symptoms of the stroke in this case are usually only short lived, lasting for a few minutes to hours. Such episodes are called transient ischaemic attacks (TIA). Symptoms caused by transient ischaemic attacks (and strokes) include weakness or numbness in an arm or leg, blurred or double vision, speech disturbances, dizzy turns or unsteadiness in walking. If you experience an episode like this, you should contact your GP or hospital immediately as it is a warning that you are at high risk of having a significant stroke and require urgent assessment and treatment.

Very occasionally, emboli causing strokes or TIAs can come from clots that have formed in the left atrium part of the heart. This mainly occurs when a person has a special type of abnormal heart rhythm called atrial fibrillation. Emboli can also, more rarely, happen if the heart valves become infected.

Stroke prevention

As the majority of strokes are caused by vascular disease, prevention relies on looking after your vascular disease risk factors. Hypertension is especially important as it is implicated in causing both types of strokes. As is the case with prevention of coronary artery disease, optimum stroke prevention requires looking after your risk factors throughout your life, not just later in life when your friends are starting to be affected. (You might be first!)

People who have already had a stroke or a TIA, or who have evidence of vascular disease in the arteries leading to the brain, are sometimes put on drugs, such as aspirin or warfarin, to stop clots forming over these vascular lesions. This is called anticoagulant therapy.

Aspirin therapy

In the above discussion on coronary artery disease and stroke, the role of aspirin in reducing the occurrence of these problems, especially in at-risk people, has been mentioned several times. It can reduce the inflammation in vascular lesions and can reduce the likelihood that clots will form over breaks in vascular lesions, preventing further obstruction of the vessel at the site of the lesion and the production of emboli.

So, as aspirin is a cheap drug, why isn't everyone with risk factors given it? The reason is that its property of reducing clot formation means people who take it are also more likely to bleed. This bleeding can at times be serious, with the most common problems being significant bleeding from the stomach, bleeding at operations and, rarely, strokes due to bleeding into the brain. As aspirin therapy would need to be taken continually to be effective, the risk from these side effects is unacceptably high compared to the benefit the person receives. Thus, only patients at a significantly increased risk of vascular disease, especially stroke, are thought to gain enough overall benefit to use this therapy continually. If you are taking aspirin, you should always make sure your surgeon (or dentist) knows before you have a surgical procedure.

Further information

National Heart Foundation

The 'Heart line' information service can be contacted on Ph 1300 362 787 or at website www.heartfoundation.com.au

Lowering blood cholesterol and other lipids

Elevated blood cholesterol has been recognised as a major risk factor for cardiovascular disease for many years. With this in mind, it is unfortunate that over the past 20 years there has been little change in the cholesterol level of the average Australian. High cholesterol levels occur in 51 per cent of the adult population overall and reach 70 per cent in women 70 years of age. This chapter details the causes of raised blood lipids and explains how diet and medication can be used to reduce lipid levels.

The causes of raised blood lipids

As stated previously, vascular disease depends on both LDL and HDL levels. (As LDL is the largest component of the total cholesterol reading, a high LDL level is usually associated with a high total cholesterol level.) While triglycerides do not cause vascular disease, they are usually high in people who get vascular disease because people with high triglycerides also tend to have low HDL levels.

There are numerous factors that can alter the levels of these lipoproteins. The effects of dietary factors are summarised in Appendix 9.

High LDL and high total cholesterol

The vast majority of people with a high total cholesterol are grouped into a condition called polygenic hypercholesterolaemia. This condition is thought to be caused by a combination of dietary and unidentified genetic factors. It is usually associated with an elevated LDL level and normal levels of HDL and triglycerides. At present it is estimated that over six million Australians have a cholesterol level of over 5.5 mmol/L and about three million have a level of over 6.5 mmol/L.

The most important contributing factor to raised total and LDL cholesterol is excess saturated fat in the diet. Part of the process of regulating LDL blood levels is the removal of excess LDL from the blood by the liver. While the whole story regarding how dietary fats affect cholesterol is not fully known, it is thought that the dietary intake of saturated fats increases blood LDL levels by reducing this LDL liver uptake and that it does this by altering the LDL receptors on the membranes of liver cells. The mechanism is described more fully in Appendix 14. Unsaturated fats are thought to do the opposite. They may also reduce LDL levels by influencing cell membrane stiffness, which in turn alters the amount of cholesterol incorporated into cell membranes.

Excess cholesterol consumption increases LDL by increasing the production in the liver of the LDL precursor, VLDL. (See Appendix 14.) While this is a much less important factor in raising LDL, you should still make sure your total cholesterol intake is not excessive.

Other common causes of increased blood cholesterol levels include obesity, diabetes and excess alcohol intake. Less common causes of raised cholesterol include diseases such as hypothyroidism, obstructive liver disease, nephrotic syndrome, acute intermittent porphyria and anorexia nervosa. Pregnancy also raises blood cholesterol and drugs, such as progesterones, cyclosporin and thiazide diuretics, are also causes. A variety of rarer inherited diseases that interfere with cholesterol metabolism in the body can also raise blood levels of cholesterol or triglycerides or both.

The major causes of low HDL are the same as those causing raised triglycerides, namely diabetes and obesity. Others include polycystic ovarian syndrome, cigarette smoking, malnutrition, lack of oestrogen, genetic factors and drugs, such as betablockers and anabolic steroids.

Dietary and other factors affecting LDL and HDL levels are summarised in the diagram in Appendix 9.

High triglycerides

Abdominal obesity and diabetes are major causes of raised triglycerides, with both conditions on the increase in Australia. In people with diabetes, an increased triglyceride level is a very important contributor to their overall increased risk of vascular disease.

Excess alcohol intake and stress, drugs (betablockers, oestrogens including HRT, corticosteroids, thiazide diuretics, isotretinoin) and other diseases, including renal (kidney) failure, infection, acute hepatitis, ileal bypass surgery, systemic lupus erythematosis, lymphomas, and glycogen storage diseases, also raise triglyceride levels.

Recent dietary fat intake increases blood triglyceride levels and individual readings can vary significantly with diet. This variation can occur in a short time period and thus, to obtain an accurate triglyceride reading, it is important to be fasting for 12 hours before a blood sample is taken. In the longer term, dietary triglycerides actually act to reduce overall triglyceride levels by reducing triglyceride synthesis in the liver. The longer the dietary fatty acid and the more double bonds it has, the greater is the reduction in blood triglycerides levels. Omega-3 fatty acids fit both these criteria very well and are often prescribed, in the form of fish oil capsules, to reduce high triglyceride blood levels.

Investigating blood lipids

There is no question that the elevation of blood lipids is a major risk factor in the development of cardiovascular disease. For this reason, all adults should have their blood lipid levels assessed. This should commence at 45 years if you are at low risk or have no risk factors for heart disease, or earlier when you develop an increased risk. Assessment is usually not needed before 20 years of age.

The measurement of blood lipids is done by analysing a blood sample. Usually several blood lipids are assessed. The minimum information required for proper assessment is your total cholesterol, HDL, triglycerides and LDL. The first three are measured and the LDL is calculated from them as follows:

$$\text{LDL} = \text{Total Cholesterol} - \text{HDL} - (\text{Triglycerides} \div 2.2)\ \text{mmol/L}$$

This equation is accurate only if triglycerides are less than 4 mmol/L. If you have high triglycerides, the measurement of your LDL apolipoprotein B level gives a more accurate indication of the LDL level. There is always one apolipoprotein B for each LDL.

A 'pin prick' cholesterol test usually gives only your total cholesterol and triglyceride levels, which is not sufficient information to adequately assess the risk of vascular disease.

From the previous discussion it should be obvious that LDL and HDL levels are at least as important as the level of total cholesterol in assessing your risk of vascular disease. Target levels for blood lipids are shown in table 22. As can be seen, the levels vary according to whether you have a past history of vascular disease.

Table 22 Blood lipid level targets

Initial problem	*Total cholesterol*	*LDL cholesterol*	*Triglycerides*
Raised cholesterol with no prior history of coronary artery disease	Less than 5.0 mmol/L	Less than 3.0 to 3.5 mmol/L	Less than 2.0 mmol/L
Raised cholesterol with a prior history of coronary artery disease or other vascular disease or with diabetes	Less than 4.0 mmol/L	Less than 2.6 mmol/L	Less than 2.0 mmol/L
Triglycerides greater than 10.0 mmol/L			Less than 4.0 mmol/L

Before deciding to initiate long-term drug therapy, tests should be repeated to guard against random error, for example, tests being mixed up. Repeat tests also avoid the selection for treatment of people who have only a temporarily elevated level or whose levels fluctuate widely. (If levels vary markedly, a third level may also be needed.) If you are commenced on either diet therapy or therapy with statin drugs, you should wait at least three weeks before being retested as it takes this length of time for your cholesterol levels to stabilise.

Factors interfering with lipid test results

- Ill health tends to reduce total cholesterol in proportion to the severity of the illness.
- Food intake can affect triglycerides and to a lesser extent HDL. It doesn't affect total cholesterol and LDL. Ideally you should have fasted for 12 hours before your blood sample is taken to avoid inaccurate readings.
- Alcohol intake can increase triglyceride levels. If there is a chance that a high triglyceride level is due to alcohol, it is worth repeating the triglyceride level after five days of abstinence to identify the contribution that alcohol consumption had on the raised triglyceride level.
- Prolonged tourniquet application and upright posture can increase levels determined from samples taken by syringe. Squeezing of the finger when taking pin prick samples can also increase levels.
- Measuring lipid levels during pregnancy is not recommended as total cholesterol and LDL increase significantly at this time.

Reducing blood cholesterol and triglyceride levels

Reducing your total cholesterol, LDL cholesterol and triglycerides can be accomplished in two main ways:

- Reducing lipid levels by modifying your diet. This involves altering the type and reducing the amount of fats present in the diet and adopting other dietary habits that aid in reducing blood total cholesterol, LDL cholesterol and triglycerides.
- Using medication. The principal group of drugs used is the statins.

Reducing lipid levels by modifying your diet

MODIFYING FAT INTAKE

Initially, you should try to achieve these optimum lipid (cholesterol) levels through dietary change. If you adhere to a diet low in saturated fat and cholesterol, you can theoretically lower your total cholesterol by 10 to 20 per cent and reduce your weight and your risk of developing diabetes. These dietary changes should aim to:

- *Minimise saturated fats.* This is by far your most important task if you are to have any hope of significantly reducing your cholesterol through diet alone. Table 9 on page 109 shows the main food groups containing saturated fatty acids. Your saturated fatty acids should not comprise more than 30 per cent of your total daily fat intake.
- *Reduce cholesterol intake.* Foods especially high in cholesterol include lambs brains, offal, tripe, liver, pâté, fish roe and egg yolks. Other major sources are meats and to a lesser extent dairy produce and some seafoods, such as prawns.
- *Substitute unsaturated fats for saturated fats.* Omega-3 and monounsaturated fatty acids provide the best defence against vascular disease. The sources of dietary unsaturated fatty acids are shown in table 10 on page 113.
- *Reduce your energy intake from fat.* Your fat intake should be no more than 25 to 30 per cent of total energy intake, as discussed in Part 4. This is a less important factor than altering the type of fat you eat, especially if you are not overweight.

A summary of the effects of these dietary changes on cholesterol can be found in Appendix 9. Your optimum fat intake is best achieved by adopting the following measures:

- Eat more fish, two or three serves per week.
- Eat red meat that is lean and trimmed of all fat. Two to three servings a week is optimal. Servings should be about the size of a pack of playing cards or weigh about 80 grams.
- Use unsaturated oil for cooking. Extra virgin olive oil is a good choice as it contains numerous antioxidants and other nutrients and contains mostly monounsaturated fat.

- Use reduced-fat or low-fat dairy products. Do not eat butter or cream and go easy on the cheese.
- Do not eat fried takeaway foods and do not fry foods at home.
- Eat minimal amounts of biscuits, cakes, pastries, chocolate products, potato crisps etc.
- Use monounsaturated spreads, such as canola and olive oil based products, or no spreads at all (or try mashed avocado). Sterol-containing margarines are also an option that you should consider.
- Consume five to seven servings of a good variety of fruit and vegetables each day.
- Eat plenty of wholegrain bread.
- Eat a small handful of nuts regularly (a few times a week).
- Consume more legumes, such as peanuts, beans and lentils.

The advantages of unsaturated fats

When substituted for saturated fats, all dietary unsaturated fats help improve your vascular disease-risk level. However, they achieve this in different ways.

Replacing saturated fats with monounsaturated fats decreases your total cholesterol and LDL cholesterol and increases your HDL cholesterol.

Replacing saturated fats with omega-6 polyunsaturated fats decreases your total cholestereol and LDL cholesterol.

The benefits of increasing your omega-3 polyunsaturated fats include lowering your blood triglyceride levels, helping prevent blood clotting, and reducing the likelihood of harmful irregular heart rhythms occurring. They also help reduce high blood pressure and make arteries more elastic. Omega-3s have an anti-inflammatory action that may help in preventing diseases such as arthritis and there is some evidence that they protect against prostate cancer. Finally, omega-3s are thought to improve brain function and may have a role in helping prevent diseases such as depression. Such benefits are yet to be proven.

CHOLESTEROL REDUCTION USING PLANT STEROLS AND STANOLS (PHYTOSTEROLS)

Plant sterols and stanols are natural compounds similar in structure to cholesterol. When added to foods in appropriate amounts, they can help reduce the absorption of cholesterol from your bowel. This in turn reduces your blood cholesterol. An intake of about three grams per day is optimal and is provided by about 25 grams of sterol-enriched margarine. This equates to about one and a half teaspoons or enough to cover about four slices of bread. This amount should not be exceeded as larger intakes may interfere with the absoption of other nutrients. (See Part 3 'Nutrition and illness prevention' for further details.)

CHOLESTEROL REDUCTION USING SOLUBLE FIBRE

Foods rich in soluble fibre reduce plasma cholesterol levels by binding to cholesterol in the gut. This prevents the cholesterol from being reabsorbed back into the body from the small intestine. (It is excreted in the faeces attached to the soluble fibre.) Foods containing soluble fibre include oat bran, barley bran, rice bran (less than oat and barley bran), lentils, dried beans, fruit and vegetables. Insoluble fibre, such as wheat bran, does not bind cholesterol so it does not help reduce cholesterol levels. However, it is the better fibre for your bowel. A high intake of fibre, especially cereal fibre, has been shown to reduce the risk of coronary heart disease for the reasons stated above. A diet containing 30 grams of fibre a day is optimal, preferably a mixture of soluble and insoluble. This can be gained from a daily intake of:

- a bowl of bran cereal
- three slices of multigrain bread
- two pieces of fruit
- two servings of vegetables
- a serving of beans.

DIETARY CARBOHYDRATES (SUGARS AND STARCHES)

Recent evidence suggests that the type of carbohydrate you eat may also play a part in vascular disease, especially in people who are overweight. High intakes of carbohydrates that are digested quickly and therefore raise blood sugar quickly are associated with a significant increase in the risk of cardiovascular disease—up to twice the incidence.

The glycaemic index (GI) rates foods according to the speed in which they raise blood sugars. Foods with a high GI raise blood sugars more quickly. People should try to include a large portion of at least one starchy food with a low GI in each meal and include as many other low GI foods as possible. A more detailed discussion on the GI occurs in Part 3 and a table with the GIs for various foods appears in Appendix 6.

Reducing lipid levels by medication

Until recently, the National Heart Foundation (NHF) guidelines for commencing lipid-lowering drug therapy were determined by examining both your lipid level and your overall risk of coronary artery disease. This view has been changed and the NHF (Barter 2001) now base their decision to recommend drug treatment solely on your risk of developing coronary artery disease. An important reason for adopting this view is that the majority of people who develop coronary artery disease do not have markedly elevated blood lipid levels. Thus, it is better to base drug treatment decisions on whether you are in a specific high-risk group rather than just on your lipid levels.

Their view is that there are nine specific groups who would benefit significantly from lipid-lowering drugs. There is good evidence that all the people in these groups who have a total cholesterol greater than 4.5 will benefit from a reduction in their blood lipids. It has been shown that a 1.0 mmol/L drop in total cholesterol equates to a 20 per cent reduction in the risk of symptomatic coronary artery disease, whether you have had previous coronary artery disease or not.

Treatment targets for drug therapy were shown previously in table 22. As a general rule, the more risk factors present, the more aggressively raised total cholesterol and LDL need to be treated. It is especially important to get lipid levels to these target levels if you already have established vascular disease.

As stated previously, dietary therapy to lower lipids should be tried first. As poor compliance is the main reason diet fails to lower cholesterol, please make sure you give your diet a proper chance. If you don't try the diet properly, you will never know if it works, and diet is much cheaper than medication. It also has no side effects.

If your diet does not achieve the desired lipid levels as set out in table 22, then drug therapy needs to be commenced. The exception to this rule is people who have already had coronary artery disease and have a total cholesterol greater than 4.0 mmol/L. These people are at a much greater risk and should be commenced on drug and dietary therapy at the same time. Unfortunately, the number of people in the NHF 'at risk' groups is large and, due to cost considerations, not all people in these groups qualify for subsidised drug treatment.

Drug therapy is not recommended for people under 18 years of age and for young adults its use is usually restricted to males with severely raised lipids. For the aged, lipid-lowering therapy is warranted in all patients with evidence of coronary artery disease and a reasonable life expectancy. It is probably not necessary in those over 70 to 75 years with no evidence of vascular disease.

DRUG SELECTION

Before drug therapy is commenced, it is necessary to categorise the type of lipid problem you have as different problems require different medications. The three categories are raised cholesterol alone, raised triglycerides alone and a combination of raised cholesterol and raised triglycerides. Detailed discussion regarding the appropriate drug for you should be done in consultation with your medical practitioner. As the vast majority of patients use statin drugs, they are discussed below.

A recent study of people commenced on lipid-lowering medication showed that a significant minority had stopped taking their drug after only six months. Those most likely to stop were people under the age of 65 years and those living outside capital cities. The most common reasons for ceasing medication were being uncertain regarding the need for treatment and poor response to medication. It is very important to stress that this medication needs to be taken for life if it is to be of value. Do not just stop if there is a problem. Discuss your problem with your GP.

STATIN DRUGS

Statin drugs account for 90 per cent of lipid-lowering medications prescribed in Australia. This is because they achieve target LDL levels in most people, they significantly reduce coronary artery disease, they work well in lowering moderately elevated triglycerides (between 2 and 4 mmol/L) and they have few side effects.

Statins work in a number of different ways. Some of their effect comes from reducing cholesterol. They do this by inhibiting an enzyme called HMGCoA Reductase, which is important in cholesterol synthesis in the body. The resultant reduced cholesterol synthesis causes an increased uptake of LDL cholesterol by the liver, thus lowering blood LDL levels. Other important effects include stabilising fatty lesions in vessel walls (fatty plaques) and reducing clotting.

There are a variety of statins on the market and newer, more potent ones are on the way. The main criterion for choice is the severity of the LDL elevation. Statins vary in their potency as follows (in descending order of potency): atorvastatin (the most potent), simvastatin, pravastatin and fluvastatin (the least potent). Patients with moderately to severely raised LDL may require the more potent drugs.

Drug interactions and side effects, which vary with different statins, are also a consideration in choice. These need to be discussed with your prescribing medical practitioner.

Statins also work well in lowering moderately elevated triglycerides (between 2.0 and 4.0 mmol/L). Where triglycerides are above this level, the statins do not work as well and better choices are gemfibrozil alone, where only triglycerides are raised, or gemfibrozil with a statin if both triglycerides and cholesterol are raised. (The use of this combination of drugs requires special care as significant muscle side effects are more likely.) It is important to treat other causes of raised triglycerides at the same time, such as excess alcohol intake and diabetes.

Statins are usually well tolerated and safe to use. Muscle pain is occasionally a problem and, very occasionally, more severe muscle damage can occur. (There have very rarely been deaths from this problem. This occurred mostly with Cerivastatin, which has been removed from sale.) This problem can be minimised by checking the blood creatine kinase level before and after treatment commences. A significant rise indicates muscle damage may be occurring. (Muscle symptoms while on statins should be reported to your doctor.)

Mildly elevated liver enzymes are not uncommon initially and only occasionally require ceasing of the drug. (People with active liver disease should not take statins.) If side effects are a problem, it is worth trying another type of statin unless the problem is significant. No long-term side effects have been found to date.

EFFECTIVENESS OF DRUG TREATMENT

The evidence to date suggests that statin drugs are beneficial both in patients with vascular disease risk factors but no pre-existing cardiovascular disease and in those who already have cardiovascular disease.

There have been four major trials on the ability of statin drugs to lower cholesterol and reduce coronary artery disease. In summary, these trials show that statin drugs can be expected to reduce LDL by about 25 per cent and this has provided a 24 to 30 per cent reduction in the incidence of significant heart disease in these patients. This has been achieved in patients with and without pre-existing coronary artery disease. Recent evidence (Aronow 2001) has indicated that statin drugs used immediately after heart attacks can improve outcomes within as little as four weeks of treatment. (Both death rates and future heart attack rates were reduced by about 15 per cent.)

It has also been shown that significantly lowering elevated triglycerides reduces coronary artery disease. The results from one large trial (Veterans Affairs High-Density Lipoprotein Cholesterol Intervention Trial) studied the effect of lowering triglycerides (by the fibric acid group of drugs) on secondary prevention of heart disease (i.e. its effect in reducing further heart disease incidence in patients with pre-existing heart disease). This trial showed that a 31 per cent lowering of triglycerides was accompanied by a 22 per cent lowering in coronary events (heart attacks).

How much can diet and medication reduce your cholesterol?

A diet low in saturated fat and the use of spreads containing plant sterols can reduce total cholesterol and LDL by 10 to 15 per cent and the use of medication should reduce cholesterol by a further 25 per cent. Additional reductions can be achieved by consuming a diet high in soluble fibre. For healthy Australians, the desired total cholesterol level is 5.0 mmol/L or less and the desired LDL level is 3.0 mmol/L or less. Using the above figures, most people with a total cholesterol up to 6.7 and a LDL up to 4.0 should be able to achieve these optimum levels with diet and the use of sterols (if needed). The addition of medication should mean that those with total cholesterol levels of 6.7 to 8.9 mmol/L and LDL levels of 4.0 to 5.3 can also achieve desired levels. Very few Australians have a total cholesterol level above 8.9 mmol/L.

Any drop in cholesterol significantly reduces the risk from vascular disease and, with some effort, most Australians should be able to achieve a normal cholesterol level. It is therefore unfortunate that about 50 per cent of adults still have a total cholesterol over 5.5 mmol/L. Are you one of them?

Hypertension (high blood pressure)

High blood pressure or hypertension is a common condition occurring in about 25 to 30 per cent of the Australian adult population. The incidence is similar in both sexes. It affects numerous organs in the body, with the effects on the blood vessels, heart muscle and the kidneys being particularly important. The effects of hypertension are worsened by all other risk factors for vascular disease and by other factors, including excess alcohol intake, a young age at onset of the condition, and the severity of the disease.

Blood pressure is the measurement of the pressure of the blood in large arteries. (Arteries are the vessels that take blood from the heart to the other body organs.) This pressure is provided by the pumping of the heart. It is needed so blood can be forced through the arteries that progressively decrease in size from the heart to the body tissues they supply.

Blood pressure readings are measurements of pressure experienced by blood in the main artery in the upper arm. The higher level, called the systolic blood pressure, is read just after the heart has pumped, when the pressure is at its greatest. The lower level, called the diastolic blood pressure, is read just before the heart pumps again, when the pressure is at its lowest. Both readings are important in assessing blood pressure.

The National Heart Foundation's optimum blood pressure level is 130/85 or less for those under 65 years and 140/90 or less for those over 65 years (NHF 1999). A diagnosis of hypertension should not be made on a single reading (unless it is very high). As a rule, several readings should be taken over a period of time.

It is also worth noting that up to 25 per cent of people with normal blood pressure will have a raised blood pressure reading in the doctor's surgery (Brown 2001). For this reason, taking additional blood pressure readings at home should be considered before hypertension is diagnosed. Such readings are also very useful in monitoring the treatment of people with hypertension. (Twenty-four-hour ambulatory monitoring of blood pressure is another useful option.)

All people diagnosed with hypertension need to be investigated by a doctor to find any underlying cause for their high blood pressure. Such a cause is only found, however, in about 5 per cent of cases. In the other 95 per cent of people with hypertension, no identifiable cause can be found.

Coronary artery disease (heart attack) is significantly increased by hypertension. Hypertension also causes increased thickness of the heart muscle wall, which eventually leads to problems with the heart's pumping ability and heart enlargement (heart failure). The risk of incurring a haemorrhagic stroke (bleeding into the brain) is related to age and hypertension, with prevention relying on good blood pressure control.

Prevention of hypertension

As hypertension is a very common disease in Australian adults, everyone needs to adopt the measures mentioned below to prevent this disease. These measures are, however, especially important for those with an increased risk of developing hypertension, including:

- people of increased age
- people with a family history of hypertension
- obese people
- smokers
- inactive people
- people consuming excessive alcohol
- people with a high cholesterol
- people with diabetes
- people with sleep apnoea.

Hypertension can be prevented or reduced in several ways, including the restriction of sodium intake (mostly as salt), eating more vegetables and fruit and less saturated fat, reducing alcohol consumption, maintaining a normal weight, and increasing physical activity.

Dietary sodium

There is no doubt that excess sodium in your diet increases your risk of developing high blood pressure. Much of this sodium is added to food as normal salt (i.e. sodium chloride) with other sources being MSG (monosodium glutamate), baking powder (sodium bicarbonate), sodium salts used in emulsifiers, and preservatives, such as sodium metabisulphite.

To maintain normal body function, you only need an intake of 8.5 mmol/day (200 mg/day) of sodium. To prevent hypertension, the National Health and Medical Research Council recommends a maximum daily intake of sodium for adults, of 40 to 100 mmol/day (or 920 to 2300 mg/day). In Australia, only about 6 per cent of males and 36 per cent of females have sodium intakes less than 100 mmol/day (National Heart Foundation, n.d.). The average Australian diet contains about 100 to 200 mmol/day (or 2300 to 4600 mg/day) of sodium.

About 90 per cent of the sodium you consume in your diet is excreted in your urine. Thus, your daily sodium intake can be determined by collecting your urine for 24 hours and measuring the sodium content.

REDUCING DIETARY SODIUM

A major problem associated with reducing sodium intake is that in an average Australian's diet, only 20 per cent of the sodium consumed is added by the consumer. The other 80 per cent is already added to the foods you buy (70 per cent) or is naturally occurring in food (10 per cent).

The main foods that contribute to sodium in your diet are bread, spreads such as butter and margarine, cheese, biscuits, takeaway foods and sauces. (A list of the foods you need to monitor if you are to reduce your sodium intake can be found in the boxed section below.) The contribution of each food to your sodium intake depends on the amount of the food you eat as well as the sodium content of the food. For example, the Vegemite in a Vegemite sandwich has a higher salt content than the bread, but the bread gives you more sodium because there is much more of it.

Some foods with large amounts of salt

Very high content (over 1000 mg of salt in 100 grams of food)
Anchovies, meat tenderisers, MSG, soy sauce (even the low-salt varieties), gravy powder, normal salt, stock cubes, meat extract, ham, salami, corned beef, meat pies, bacon, sausages, spring rolls, dim sims, smoked salmon, salted pretzels, parmesan cheese, blue-vein cheese, cheese spread, processed cheddar cheese, olives, kelp, normal baking powder, crumpet, flavoured cracker biscuits.

High salt content (400 to 1000 mg of salt in 100 grams of food)
Bread, luncheon meat, pâté, potato crisps, frankfurts, pizza, hamburger, fried takeaway foods, canned/packet soups, canned fish (salmon, tuna), butter, hard cheeses, pies, sausage rolls, Chinese and Lebanese foods, savoury biscuits, some cereals (Corn Flakes, Rice Bubbles, Special K, Coco Pops, Frosties, Nutri-grain, Fruit Loops, Weeties, Lite Start), some soda waters, most sauces (excluding mayonnaise, coleslaw dressing, Italian dressing).

Medium salt content (120 to 400 mg of salt in 100 grams of food)
Sweet biscuits, salted nuts, canned vegetables, toasted muesli, cheesecake, cottage cheese and ricotta, mozzarella cheese, hot chips, caramels, toffee, pastry, cakes.

Many of the above products do come in salt-reduced/low-salt varieties. This should be evident from the product information on the label.

Some foods taste salty, making their high-salt content obvious. However, many foods are able to hide their added salt well so that it is difficult to taste. The sugar in sweet, processed foods hides the taste of salt very well; for example in cakes, biscuits and some breakfast cereals. The salt added to cakes and biscuits comes mainly from the baking powder and self-raising flour used in their preparation.

Bread is a very common source of salt and contributes about 25 per cent of daily salt intake. There are some salt-reduced breads and it is important to purchase these types of bread if you are serious about reducing your salt intake. You can also make your own 'no added salt' bread at home. The sodium content of 'normal breads' does vary, so if a low-salt variety is not available, look at the product information on the packaging. Similarly, breakfast cereals vary widely in their sodium content, so try to choose one with a low level.

With regard to the rest of your diet, the best way to reduce salt intake is to reduce the quantity of prepared foods you purchase. Try to prepare as many meals as possible at home from fresh ingredients or ingredients that are salt reduced or have no salt added.

Many brands of packaged products used in home cooking, such as tomatoes and stocks, have no salt added. There are even unsalted peanut butters. Look for these rather than the ones with added salt. They will normally have 'no added salt' displayed on the label. You can also tell by looking at sodium content data displayed in the 'nutritional information' label.

If your family is used to having salt added to their food, ask them to be patient. Although their food will initially taste different, they will usually get used to the difference in about two to three weeks and eventually they will prefer their food without salt. The impact of reducing salt in your meals can be lessened by adding flavour substitutes, such as herbs, curry spices, garlic, onion, lemon, lime, vinegar, plum jam etc.

If you are an adult trying to reduce your blood pressure by reducing salt intake, please remember that it takes about three months for any effect on blood pressure to occur. A low-salt diet in a person with a normal blood pressure does not usually decrease their blood pressure.

Salt and food labels

There are now low-salt alternatives for many foods traditionally high in sodium, such as sauces and spreads. There are several different label wordings that indicate a reduced-salt level. These are:

'Low salt': indicates the product contains less than 120 mg of salt per 100 grams of food. (This is equal to 0.3 per cent salt content.)

'Salt free' or 'unsalted': indicates the product contains no added salt and has been made from products that have not had any salt added.

'Salt reduced': indicates the product contains at least 25 per cent less salt than its regular counterparts.

WHO SHOULD BE CAREFUL ABOUT GOING ON A LOW-SALT DIET?

You should consult your doctor before commencing a low-sodium diet if you have a kidney or gastrointestinal disease that causes you to lose sodium or if you are on any of the following medications: blood pressure medication, fluid tablets (diuretics) or lithium. Women who are pregnant should keep to their usual sodium intake.

You should not use potassium chloride 'salt substitutes' if you have kidney disease or with certain fluid tablets (ask your doctor).

More vegetables and fruit, less saturated fat

Increasing the amount of fruit and vegetables and reducing the intake of foods high in saturated fats (and limiting sugar) in your diet can significantly lower blood pressure. One study (Conlin 2000) showed that such a diet resulted in 70 per cent of people with hypertension having their blood pressure returned to normal. (When there was no change in saturated fat intake, this figure decreased to 45 per cent.) These blood pressure changes occurred with no reduction in body weight.

When salt reduction is added to this diet, the reduction in blood pressure is understandably even greater. The fact that this type of diet can also significantly reduce coronary artery disease and several important types of cancer, and helps maintain a normal weight, which in turn helps reduce diabetes type 2, makes a compelling argument for its adoption.

Other preventative measures

Maintaining an optimal alcohol consumption of a maximum of two standard drinks per day can help reduce your blood pressure. Any increase above this level can result in an increase in blood pressure and an increase in the incidence of strokes.

Being overweight is a significant cause of high blood pressure. The cornerstones in treating excess weight are reducing dietary energy consumption and increasing physical activity. As well as reducing blood pressure through weight loss, increased physical activity can significantly reduce blood pressure by itself.

Caffeine

Caffeine is an addictive drug and may cause increased stiffening of your arteries, which can increase your blood pressure. If you have high blood pressure, you may be well advised to restrict coffee intake to one or two cups per day or use decaffeinated coffee.

Some coffees, such as unfiltered Arabic or Robusta, can raise your cholesterol slightly. The responsible ingredient is not caffeine but a compound in coffee called cafestol. Filtered and instant coffees appear not to have this effect.

The commonest sources of caffeine are, in order of content per serving, fresh coffee (80–90 mg of caffeine), energy drinks (80 mg), instant coffee (60–90 mg), strong tea (50–60 mg), 375 ml cans of cola drink (30–50 mg), weak tea (20–30 mg) and chocolate products, including cocoa, hot chocolate and chocolate bars (Stanton 2001). Coffee is discussed in more detail in the 'Caffeine' section on page 125.

Treatment of hypertension

As stated before, the National Heart Foundation's optimum blood pressure level is 130/85 or less for those under 65 years, and 140/90 for those over 65 years. It is recommended that treatment be commenced at blood pressures over 140 systolic or 90 diastolic for normal people and at blood pressures over 130 systolic or 85 diastolic for those with diabetes or significant kidney disease.

The treatment of hypertension beyond the dietary measures mentioned above consists of a wide variety of medications and is beyond the scope of this book. Everyone should have their blood pressure measured on a regular basis by their doctor. Once on successful treatment, it is important your blood pressure is monitored regularly to ensure the levels remain satisfactory. Treatment is required for life, although in some people significant weight reduction and an increase in physical activity can allow medication to be reduced or even ceased, but only under medical supervision.

Further information

National Heart Foundation
Website: www.heartfoundation.com.au

Diabetes

In Australia today, the incidence of diabetes is rising rapidly (see figure 18). This fact is supported by the recent initial findings from the Australian Diabetes, Obesity and Lifestyle Study (AusDiab), which has suggested that as many as 7.8 per cent of Australian adults over 25 years have diabetes (Colagiuri 2001). This is a huge number of people! Are you one of them? The following statistics are equally disturbing.

- Half of the people with diabetes in Australia do not know they have the disease.
- 20 per cent of elderly Australians have diabetes.
- About 16 per cent of adults have impaired glucose handling by the body (or precursor of diabetes). This impaired glucose handling is appearing at much earlier ages (even in adolescents) than has previously been the case and Australia may be headed for an even worse diabetes epidemic than it is already experiencing.

What is diabetes?

Diabetes is a condition in which your blood sugar (blood glucose) level remains higher than normal. The hormone insulin is responsible for regulating the blood sugar level in your body. Diabetes can be due to your body producing less insulin than normal and/or an inability of your body to use insulin properly.

There are several types of diabetes and several conditions that can lead to diabetes.

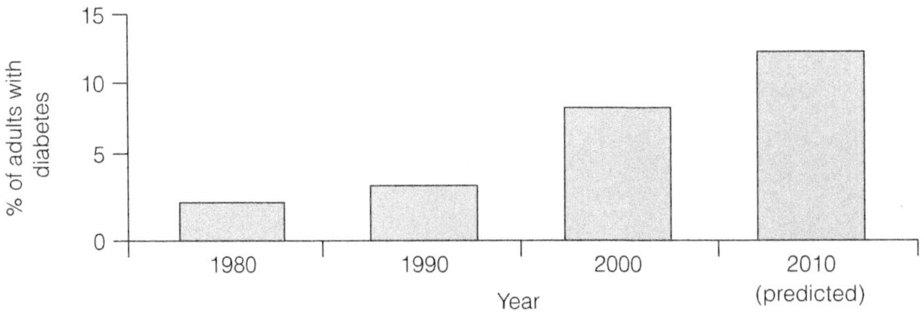

Figure 18 Diabetes incidence in Australian adults

Type 1 diabetes

In this condition, people produce very little or no insulin. It starts mainly in the young and is responsible for about 10 per cent of diabetes. Most are diagnosed quickly as symptoms are obvious at the onset.

Type 2 diabetes

Type 2 diabetes accounts for 90 per cent of Australians with diabetes. The major problem in type 2 diabetes is that the insulin you produce does not work as well at reducing your blood glucose. This abnormality is termed 'insulin resistance'. It is usually caused by abdominal obesity, although some races have a genetic predisposition to this problem. It can also be caused by low weight at birth. Early on in life the body can compensate for insulin resistance by producing more insulin. However, as you get older, your capacity to produce insulin decreases and eventually you cannot produce enough to meet the increased requirements generated by your insulin resistance. This situation is compounded by the fact that abdominal obesity usually increases with age, thus increasing the level of insulin resistance. (It is worth noting that it is rare for type 2 diabetes to occur in a person with a BMI of 22, i.e. a weight in the middle of the healthy range.)

Figure 19 shows how insulin resistance and insulin production vary throughout life. In normal people production levels never fall below requirement levels. However, people with significantly increased insulin resistance will eventually require more insulin than they can produce and thus develop diabetes. The higher the level of insulin resistance, the sooner diabetes occurs. The fact that the causes of type 2 diabetes get worse as you get older usually means the disease tends to get worse also and treatment usually needs to be increased as time passes.

Whilst most type 2 diabetes occurs in older people, some obese young people are now developing the disease. About 50 per cent of people with type 2 diabetes remain undiagnosed because the onset is slow and the symptoms are non-specific, such as blurred vision, skin

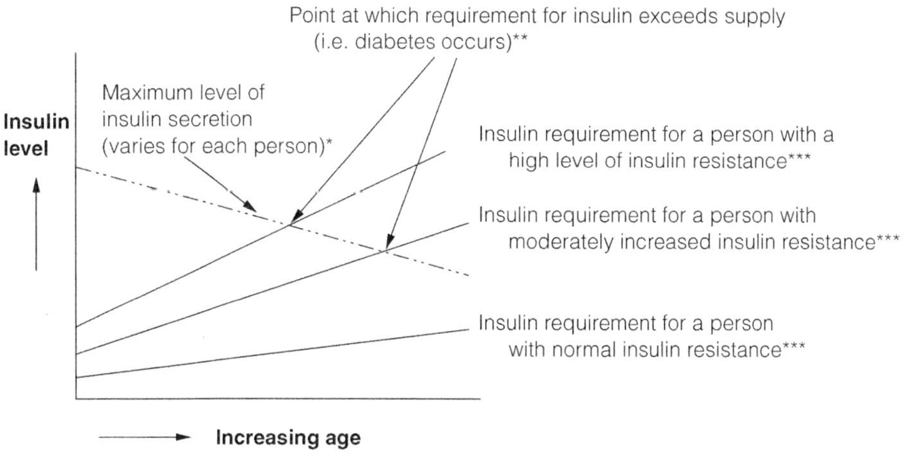

* Insulin secretion levels vary from person to person. A person able to produce larger quantities of insulin would have a higher dotted line than that shown in the figure and would be less likely to develop diabetes (and vice versa).

** By reducing your obesity level, you reduce your level of insulin resistance and thus your insulin requirement. This delays the age at which your maximum insulin secretion becomes less than your insulin requirement (i.e. delays diabetes). In some people, the delay is long enough so that diabetes does not occur at all.

*** Insulin resistance tends to increase with age and increasing weight, especially if the obesity is central (around your waist). Some races also have a higher level of insulin resistance. The higher your insulin resistance, the higher is your 'insulin requirement' line on the graph and the more likely you are to develop diabetes.

Figure 19 Insulin secretion and requirements with age

infections, slow healing, tiredness and numbness in the feet. Many people with type 2 diabetes have 'metabolic syndrome' or 'syndrome X'.

Type 2 diabetes is also termed non-insulin-dependent diabetes. However, as many people with type 2 diabetes need to be treated with insulin, this name is a bit misleading and is being used less often.

Gestational diabetes

About 4 to 6 per cent of women develop diabetes during their pregnancy. They usually return to normal after the pregnancy but do have an increased risk of type 2 diabetes later in life with over 30 per cent developing the disease within ten to twenty years of their pregnancy. Thus, they need to be regularly screened for diabetes. Women at risk of diabetes in pregnancy include those with:

- a maternal age of 30 or more
- a first-degree relative with diabetes
- a past history of diabetes in pregnancy
- obesity
- a poor obstetric history (problems during childbirth)
- a specific ethnic background, including those who are Aborigines, Torres Strait Islanders, Pacific Islanders, southern Asian or Mediterranean
- glucose in their urine already
- multiple pregnancy
- high-risk pregnancies, such as those where high blood pressure occurs.

Insulin resistance (or impaired glucose tolerance)

Many people suffer from a mild form of insulin resistance that is not yet serious enough to cause diabetes (a form of 'pre-diabetes'). This impaired glucose tolerance is often genetically determined, occurring in around 30 per cent of Caucasians and at much higher levels in other races, including Aborigines and Pacific Islanders. Some of these people will go on to develop type 2 diabetes and, even if they do not, they still have an increased risk of developing vascular problems such as heart attacks.

At present it is thought that about 16 per cent of adult Australians have impaired glucose tolerance. When added to those with diabetes, this presents a huge problem and one that is going to be a massive financial burden for Australia.

Diabetic complications

There are numerous serious complications caused by diabetes and about 66 per cent of people with diabetes suffer from the complications of their disease. These complications are due mainly to damage to blood vessels from vascular disease and they can be divided into two main groups according to the type of vessels that are affected.

Those caused by damage to large blood vessels (macrovascular complications) include coronary artery disease (heart attacks), strokes and peripheral vascular disease (this mainly affects the lower legs and can cause gangrene and loss of part of the limb). These are more common in type 2 diabetes and over 50 per cent of people with type 2 diabetes have at least one macrovascular complication.

Those caused by damage to small blood vessels (microvascular complications) include blindness, kidney disease and nerve damage. Small blood vessel complications are equally common in type 1 and type 2 diabetes. Over 66 per cent of people with type 2 diabetes have at least one microvascular complication.

A major factor causing these complications is the raised triglyceride and lower HDL cholesterol levels that usually accompany the disease. In people with diabetes, these lipid abnormalities usually require drug therapy. Complications usually occur about ten years after the onset of the disease. However, as diagnosis is often delayed, complications need to be looked for at diagnosis.

Postmenopausal women with diabetes also have a significantly higher rate of fractures associated with osteoporosis than other postmenopausal women (Nicodemus 2001) and they need to be assessed and treated for osteoporosis early in menopause.

Some facts about diabetes

- Diabetes is the most common cause of blindness in Australia.
- Diabetes is the second most common cause of kidney failure in Australia.
- A person with diabetes has the same chance of having a heart attack as a person who has already had one.
- Diabetes also causes impotence, peripheral vascular disease that can result in foot ulcers and even lower limb amputations, peripheral nerve damage and strokes.
- Fifty per cent of those with undiagnosed diabetes already have significant complications from the disease that can lead to the above-mentioned problems. In the case of visual complications, 37 per cent already have eye damage at diagnosis. Thus, even though undiagnosed people with diabetes may not have symptoms, the disease is still doing them long-term harm.
- There is very good evidence (Pepys 2001) that early treatment of diabetes reduces death and ill health from all types of diabetic complications and especially those associated with the eyes and the kidneys (microvascular complications).

Prevention of type 2 diabetes

Through weight loss and exercise

A word of warning before we discuss this topic: anyone taking oral medication or insulin to treat existing diabetes needs to consult their doctor before altering their diet or exercise program. Such changes may cause blood sugars to go too low (a 'hypo') if medication levels are not adjusted beforehand. Anyone with diabetes should carry a source of sugar with them at all times to consume if they feel a 'hypo' coming on.

As stated previously, type 2 diabetes is by far the most common type of diabetes and excess weight is a significant causal factor. A BMI of between 25 and 30 gives you a threefold increase in risk of developing the disease; a BMI of over 35 increases your risk twentyfold (Field 2001). Luckily, there is good evidence to show that the onset of this type of diabetes can be delayed in the majority of people (in many people permanently) by lifestyle modification, including exercise and maintaining a healthy weight; that is, a BMI between 20 and 25. As stated above, abdominally obese people, particularly men, have a significantly increased risk of developing diabetes and need to be especially focused regarding weight loss. Abdominal obesity is best measured by waist circumference and males should aim for a waist circumference of less than 95 centimetres and females less than 80 centimetres (for Europeans).

For lifestyle interventions to be successful, people need good initial education regarding their risk of developing diabetes, an individual management program emphasising the long-term nature of dietary and physical activity change, and individual long-term management with regular (say monthly) follow-up. The use of such programs in people with insulin resistance (glucose intolerance) has been shown to delay the incidence of developing diabetes in about 65 per cent of these individuals (Kramer 2001). Such evidence indicates that you should adopt a healthier lifestyle with respect to diet and exercise to prevent the onset of type 2 diabetes, especially if you are at increased risk of developing the disease. Advice regarding suitable diet and physical activity programs appears in Parts 3 and 4.

EATING FOODS THAT HAVE A LOW GLYCAEMIC INDEX

Carbohydrates are the food compounds responsible for the glucose that enters the blood from our diet. Recent research has shown that categorising carbohydrates according to how quickly they release glucose into the blood following digestion is very helpful in determining which are the most beneficial.

The glycaemic index (GI) of a carbohydrate-containing food is a measure of the extent and the duration of the rise in blood glucose (sugar) that occurs following the consumption of a particular food. A low GI food causes a lower and slower increase in blood sugar. (This topic was dealt with in detail in Part 3 in the section 'Carbohydrates and low-glycaemic index foods' on page 117 and should be studied as the inclusion of low GI foods should be an integral part of everyone's diet.) The health advantages include:

- weight loss
- improved blood lipids
- reduced glucose intolerance and less risk of developing diabetes

- better control of diabetes in those with the disease
- reduced risk of coronary heart disease (heart attacks).

Remember, because of the interactions of different foods in a meal, these GI levels can only act as an approximate indication of glucose response. Thus, foods with a small GI difference of say 10 are not likely to have significantly different effects. It is more important to make changes in food choices where the difference in GI levels is large, say 30. (Appendix 6 has a list of low GI low fat foods.)

At-risk groups

Some population groups are at increased risk of developing diabetes. All these people should be actively encouraged to maintain a healthy weight (a BMI between 20 and 25), maximise their physical activity, and have a diet with a low glycaemic load. They also need to be regularly screened for diabetes (see the boxed section below for Australian diabetes screening guidelines). These groups are as follows:

- People with a family history of type 2 diabetes (especially before 60 years).
- Indigenous Australians and those from high incidence countries, such as Pacific Islanders and those from Indian subcontinent.
- Women with a history of gestational diabetes—30 per cent go on to have impaired glucose tolerance or diabetes within 10 to 20 years. (The sisters of women with gestational diabetes are also at an increased risk of gestational diabetes.)
- People with hypertension or blood lipid problems.
- People with impaired glucose tolerance.
- People with a recorded borderline blood sugar.
- Women with polycystic ovary syndrome and obesity.
- People over 55 years of age (risk starts increasing over the age of 40 years).
- Obesity is a lower risk factor, but still very important. People with abdominal obesity are especially at risk.

Screening for diabetes

As stated previously, half the diabetics in Australia remain undiagnosed. This is despite the fact that 90 per cent of this group visited a doctor within the last year. A comprehensive screening program targeting at-risk groups has been introduced to overcome this problem and is outlined in the box below. It is estimated that 80 per cent of undiagnosed people with diabetes are in these groups.

Type 2 Diabetes Screening Guidelines

The incidence of diabetes does not warrant screening all Australians. However, with the increase in diabetes incidence, the following screening guidelines have been recommended by the Royal Australian College of General Practitioners and the National Health and Medical Research Council (NHMRC). Those requiring screening include:

- People with clinically evident cardiovascular disease, including heart attacks, angina, strokes and peripheral vascular disease.
- Women with polycystic ovary syndrome who are overweight.
- Women with a past history of gestational diabetes.
- Those with previously diagnosed glucose intolerance or a borderline blood sugar.
- Everyone over the age of 55.
- Those aged 45 and over with one or more of the following risk factors:
  —obesity (BMI greater than 30)
  —hypertension (high blood pressure)
  —a first-degree relative (sibling or parent) with diabetes.
- Aborigines, Torres Strait Islanders, Pacific Islanders, those from the Indian subcontinent and those of Chinese origin once they are 35 years old.

While smokers and those with lipid abnormalities, either high triglycerides or high LDL cholesterol, are not at increased risk of diabetes, they are at increased risk of vascular disease and should perhaps also be tested earlier than 55 years of age. (This is not an official recommendation of the NHMRC.)

After initial screening, testing should be done every three years if the result was normal, or yearly if the person was shown to have impaired glucose tolerance but not actual diabetes.

Screening should be done by measuring fasting blood sugars using blood taken by a syringe. Blood glucose testing using a home glucose monitor is not accurate enough for the diagnosis of diabetes. A fasting blood glucose below 5.5 mmol/L means diabetes is unlikely and a repeat test should be done in three years. A fasting blood glucose reading between 5.5 and 7.0 mmol/L requires further investigation, usually with an oral glucose tolerance test. If the glucose tolerance test doesn't indicate diabetes, a blood sugar test should be repeated in one year. A level above 7.0 mmol/L indicates diabetes is likely. However, another test should be done to confirm the diagnosis. (See Appendix 10 for further testing details.)

Screening blood sugar tests are ordered by your medical practitioners when you present for routine check-ups and check-ups associated with pregnancy. You may also be tested if you present with symptoms caused by diabetes, including blurred vision, skin/other infections, slow wound healing, numbness in the feet, foot ulcers, passing excess urine, passing urine at night and loss of weight. (Weight loss occurs only in very obvious diabetes and is due to water loss associated with excess urine output. Most people with diabetes are overweight.)

Prevention of diabetic complications

An integral part of reducing diabetic complications is treating conditions that worsen these complications. This includes decreasing weight by appropriate diet and exercise, stopping smoking, reducing alcohol intake to 20 grams per day or less (two standard drinks), and aggressive treatment of any lipid problems and elevated blood pressure. People with diabetes should have a total cholesterol less than 4.0 mmol/L, an LDL less than 2.5 mmol/L, triglycerides less than 2.0 mmol/L, and a blood pressure less than 130/80 mmHg. (Blood pressure should be 120/70 or less in people with diabetes who have over 1.0 g of protein per day in their urine.)

Good control of blood sugars, achieved via regular blood sugar monitoring, benefits all diabetic complications, but especially microvascular complications, such as those affecting the eyes and kidneys. Methods of monitoring include home blood glucose monitoring, regular checking of Hb A1c levels to assess longer-term blood glucose control, and regular check-ups with a GP.

Table 23 Target levels for diabetic control

Level of control	*Blood glucose before meal (mmol/L)*	*Blood glucose after meal (mmol/L)*	*Hb A1c (%)*	*Comment*
Ideal	4.0 to 5.4	4.0 to 7.7	Less than 7	Normal levels
Moderate	4.0 to 7.7	4.0 to 11.0	7 to 9	Associated with macrovascular complications (minimises microvascular complications)
Poor	Greater than 7.7	Greater than 11.0	Greater than 9	Associated with microvascular and macrovascular complications

Assessment for diabetic complications needs to be done regularly by both GPs and specialist medical practitioners. This includes yearly eye checks with an opthalmologist. At present, about 50 per cent of Australians with diabetes have not seen an opthamologist in the past two years, significantly increasing their risk of retinopathy and resultant blindness (McKay 2000).

Further information

Diabetes Australia
Website: www.diabetesaustralia.com.au

Other influences on vascular disease

Raised homocysteine levels

Homocysteine is an amino acid that occurs naturally in the body. Increased levels are due to abnormalities in the way homocysteine is metabolised and are associated with an increased incidence of coronary artery disease. Homocysteine causes injury and inflammation in the lining of the vessel walls, helping cholesterol gain entry. It may also increase blood clotting.

Mildly raised levels of homocysteine are relatively common, occurring in up to 10 per cent of the population. High levels are relatively rare and occur in classical homocysteinuria, which is an inherited deficiency in the enzyme cystathionine-b-synthetase (CbS). In severe cases (the homozygous state), 50 per cent of those affected have significant vascular problems by the age of 30. Less severe cases (the heterozygous state) are associated with only slightly elevated homocysteine levels.

Homocysteine levels can be measured by a blood test. At present, there is no evidence to support routine screening for this condition in normal people and testing should be limited to patients with unexplained vascular events, such as a heart attack with no obvious risk factors. (This is especially so if the person is young or has a strong, unexplained family history of coronary artery disease.)

Lowering homocysteine levels

Reducing homocysteine levels can be achieved through supplements of vitamin B6 (25–50 mg/day) and folic acid (0.5 mg/day). Vitamin B6 acts as a co-factor (a helper substance) for the enzyme CbS, which breaks down 50 per cent of homocysteine. A form of folic acid acts as co-factor in the conversion of the remainder of homocysteine to other compounds. At present, few patients with raised homocysteine levels are diagnosed, thus few benefit from such treatment.

Some research is being conducted at present into whether dietary folate supplements will help reduce vascular disease in the general population. There is no evidence at present that they do.

Type A personality, stress and depression

The role of stress and Type A personality (anxious, 'highly driven' people) in causing coronary artery disease has always been controversial. There have been many studies into whether those who are exposed to high levels of stress or prone to angry outbursts are more likely to have heart attacks. While a recent analysis of the most accurate studies (Myrtek 2001) found no significant increase in risk for this group, this is still an undecided issue. One thing that is certain, however, is that it is still not the best personality to adopt.

More recently, depression has also come under suspicion as a possible cause.

Lipoprotein(a)

Higher than normal blood levels of lipoprotein(a) increase coronary artery disease by increasing atheroma lesions and by helping prevent clot breakdown. Lipoprotein(a) levels are genetically determined and vary little throughout life. High levels can double the risk of coronary artery disease (Seed 2001). If your family has a high incidence of coronary artery disease or you have numerous risk factors, you should have your level checked. While there is no specific treatment, a raised level means you will need your other risk factors for vascular disease treated more vigorously.

Antioxidants

The concepts involving the oxidation of important body compounds by free radicals and its prevention by antioxidants was dealt with in detail in Part 3 and earlier in Part 5, and these sections should be re-read in conjunction with the following information.

The effects of antioxidants on the body are complex and still poorly understood. However, it is generally believed that foods rich in antioxidants, particularly fruit and vegetables, may be helpful in the prevention of vascular disease. This is probably mediated through preventing the oxidation of LDL cholesterol. However, not all antioxidants appear to be effective in reducing vascular disease. Antioxidant supplements, unfortunately, have not been shown to achieve the same beneficial effects (Woodhead 2001).

Alcohol

Discussing the health benefits of alcohol is somewhat of a paradox as, apart from tobacco, alcohol causes more physical and mental illness than any other drug or substance. Particularly underestimated are the less obvious behavioural effects that excess alcohol has on many people, often on a daily basis. These include workplace injury and under-performance, as well as the changes in personality that are so detrimental to long-term personal relationships.

Table 24 Additional beneficial dietary influences on vascular disease

Food	*Effects*
Vegetables and fruit	• The numerous antioxidants present, such as carotenoids, polyphenols and catechins, help prevent harmful oxidation of LDL, thus reducing vascular disease. Tomatoes have powerful antioxidants, such as lycopene, which can reduce LDL oxidation and there is evidence they can reduce the incidence of prostate cancer. • Green, leafy vegetables provide folate which helps reduce homocysteine levels. This may prove to be important in reducing vascular disease. • Avocados contain high levels of plant sterols and folic acid and their fat is monounsaturated (i.e. good fat). • Vegetables contain soluble fibre that can help reduce cholesterol levels.
Nuts	• Nut fat content is mostly monounsaturated and this reduces blood total cholesterol and LDL. • Nuts also have antioxidants, such as vitamin E, to help prevent LDL oxidation. • Nuts are high in an essential amino acid called L-arginine. This is converted in the body to nitric oxide, which helps open up blood vessels and thus reduce vascular disease. • For these reasons, nuts in small quantities are excellent in a healthy diet. However, do not give to young children.
Tea	• Both green and black tea have a high content of antioxidants, especially theaflavins. There is also evidence that these antioxidants may be protective against some types of cancer.
Soy products	• Soy products reduce total cholesterol and LDL. This effect is seen with eating as little as 20 g per day of soy protein. However, levels of 30 to 50 g per day are better at lowering cholesterol. • Part of the effect of soy protein on lipids may be associated with their plant sterols. Therefore, people should eat whole-soy foods, not just the proteins. • The cancer protection properties sometimes attributed to soy products are still inconclusive.

It must therefore be stressed that any overall benefit relates to the consumption of minimal quantities of alcohol. One to two standard drinks per day is optimal (10 to 20 grams of alcohol). Any intake above two drinks per day (20 grams) has no overall beneficial effect.

With these limits in mind, there is good evidence that low-level consumption has beneficial effects for vascular disease, especially when the alcohol is taken with food. Alcohol on its own has several recognised beneficial effects for vascular disease, including increasing HDL, perhaps decreasing LDL and, when consumed in low amounts, a slight reduction in blood pressure. Higher intakes increase blood pressure and the incidence of strokes.

Red wine has the added benefit of possessing antioxidants (polyphenols and anthocyanins). These antioxidants are the red pigments from the grape skins and they may help reduce vascular disease by preventing the oxidation of LDL and reducing clot formation. White wine also has antioxidants but to a much lesser extent.

Beneficial dietary influences on vascular disease

In addition to foods rich in antioxidants, studies have shown that other foods are also beneficial with regard to reducing vascular disease. These are shown in table 24 on page 245.

Part 6

Cancer prevention

Understanding how to prevent cancer

The growth of cells in the body and their rate of reproduction are tightly controlled by genes contained in the cells. A cancer occurs when there is a malfunction in the genetic control of this process. This allows cells to grow faster and reproduce more rapidly than would normally be the case.

Cancers may grow locally without spreading to other places in the body, termed a benign tumour, or they may grow locally and spread to other tissues where they start new deposits of the same type of cancer. This process is called metastasising and it is also thought to be due to a gene abnormality.

Illness and death from cancer are due to damage to normal parts of the body caused by abnormal cancer tissue.

Death and disability from cancer

Most of the burden of disease attributable to cancer comes from cancers that can to a large extent be prevented. The most important of these are breast, lung and colorectal cancers. A large fall in the incidence of these common cancers will need to occur if there is to be a significant reduction in the premature loss of life from cancer. The incidence and years lost due to disability and death from these cancers are shown in figures 20 and 21. While there are relatively few deaths from melanoma, it is important because it is a major cause of cancer in young people (especially males) and is almost always preventable. Other cancers that can be almost completely prevented include lip and cervical cancer.

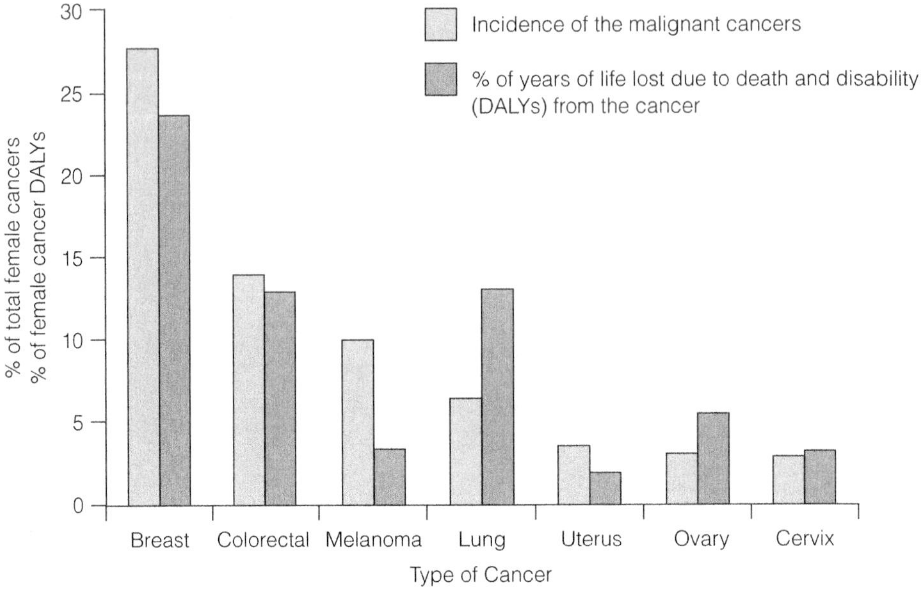

Sources: Adapted from Australian Institute of Health and Welfare: Mathers, 1999, and Australian Institute of Health and Welfare, 2000.

Figure 20 Cancer incidence and years of life lost due to death and disability (DALYs) in Australia (1996)—females

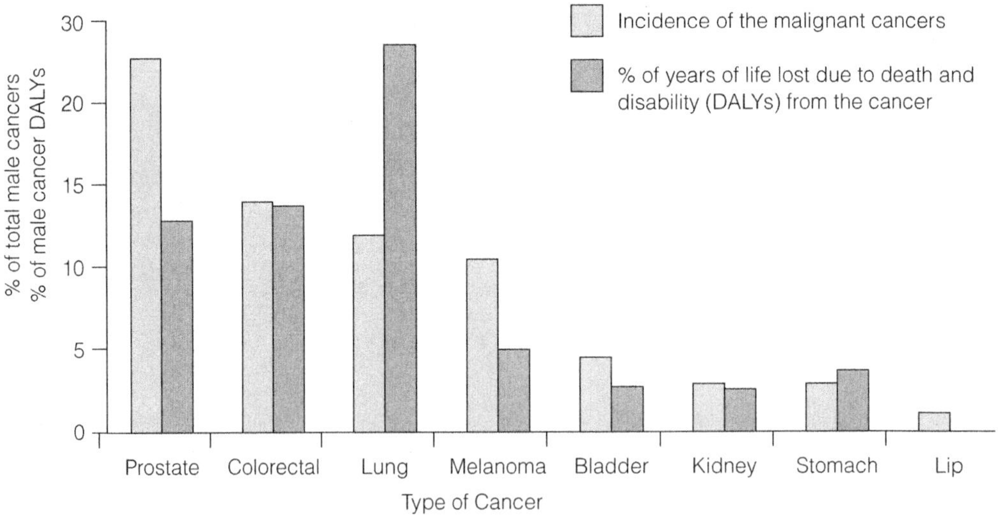

Sources: Adapted from Australian Institute of Health and Welfare: Mathers, 1999, and Australian Institute of Health and Welfare, 2000.

Figure 21 Cancer incidence and years of life lost due to death and disability (DALYs) in Australia (1996)—males

Healthy life options can have a huge effect on reducing cancer deaths. Adhering to the recommendations made in these sections can reduce your overall risk of death from serious cancers by well over 50 per cent, as can be seen in table 25. The two main ways of preventing deaths from cancers are preventing cancers from occurring, and finding and treating early cancers before they become incurable. This involves screening for cancers and identifying and treating cancer symptoms as soon as possible.

Table 25 Effect of cancer prevention

Improvement	*Reduction in mortality* %
Better diet	30
Better screening and early detection	25
Avoiding cigarettes	20
Overall reduction in death rate	Well over 50

Preventing the initiation of cancer

Many cancers are environmental in origin and while not all the causes of cancer are known, many important ones are. Avoiding these causes significantly reduces cancer incidence. The prime example is lung cancer, which can be prevented in 90 per cent of cases by avoiding smoking. Most people who develop lung cancer die from the disease and prevention is therefore imperative.

Less well known is the association between diet and many types of cancer. Dietary modification can reduce your overall incidence of cancer by about 30 per cent. When this figure is added to the cancers eradicated by avoiding cigarettes and excessive sun exposure, it can be seen that avoiding exposure to cancer-causing agents can reduce your cancer incidence by nearly 50 per cent. This figure does not include the additional benefits of cancer screening that will be discussed later.

As stated above, cancers occur because a change in the genes of a single cell allows that cell to grow and multiply more quickly than a normal cell. The actual mechanism is likely to be quite complicated and involves the interplay of numerous factors, such as a genetic predisposition to the cancer, exposure to cancer-causing substances etc. While we know important causal factors in many cancers, just how long we need to be exposed to these factors for cancerous change to occur is often uncertain and varies between different cancers.

With this degree of uncertainty, it is important that cancer prevention strategies, such as reduced sun exposure, smoking cessation, and increased fruit and vegetable intake, are adopted as early in life as possible. It is likely that for many cancers the most vulnerable time for initiation is childhood. It is therefore particularly important that exposure to known cancer-causing substances (carcinogens) is avoided from childhood onwards.

There are numerous other substances that have been found to initiate cancer in humans, probably the most significant being asbestos.

Medical intervention

Most of the cases of cancer presented in figures 20 and 21 would cause death without medical intervention. The percentage of people that die from each type of cancer varies greatly. Lower death rates among certain cancer types are due to four factors.

- Effective screening for the cancer before symptoms occur, such as programs used in cervical and breast cancer prevention.
- Early detection of symptoms and treatment before the cancer spreads (metastasises). More effective screening and early intervention could reduce cancer death rates by at least 25 per cent in the following 25 years. (To maximise your benefits from screening and early intervention, you need to be aware of screening programs relevant to you and know the early signs of various types of cancer. Early detection is effective in reducing deaths from many cancers including colorectal, bladder and kidney cancers and melanoma.)
- More effective treatments for cancers that have metastatised, such as those used for lymphoma and leukaemia.
- Late onset/slow progression of the disease. For example, most males with prostate cancer die from another disease.

Screening to diagnose cancer before symptoms occur

Screening for cancers involves performing a procedure on selected at-risk individuals with no existing symptoms to see if there is any indication of the presence of an early cancer. Most people (85 per cent) who die from cancer die from the spread of the cancer to other parts of the body (metastatic disease). For most cancers, the pathway from cancer initiation to local invasion (local spread) to metastatic disease takes a long time. For example, the initiation of malignant melanoma often occurs by the age of 15 but most Australians are over 40 when the disease is diagnosed. In bowel cancer, the progression from a non-cancerous polyp lesion to invasive cancer is thought to usually require at least ten years.

This timelag between cancer initiation and spread allows diagnosis of the cancer before it has had time to spread and this prevents death in many cases.

Deciding on whether you will benefit from being screened for a particular cancer is a matter of balancing three factors: the risk you have of contracting a particular cancer, the risk of the screening technique involved, and the benefit early detection will provide you. Screening recommendations are also based on economics and you may wish to take this into consideration when deciding on your screening options.

Different 'levels' of screening are appropriate according to your risk level. For example, testing the faeces for blood is an easy non-invasive screening test for bowel cancer that is suitable for everyone over the age of 50. Colonoscopy is a more complicated procedure that is usually recommended only if you have a higher risk of bowel cancer. These types of more invasive screening techniques are not without risk (or expense) and should therefore be restricted to those who would definitely benefit. For example, bowel perforation is a recognised complication of colonoscopy that can cause serious illness. This risk would probably be too great to recommend its use as a screening procedure for the whole population. However, a colonoscopy is quite suitable for people at higher risk of bowel cancer who would gain greater benefit.

Screening to find a cancer early is of little use if this early detection does not improve the treatment outcome. This is one of the pertinent issue surrounding the present debate about routine screening for prostate cancer. About 15 per cent of prostate, breast and bowel cancers and melanomas tend to cluster in families. At present, nine genes that can transfer an increased risk of cancer between family members have been found. While these genes can be tested for, it is important that proper genetic counselling occurs beforehand so that the implications of finding a family genetic problem are fully understood.

Recently, full-body CT scans have been promoted as a means of screening healthy people for early cancers. There is no evidence that such scans are helpful in increasing life expectancy and they may be giving false reassurance as early cancers may well be missed. They may also discover abnormalities that may never give any problem and thus cause unnecessary worry. The dose of radiation involved is also excessive and may cause long-term harm. These scans are not recommended as a form of screening.

The importance of early recognition of cancer symptoms

Finding a symptom that may indicate the presence of a cancer is not the end of the road. It is most likely your symptom will not actually be due to a cancer. If a cancer is uncovered, proper treatment will allow you a complete cure if the cancer is found early enough. Do not delay! Many common cancers have death rates less than half their incidence rates, indicating that over 50 per cent have been cured once found.

Early diagnosis also allows early treatment. This reduces the disability you may suffer as less extensive treatment will be required and there will be less disability from the actual disease. Proper early treatment is also very likely to increase your life expectancy, even with serious metastatic disease. Sixty per cent of all Australians with serious cancer will survive at least five years. This is a much better life expectancy than a person with significant heart failure can expect.

Thus, it is essential to report any symptoms of cancer as early as possible.

Cancer and diet

Environmental factors, a large percentage of which are dietary related, account for about 50 to 80 per cent of all cancers. Dietary modification can play an important part in cancer prevention, with a reduction in cancer deaths of 30 to 40 per cent being achievable in Australia through dietary change alone. This equates to about 30 000 lives saved each year. Well over half of this benefit originates from the consumption of at least 400 grams per day of vegetables and fruit.

This topic is a very important one and is covered in detail in Part 3 in the section on 'Diet and cancer prevention'.

Cancer risk website

Harvard University in the USA has an interesting website (www.yourcancerrisk.harvard.edu) that allows you, by answering a variety of questionnaires, to calculate your personal risk of developing different types of cancer, including breast, colorectal and prostate cancer. It also helps you identify factors that you can modify to reduce your overall chance of contracting the particular cancer you are looking at.

Further information

NSW Cancer Council
For information about any cancer topic see the Council's website: www.nswcc.org.au

Cancer Info Service
Ph: 13 11 20

American Institute For Cancer Research
Website: www.aicr.org

Harvard University cancer risk assessment
Website: www.yourcancerrisk.harvard.edu

Prevention of lung and other smoking-related cancers

Smoking is responsible for 20 per cent of all deaths and 30 per cent of all cancer deaths. Fifty per cent of regular smokers die of smoking-related causes with tobacco causing more mortality and illness than any other drug. Approximately 80 per cent of all drug-related deaths are due to smoking. Unfortunately, the effect of smoking on mortality is even greater in younger age groups.

The good news is, most of this mortality can be prevented if smoking is given up early. Stopping smoking before middle age (say 45) reduces disease due to smoking by 90 per cent.

At present in Australia approximately 21 per cent of women and 27 per cent of men over 18 years of age smoke regularly. It is more common in Aborigines, people of Arabic decent and in those with mental illnesses. It is a problem that starts in adolescence with 16 per cent of 14 to 19 year olds smoking. Eighty per cent of smokers have started by the age of 18 years. The incidence of smoking is seen in figure 22.

Cigarette smoke contains over 400 pharmacologically active chemicals that are harmful. They can be carcinogenic (cause cancer), irritant (harm living cells), cytotoxic (kill living cells), antigenic (cause allergic reactions) or mutagenic (cause changes to cell genes).

Death and disability from smoking

Smoking is the leading cause of cancer in men and women in Australia. Smoking causes 85 per cent of lung cancers. In males, lung cancer is the most common cause of cancer and causes the most deaths from cancer. In women, it is the fourth most common cancer and the third

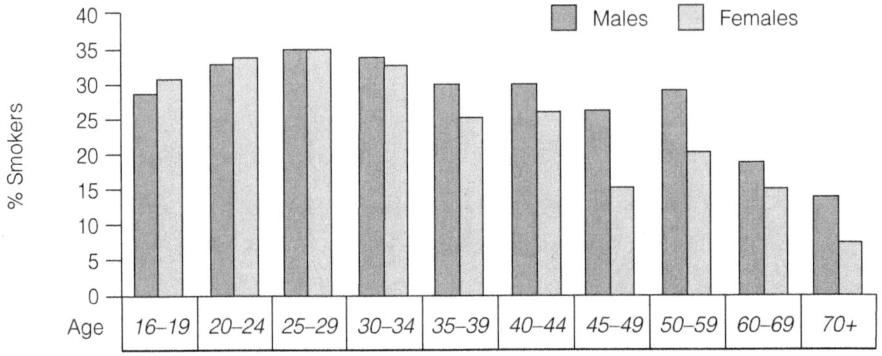

Source: Australian Institute of Health and Welfare, 2000.

Figure 22 Smoking rates in Australia by age in 1995

most common cause of cancer deaths. Many of these cancers and deaths unfortunately occur in relatively young people. Just one pack of cigarettes per day increases lung cancer risk by 10 times, and two packs per day increases it by 25 times.

At present lung cancer is significantly more common in males. However, this reflects past smoking habits. The increase in female smokers and reduction in male smokers over the past 25 years has caused the lung cancer rate between 1990 and 1996 to decrease by 2 per cent per year in males and increase by 1.6 per cent per year in females.

Other cancers caused by smoking are shown in table 26.

Other diseases associated with smoking—a long list!

- Respiratory diseases, including chronic obstructive lung disease, exacerbations of asthma and an increased incidence of pneumonia and other respiratory tract infections. Chronic obstructive lung disease (chronic bronchitis and emphysema) is responsible for a huge amount (about 3.7 per cent) of the total burden of disease. Unfortunately, many people with milder disease remain undiagnosed as they accept their symptoms of cough and shortness of breath as a normal part of ageing.

Table 26 % Cancers caused by smoking

Cancer type	*Male (%)*	*Female (%)*
Lung	84	77
Mouth and pharynx	57	51
Oesophagus	54	46
Larynx	73	66
Bladder	43	36
Kidney (parenchyma)	28	21
Kidney (pelvis)	55	48
Pancreas	24	19
Stomach	14	11
Cervix	-	19
Vulva	-	40
Penis	30	-
Anus	48	41
Bowel		

Source: Kindly supplied by the Cancer Council of NSW. Website: www.cancercouncil.com.au

Screening smokers at an early age (say 35), using tests that assess their lung function, could help identify this condition early on and hopefully prevent its progression in many people. If you are a smoker and are 35 or over, ask to have your lung function checked next time you see your GP.

- Vascular disease, including coronary artery disease, strokes and peripheral vascular disease.
- Hypertension.
- Loss of vision due to vessel disease in the eyes.
- Maternal smoking causes adverse effects on the foetus, including smaller babies and an increased incidence of miscarriage and neonatal death.
- Rheumatoid arthritis.
- Osteoporosis.
- Premature ageing (wrinkling) of the skin, especially the face. The skin also becomes drier and has a grey appearance. It is not a good look!
- Impotence in men.

The contributions that these diseases make to the burden of disease caused by tobacco are shown in figure 23.

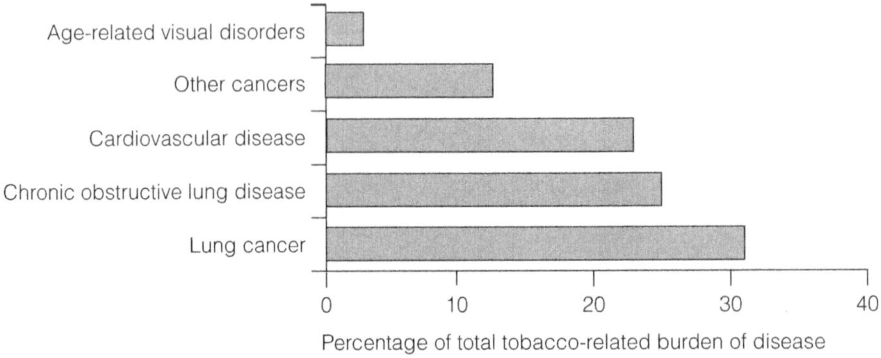

Source: Adapted from Australian Institute of Health and Welfare: Mathers, 1999.

Figure 23 Distribution of burden of disease caused by tobacco (1996)

Types of smoking and disease

The smoking of light (low tar/low nicotine) cigarettes does not reduce the incidence of smoking-related disease. The reason for this is that, to compensate for getting less nicotine per cigarette, smokers actually inhale deeper, which increases the amount of particulate matter inhaled into the lungs. Another problem with this type of cigarette is that people just smoke more of them to maintain their usual nicotine levels.

Pipe and cigar smokers inhale less and therefore have a slightly lesser mortality from smoking cigarettes (except in upper airway cancers). However, they do get high levels of nicotine and are likely to be very nicotine dependent, making cessation more difficult.

Passive smoking causes respiratory illnesses including lung cancer. The risk of lung cancer in passive smokers is about 1.5 times that of 'unexposed' non-smokers. Children with parents who smoke are more likely to get pneumonia and bronchitis and the smoke makes asthma worse.

Genetic predisposition to nicotine addiction

There is good evidence to support a genetic cause for nicotine dependence, which may be a significant factor in the failure of long-term users to quit. This genetic predisposition is due to several factors.

An enzyme that breaks down nicotine, called cytochrome P450 2A6, has three different forms and possessing the form that breaks down nicotine more quickly leads to an increased risk of addiction.

Smoking also has an antidepressant effect on the brain. This is caused by the lowering of a brain enzyme called monoamine oxidase, and this change makes depressed people feel better when smoking. Thus they are more likely to become addicted. Many cases of depression are inherited.

Finally, there are inherited differences in the way nicotine acts on the nervous system.

Quitting smoking

People who smoke can be divided into three groups with respect to their views on quitting—the 'not ready' group, the 'unsure' group, and the 'ready' group. Where do you fit in after reading this chapter? If you're in the unsure or ready groups, phone your GP for an appointment. Here are just some of the immense benefits to be gained from quitting.

- After two days, the risk of myocardial infarct (heart attack) decreases, due to reduced vessel narrowing and reduced carbon monoxide in the blood. (Carbon monoxide decreases the blood's oxygen carrying capacity.)
- After two to three months taste and smell improve.
- After one year the risk of myocardial infarct (heart attack) is halved.
- After 15 years overall risk levels have almost returned to normal unless permanent lung damage is already present.
- Stopping prior to pregnancy eliminates the risk of having a low birth-weight baby.
- Children of non-smokers are less likely to smoke and children affected by asthma and bronchitis are likely to improve if their home becomes smoke free.
- Fitness levels will improve.
- A person smoking 25 cigarettes per day will save at least $3000 a year (after tax) by giving up smoking.
- Skin may improve to a degree.
- Stopping smoking before middle age reduces disease due to smoking by 90 per cent, including most of the lung cancer and cardiovascular effects (i.e. most smoking-related deaths). Some changes, such as chronic bronchitis changes and skin changes, will remain to a degree, so the earlier you give up the better.
- Quitting by age 35 increases life expectancy by 8.5 and 7.7 years in men and women respectively; quitting by age 55 increases life expectancy by 4.8 and 5.6 years in men and women respectively.

About 40 per cent of smokers make at least one attempt to quit a year, but only 5 per cent of smokers quit without any relapses. Ceasing to smoke is a very difficult task and one that should not be underestimated or regarded lightly.

The main problem associated with quitting is that the nicotine in tobacco is an addictive substance. About 33 per cent of people who try tobacco smoking at any time during their lives become nicotine dependent. Also, smoking is often a habit that accompanies everyday activities such as eating, watching television and socialising with friends. Breaking these associations is very difficult. Weight gain may also occur with quitting, which can be a problem if not anticipated.

The five stages of quitting

There are several stages to quitting smoking (NSW Health, *Quit Because You Can*). If you are to succeed at this difficult task, it is important to go through each stage thoroughly. The reason that most people fail when attempting to quit is because they do not allocate enough time to planning and implementing their quitting strategy.

STAGE 1—DECIDE TO QUIT

You must want to quit and you must realise it is an important priority in your life. Quitting is difficult. The average number of quitting attempts before achieving success is four.

STAGE 2—PREPARE FOR QUITTING

Preparation for quitting requires an understanding of your addiction to nicotine and recognising why you smoke. Reasons include: out of habit, pleasure, social pressure, emotions such as stress, and nicotine addiction. Part of this process is assessing the level of your nicotine dependency—the questionnaire in table 27 provides a good guide to your levels of addiction.

STAGE 3—PLAN WAYS OF DEALING WITH QUITTING

There are numerous ways to make quitting easier. By far the most important is to visit your GP for general advice regarding quitting and problems that might occur, such as weight gain. Even in committed quitters, trying to quit without help only succeeds in a maximum of 15 per cent, with over 50 per cent having relapsed within a week.

The first thing you need to do is to gauge how difficult it is likely to be for you to quit. The greater the difficulty, the more intensive and frequent your support program will need to be. Several factors that help predict 'difficult quitters' include:

- having a high-nicotine-dependency level
- having tried to quit a number of times or being able to quit previously only for short periods of time. (The shorter the time, the more frequently you will need follow-up.)
- having suffered from severe withdrawal symptoms on previous attempts to quit.

By far the most successful quitting method is stopping suddenly and completely. This can be done with or without nicotine replacement therapy. Gradually reducing smoking is not recommended as it encourages smokers to compensate by inhaling more deeply and buying stronger cigarettes.

Table 27 Nicotine dependency questionnaire

Fagerstrom tobacco dependency questionnaire

Question	*Response*	*Score*
How soon after you wake do you smoke your first cigarette?	Within 5 minutes	3
	Within 6 to 30 minutes	2
	After 30 minutes	1
Do you find it difficult to refrain from smoking in places where it is forbidden?	Yes	1
	No	0
Which cigarette would you hate to give up?	The first one in the morning	1
	Any other	0
How many cigarettes do you smoke a day?	10 or less	0
	11 to 20	1
	21 to 30	2
	More than 30	3
Do you smoke more frequently in the morning than the rest of the day?	Yes	1
	No	0
Do you smoke more if you are so ill that you are in bed most of the day?	Yes	1
	No	0
Your score (out of 10)		**/10**

0 to 2: indicates very low dependence
3 to 4: low dependence
5: medium dependence
6 to 7: high dependence
8 to 10: very high dependence.
A score of 5 or above indicates the smoker will probably need drug therapy to cease smoking.

Source: RACGP, 2002.

Nicotine withdrawal symptoms that were a problem on previous attempts at quitting should be identified so they can be anticipated and treated early. Withdrawal symptoms include cravings, headaches, lightheadedness, changed sleeping patterns, cough, irritability and anxiety, constipation, mouth ulcers, lack of concentration, and temporary increase in appetite. The withdrawal period starts about two hours after stopping, is at its peak at about day four, and ceases for most people within 15 days of stopping smoking. Increased phlegm and cough can last six to eight weeks but is a good sign as it indicates your lungs are getting rid of the accumulated tar and mucous.

A weight gain of three to four kilograms is usual. This occurs because the appetite suppression and increased metabolic rate caused by the nicotine is removed when quitting. Also your taste improves, allowing you to enjoy food more, and you tend to put more food in your mouth to keep your hands busy. The use of nicotine replacement acts to delay this weight gain but doesn't usually stop it. It is important to anticipate this problem and get dietary advice before quitting.

Alcohol and caffeine intake will also need to be reviewed. In general, smokers tend to consume higher levels of these drugs as both caffeine (from coffee, tea and cola drinks) and alcohol have less effect in the presence of nicotine. Their intake should be reduced (by about half) when ceasing smoking. This is especially the case with alcohol as excess consumption can reduce quitting motivation. The side effects of caffeine, including irritability, restlessness and insomnia, are more likely to be noticed if caffeine is not reduced. Stopping caffeine can also give withdrawal symptoms, such as a headache, so reduce your caffeine level gradually.

If you have a history of depression, you will need to be aware that nicotine withdrawal can depress your mood and this may require treatment.

Exposure to other people's smoke (i.e. passive smoking) often leads to relapse. It is therefore important to try to create an environment that is as smoke free as possible while quitting. This especially applies to home and work.

The smoking of other substances also increases the likelihood of failure. Thus, all forms of smoking should be ceased when attempting quitting. Women who have significant problems with premenstrual tension symptoms may also have problems with quitting. These symptoms should be treated as best as possible before quitting.

It also helps to get support from friends and family and perhaps find a quitting partner to quit with. Printing out and displaying at work and at home a list of the reasons why you decided to quit often acts as a beneficial reminder (perhaps with a picture of loved ones, such as your children).

Finally, making a list of the activities you do when smoking will help you anticipate potential problem times while quitting.

STAGE 4—QUITTING

The first task in actually quitting is to set a specific day to quit. You should choose a low-stress day that is not too far away. The day before quitting, check your house, car, workplace etc. for cigarettes, lighters and ashtrays and throw them out.

Coping with cravings and withdrawal symptoms can be helped by having specific tasks or activities planned that you can use to distract you—short exercise routines that can be done almost anywhere are a good idea or have a good book handy. Worry beads for empty hands are sometimes a help. Drinking water or taking a few long slow breaths have also been found to help some people. (Do not take too many breaths as you may hyperventilate and become dizzy.) Eating needs to be watched as it is easy to start snacking. Be sure you have some low energy foods like fruit and vegetables around.

It is important to realise that just one cigarette will hurt your resolve and is the usual way back to regular smoking. However, it does not mean you will fail. You can learn from the mistake and avoid it next time.

Rewards for yourself during the time you are quitting (and after) should be part of your plan. Remember, you will have more money to spend!

Regular support during quitting is very important. This can be provided by visits to your doctor to monitor progress and discuss nicotine replacement if necessary. You can also call the government sponsored 'Quitline' at any time (ph: 13 18 48).

STAGE 5—STAYING A NON-SMOKER

The urge to smoke can return and this often occurs at times of stress. In the early stages of being a non-smoker, try to anticipate and reduce stress wherever possible. Use the strategies you learned while stopping smoking and don't be afraid to get support from your GP or friends as needed.

The first two weeks is the most dangerous period for failure and, without help, 62 per cent of people will relapse during this period. This is the period where intensive support is most needed. After this time, those people most likely to relapse are:

- those exposed to other people smoking
- those drinking excessive amounts of alcohol
- those who experience severe withdrawal symptoms
- those who cope poorly with life stresses.

In the past, avoiding triggers or situations associated with smoking has been advocated as a method of preventing relapse. This might include visiting clubs, seeing past smoking mates, or eating/drinking habits associated with smoking. Realistically, however, it is not possible or even beneficial to remove all these 'associations' for the long term. It is now felt that controlled exposure to these 'associations' is preferable as this helps to gradually reduce their negative effect. When confronting these situations, the help of a supportive friend or partner is of benefit. The most important cues for smoking are usually found in the smoker's own home. It is here that most support is needed, including making the home a non-smoking environment.

Frequent follow-ups for people who have a history of short quitting attempts, refraining from other forms of smoking, anticipating and treating withdrawal symptoms early, and reducing alcohol and caffeine intake all aid in preventing relapse.

Drug therapies for quitting smoking

The ability to quit seems to vary greatly between individuals. Many are able to quit fairly easily with normal 'Quit' campaign strategies. Those motivated individuals who find quitting difficult are probably in the group with a genetic basis for their nicotine dependence. These people are the ones most likely to suffer the medical problems associated with smoking. This highly addicted group often needs more intensive treatment which usually involves drug therapy.

NICOTINE REPLACEMENT THERAPY

Nicotine replacement therapy works by desensitising nicotine-sensitive receptors in the brain. It is best used in people smoking over ten cigarettes per day and must be used as a replacement for cigarettes. You should not smoke while using them!

All forms of replacement therapy are effective as long as high enough nicotine levels are attained. If they are not, then the person may smoke as well to get the extra nicotine. Some smokers attain nicotine levels in the blood of 40 ng/ml with each cigarette, while patches usually give levels of 10 to 15 ng/ml. Therefore, two patches may be required at the same time. Nicotine gum gives a level of about 15 ng/ml. Replacement therapy continues for seven to eight weeks and the dose should not be decreased during this time. The success rate is significantly less if replacement therapy is ceased early.

Nicotine replacement therapy is relatively free of side effects, the main ones being hiccups, gastrointestinal disturbances, jaw and tooth pain from over-vigorous chewing, and rashes from patches. Twenty-four-hour patches may also cause sleep disturbances and result in daytime sleepiness. Less common side effects include sweating and nervousness, muscle/joint pains, dry mouth and diarrhoea.

Nicotine replacement therapy is not recommended in pregnancy and anyone with a history of stroke, heart disease or other significant illness, or who is taking other medication should see their GP before commencing nicotine replacement therapy. In most cases it can be used safely as a replacement in patients with heart disease as it is safer than continuing to smoke (Kimmel 2001), but see your GP first! While nicotine replacement therapy is available over the counter at pharmacies, you should discuss its use with a medical practitioner as part of a total quitting strategy.

ANTIDEPRESSANT DRUGS

Bupropion (product name Zyban) has been shown to be effective alone (i.e. without nicotine replacement) in treating nicotine dependence. It takes several weeks to work and is used for about seven to ten weeks. It gives both an anti-craving effect and an antidepressant effect. This helps replace the antidepressant effect of the nicotine. Drug interactions and adverse reactions, such as rashes, insomnia, dry mouth and occasionally seizures, occur with bupropion and this issue needs to be discussed with a medical practitioner before taking the drug. It is available in Australia by prescription only as a 150 mg sustained-release tablet.

Nortriptyline, another antidepressant, has also been shown to be of benefit.

The use of both nicotine replacements and antidepressants is useful in some people.

Behavioural therapies for quitting

Behavioural therapies available to assist in quitting include stress management, managing the daily activities and rituals associated with smoking, and dealing with exposure to oral and visual stimulation associated with smoking. These have proved to be of limited benefit in initiating quitting. However, they are of considerable benefit in treating relapse.

Other therapies of dubious benefit

Both hypnotherapy and acupuncture have been shown to have little impact on nicotine addiction and their benefit is uncertain, as is the effect of aversion therapy. Anxiolytic drugs (sedatives) are not effective and should not be used. As stated before, low nicotine-tar cigarettes are not helpful as smokers just smoke more of them, giving them even higher levels of other inhaled chemicals, such as carbon monoxide.

Smoking prevention

Smoking is an issue that concerns everyone, smoker or non-smoker. The people who have been affected, are affected or will be affected may well be your children, parents, or other loved ones.

Smoking is a dependence that is usually commenced in adolescence, with 80 per cent of smokers having started by the age of 18 years. In 1999 in NSW, about 19 per cent of males and females in the 12 to 17 year age group reported smoking recently. That's about 85 000 school students.

Smoking in adolescence is encouraged by company marketing that directly targets these vulnerable young people. Techniques that are being or have been used include:

- Generous payments to actors and film companies to increase the use of cigarettes by actors in movies.
- Making cigarettes 'tasty' by including additives such as honey, chocolate, maple syrup, vanilla and fruit extracts.
- The disruption of youth smoking prevention programs and the creation of 'scampaigns' that appear to discourage youth smoking but are in fact designed to increase use by associating cigarette use with an adult world.
- Placing cigarettes in positions in stores that are easily accessible to young people. Placement in stores amongst everyday household foods, such as bread and confectionery, helps to make cigarettes appear a 'normal' product.
- The promotion of fashion parades and dance parties (through the internet) where cigarette smoking was promoted and encouraged.
- Continued 'special events' sports sponsorship in Australia, for example the Grand Prix and the 'Indy Car Race'. This is to be phased out by 2006.
- Actively lobbying politicians and political parties, and contributing to party funding.

This targeted marketing is allowed to persist because the general population does not care enough about its youth. There can be no better evidence for this than the fact that political parties in this country feel they can accept financial assistance from tobacco companies without electoral harm. Please remember, these companies (and the people who run them and work for them) know cigarettes kill. People working in the tobacco industry choose to do so and, in doing so, choose to promote your death and the death of your loved ones for financial gain.

What can be done?

Your children must receive adequate education regarding the risks of smoking and an appreciation of the way they are being manipulated and intentionally harmed. Part of this education program should include making your home a smoke-free zone as this significantly reduces the likelihood that adolescents in your household will take up smoking (Wakefield 2000). Having parents that do not smoke, not surprisingly, has a similar effect.

As an individual, it is important you do not support any organisation that accepts tobacco sponsorship and that you try to exert pressure on organisations that you are involved with to do the same. You should not purchase any products made by tobacco companies. Some of these companies have diversified away from just producing cigarettes.

You can also write to your local government member regarding tobacco marketing. Laws can be changed. If you feel strongly about this issue, become involved in the anti-smoking lobby. A good start would be to ring ASH Australia.

Recognising possible lung cancer symptoms

Reporting symptoms that may possibly indicate the presence of a lung cancer *as soon as they appear* may help detect early cancers and allow the disease to be cured in some cases. Any of the following symptoms can be an indication that lung cancer is present. (It needs to be emphasised that they also occur in many other diseases and people with these symptoms will probably not have cancer. However, you won't know until you find out!)

- Coughing up blood stained sputum.
- A respiratory infection that doesn't settle in the usual length of time.
- A cough that persists or a change to your usual cough if you are a smoker.
- Shortness of breath or an increase in your shortness of breath if you are a smoker.
- Persistent wheezing.
- General symptoms such as tiredness/lethargy, weight loss.

Smokers past and present need to be especially observant.

The future—screening for lung cancer

Most patients with lung cancer die from the disease because they are diagnosed too late for treatment to achieve a cure. However, if lung cancers can be caught early enough, cures can be achieved. Stage 1 lung cancers have a cure rate of 70 per cent.

Recent evidence from the USA (Henschke 2001) has shown that CT scans of the lung detect six times as many early lung cancers as normal chest X-rays. These may be useful for screening purposes in high-risk individuals. To date there have been no completed controlled trials of CT scan screening for lung cancer and there is no evidence that it improves survival. Until present research determines this issue, it is too early to recommend CT scanning as a screening technique.

Further information

ASH Australia
Ph: (02) 9334 1876; Fax: (02) 9334 1742; website: www.ashaust.org.au

Infact
A good website regarding all issues about smoking: www.infact.org

NSW Health
Locked Bag 961, North Sydney, NSW 2059; website: www.health.nsw.gov.au

Quitline
Ph: 13 18 48

Bowel cancer prevention

Bowel cancer is the second most common cause of death and disability from cancer in both men and women. It is also responsible for 14 per cent of all the burden of disease caused by cancer. It is therefore a cancer that all people need to make a special effort to prevent. Dietary prevention and screening are the two important strategies that you need to adopt to minimise your risk of developing bowel cancer.

Diet and bowel cancer

There is overwhelming evidence that the majority of bowel cancers occur due to environment factors and that these factors are mostly dietary in origin. A better diet and healthier lifestyle can reduce the risk of colon cancer by 65 to 75 per cent. Such reductions would make a huge difference to the burden of disease bowel cancer causes. For this reason they should be adopted by everyone.

This topic has already been fully covered in Part 3 in the section on 'Diet and cancer prevention' and this should be read in conjunction with the information presented in this chapter on screening for bowel cancer. A summary of the dietary and lifestyle recommendations by the NHMRC for reducing bowel cancer are as follows:

- Eat at least five portions of vegetables per day. A portion of vegetables weighs 60 to 90 grams.
- Eat a high-fibre diet.
- Reduce dietary fat intake to 25 per cent of total energy intake and avoid large amounts of animal fat.

- Maintain a normal weight as obesity increases the risk of bowel cancer.
- Avoid smoking.
- Partake in regular physical exercise. There is convincing evidence that regular physical exercise, especially if done throughout life, protects against bowel cancer.

Other measures not at present included in the NHMRC recommendations include avoiding excess alcohol consumption, avoiding charred foods, increasing resistant starch in the diet and avoiding large amounts of red meat and processed meats. The evidence linking bowel cancer and red meat is controversial at present.

Screening people at normal risk of bowel cancer

As 85 per cent of bowel cancers arise in patients at normal risk of developing the disease, the use of screening to reduce the overall incidence of bowel cancer in the community will require the involvement of the vast majority of these normal risk individuals. Around 98 per cent of the population is at normal risk of bowel cancer. They are those people who have no disease that predisposes them to bowel cancer and also have no family history of bowel cancer or only one first-degree relative (parent or sibling) who contracted bowel cancer after the age of 55 years.

At present, Australian government health authorities have not made a formal recommendation that the 'normal risk' population should be screened. However, there is a large body of evidence that supports such preventative measures from the age of 50 years. The options at present being discussed for such screening are:

- Faecal occult blood testing (FOBT)—testing for blood in the faeces. This is the principal screening option being assessed.
- FOBT (yearly or second yearly) with flexible sigmoidoscopy every five years.
- Colonoscopy every ten years. (At present this option is probably unrealistic for screening all the population due to lack of facilities and inadequate numbers of suitably trained practitioners.)

Faecal Occult Blood Testing

As stated above, the majority of the population has a normal risk of developing bowel cancer. If you are in this group, there is very good evidence that FOBT will reduce your chance of developing a bowel cancer by finding lesions before they become cancers. It will also reduce the chance of you dying from bowel cancer by finding early cancerous lesions while they can still be cured.

It is generally believed that FOBT of all adults over 50 years in Australia could reduce deaths from colorectal cancer by 14 to 19 per cent. A recent study from Denmark suggests this figure may be more like 30 per cent in those participating in the testing (Jorgensen 2002). Thus, most experts are recommending the adoption of FOBT, preferably yearly, as a screening procedure. There are several types of faecal occult blood screening tests available.

The established FOBT involves collecting three small specimens of your bowel motions at home on different occasions, smearing them onto a slide, and sending them to a laboratory to be checked for the presence of blood. This test requires medical and dietary restrictions prior to collection. Most studies that have shown FOBT to be beneficial used this type of procedure. (This does not mean that newer tests will be less beneficial.)

Newer FOBT involve collecting (by brush) two specimens of your bowel toilet water on consecutive occasions and sending them to a laboratory to be checked for the presence of blood. No medical and dietary restrictions are required prior to collection.

A positive result with either type of test just means that blood was found in the faeces and that this requires further investigation. There are many causes for blood in bowel motions and it does not mean cancer is present. Most people with a positive test will not have bowel cancer. For those that do, FOBT often finds cancers relatively early and bowel cancers detected early have a 90 per cent cure rate. Do not delay seeking medical attention if you do have a positive test.

DISADVANTAGES OF FOBT

False positive and negative tests are a problem with FOBT. Not all colon cancers bleed. For this reason, 50 per cent of individuals with colorectal cancer will have a negative test (i.e. FOBT misses 50 per cent of cancers). Up to 3 per cent of the general population will have a false positive test. This means that a large number of people will have unnecessary worry and an unnecessary procedure to exclude the cancer. This procedure is almost always a colonoscopy, which very occasionally has significant complications.

Also, people do not like handling faeces and the test has a record of poor compliance. Compliance should be better with the newer tests.

FOBT with flexible sigmoidoscopy screening

Flexible sigmoidoscopy can be offered as a screening procedure for individuals at normal risk of bowel cancer in addition to FOBT. This combination can be expected to pick up about 75 per cent of cancers, although there have been few studies to look at the effectiveness of this combination as a screening technique.

In this examination, a tube is inserted through your anus to examine your rectum and the last part of your bowel for cancers. It can be expected to pick up about 50 per cent of bowel cancers as about half of all bowel cancers occur in this area. Its main drawback is that it cannot disclose the other 50 per cent of cancers higher up the bowel. For this reason, it must be done in conjunction with FOBT.

Flexible sigmoidoscopy is done in a doctor's surgery, is not painful, and does not require an anaesthetic. It should be done every five years.

Screening with colonoscopy

A colonoscopy is an examination of all of the large bowel using a long fibreoptic instrument. It is inserted via your anus and can also be used to remove most small polyps and early cancers (i.e. it treats your lesions as well as finding them). The procedure is done in hospital, usually under an 'intravenous sedation' anaesthetic.

Some experts are recommending that colonoscopy should be used to screen the 'normal risk' population. It is proposed that this could be done once every ten years as it usually takes this long for a bowel cancer to develop from a non-cancerous polyp lesion. Almost all bowel cancers develop from such lesions. The cost of such a screening program would be similar to FOBT.

The main advantage of colonoscopy is that all lesions can be found as it examines all parts of the large bowel. The majority of lesions can also be treated at the same time and false positive or false negative tests are rare.

The principal disadvantage is that the procedure is associated (although rarely) with significant complications, such as anaesthetic complications, bowel perforation (about one in 4000 procedures with a skilled surgeon) and occasionally death. (The risk of significant haemorrhage or perforation increases to about one in 1000 if a polyp needs to be removed.) Also, there are not enough well-qualified doctors or enough facilities to carry out the increased number of colonoscopies that such a screening program would require. As the complication rate is to some extent related to the skills of the person performing the test, this relative shortage may present problems. For these reasons, there is still considerable expert debate about the usefulness of colonoscopy for routine screening in normal risk patients.

A negative colonoscopy does not give a 100 per cent guarantee that no cancer is present and if bowel symptoms develop, review by a doctor is required.

It should also be emphasised that expertise in performing colonoscopies comes with experience. If you need a colonoscopy, make sure that you ask your GP to refer you to a practitioner who they know well and who does lots of them, preferably a colorectal surgeon.

Screening people at higher risk of bowel cancer

Only 2 per cent of the population is at a significantly increased risk of bowel cancer. These people require more thorough screening, which should be done by colonoscopy rather than barium enema X-ray whenever possible. Barium enemas detect only about 40 per cent of the polyps that are found with colonoscopy. The frequency of screening depends on the person's risk level and all patients with an increased risk of bowel cancer need to discuss a treatment program with their medical practitioner.

Those at moderate risk

People at moderately increased risk of bowel cancer include those with a first-degree relative (parent or sibling) diagnosed with bowel cancer before age 55 years; those with two first-degree relatives with bowel cancer at any age; or those with one first-degree relative plus one second-degree relative (grandparent, aunt, uncle, niece or nephew) on the same side of the family with bowel cancer at any age. These people need regular check ups with their doctor, FOBTs each year, and colonoscopy screening starting at either 50 years of age or when the person reaches an age ten years before the first family diagnosis of bowel cancer.

Those at high risk

Individuals in this group account for less than one per cent of the population and include:

- People with three or more relatives (primary or secondary) with bowel cancer. They need to consider having genetic testing to exclude inherited bowel cancer and more frequent colonoscopy screening.
- People with inherited bowel cancer. There are two inherited bowel cancer groups and both are rare. They are familial adenomatous polyposis (FAP) and hereditary non-polyposis colorectal cancer (HNPCC).
- People with ulcerative colitis and granulomatous colitis. Colon cancer occurs frequently in sufferers of ulcerative colitis and less commonly in those with granulomatous colitis. In ulcerative colitis, the risk of cancer is minimal for the first ten years after diagnosis and then escalates continually. The chance of colon cancer is between 8 and 30 per cent 25 years after diagnosis. Treatment consists of regular check-ups and colonoscopies. Surgical removal of the large bowel is also an option in ulcerative colitis.

FAP and HNPCC—genetic testing in bowel cancer

Genetic testing for bowel cancer is usually done using a blood sample from someone in the family that definitely has the disease. Once a mutation is identified in that person, others in the family can be checked for the same mutation. (Testing is done from age 12 for FAP and age 18 for HNPCC.) The consequences of genetic testing are many and often involve all family members, not just the person being tested. For example, what should other family members be told about the results? Would they want to know? For this reason, people requesting or needing genetic testing should be referred to a specialist in genetics or a genetic clinic for counselling prior to testing.

Familial adenomatous polyposis (FAP)

This condition is due to a mutation (change) in a bowel cell gene (the APC gene). The changed gene causes many polyps to grow in the bowel, which will all turn cancerous if left untreated. The polyps develop in late teens to early adulthood and cancer is likely by the age of 40.

There is a 50 per cent chance that a person will have this disease if their parent has it. Diagnosis by gene testing is now available for this condition. (If the gene is not present, bowel cancer risk is normal.)

Hereditary nonpolyposis colorectal cancer (HNPCC)

This is due to a change in any of five known genes. Cancers associated with this condition arise from a polyp but there are not multiple polyps present as in FAP, so the problem is more difficult to diagnose. It should be suspected in families with bowel cancer in at least two generations. Genetic testing can be done but it is not possible to identify all carriers yet.

It can appear at varying ages, but most commonly in 30 and 40 year olds and older age groups. However, it can appear in people in their twenties or even younger. Women over the age of 35 with this condition should have check ups for uterine, ovarian and other cancers as they have an increased risk of these cancers also.

Recognising possible bowel cancer symptoms

Reporting symptoms that may possibly indicate the presence of a bowel cancer *as soon as they appear* can help detect early cancers and allow the disease to be cured. Any of the following symptoms can be an indication that bowel cancer is present. (It needs to be emphasised that they also occur in many other diseases and people with these symptoms will probably not have cancer. However, you won't know until you find out!)

- Blood in the bowel motion.
- Mucous in the bowel motion.
- Abdominal pain.
- Any change in bowel motion, including diarrhoea or constipation.
- General symptoms such as tiredness/lethargy, weight loss.
- Feeling a lump around your back passage.

Further information

Colonoscopies
Colorectal Surgical Society of Australasia
Website: www.cssa.org.au

Gastroenterological Society of Australia
Website: www.gesa.org.au

Breast cancer

Breast cancer is the most common cancer in Australian women (30 per cent of all female cancers) and causes the most cancer deaths (19 per cent). About 10 000 new cases of breast cancer are detected in Australia each year and about 2500 deaths occur. It will affect one in 12 women during their lifetime, with the risk increasing with age.

As well as being the most common female cancer, breast cancer also occurs relatively early. Overall breast cancer accounts for 24 per cent of the female cancer disease burden, but in the 35 to 54 year age group it accounts for a massive 37 per cent. For these reasons, decreasing the incidence of breast cancer is of paramount importance in reducing overall female cancer death and disability in Australia.

Breast cancer initiation

Like all cancers, breast cancer is caused by a single cell that is transformed by a series of gene changes (mutations). This transformation disrupts normal genetic control of the cell's growth, allowing it to grow abnormally. These genetic changes can be inherited or acquired.

The large majority of these changes are acquired during life due to damaging influences, such as cancer-causing chemicals, on the cell's genes. These acquired changes occur more commonly with increasing age. Gene changes acquired through life occur only in the

Table 28 Incidence of breast cancer in Australian women with no family history of breast or ovarian cancer

Age	*Risk of developing breast cancer in the next 10 years*
20	1 in 2000
30	1 in 250
40	1 in 70
50	1 in 40
60	1 in 35
70	1 in 30

cancerous cells and cannot be passed on to children. For this reason, most women with a family history of breast cancer do not inherit any predisposition to cancer from their parents.

In a small percentage of cases (less than 5 per cent of breast cancers), cancerous gene changes are 'handed down' from parents (i.e. inherited) as the gene changes are present in every cell of the person's body. Inherited genetic mutations can be from the woman's father or mother, so it is important to look for breast cancer in both sides of the family, including breast cancer in males. Your family history is more significant in increasing your risk of having inherited breast cancer in your family when:

- more relatives are involved
- the relatives involved come from the same side of your family
- the relatives developed their cancer at a younger age, especially under 40 years
- the relatives are genetically closer to you, especially parents and siblings
- a family member has had a genetic test showing they have a genetic abnormality associated with breast cancer (or ovarian cancer)
- there is a family history of ovarian cancer, as this may also increase the risk of developing breast cancer, especially if it occurred at less than 50 years of age
- you are of Jewish descent—the breast cancer genes BRCA-1 and BRCA-2 are more common in people of Jewish descent.

While most women with a family history of breast cancer will not develop the disease, all women with any family history should discuss the matter with their GP.

You can determine your risk of having breast cancer in the family by answering a questionnaire produced by the National Breast Cancer Centre called 'Do you have breast cancer in your family?'. It is available at: www.nbcc.org.au/pages/info/resource/nbccpubs/nbccpubs.htm—look in the section on consumer booklets, audio etc.—or it can be sourced from the National Breast Cancer Centre through your GP.

Breast cancer genes

Several genes have been identified as being associated with an increased risk of breast cancer. The two main inherited genes are the BRCA-1 gene and the BRCA-2 gene, both of which occur in about 1 in 1000 people. (The rate is about 1 in 100 in people of Jewish descent.) Together, these mutated (genetically changed) genes are responsible for about 1 to 5 per cent of breast cancers and are also associated with an increased risk of ovarian cancer.

Women with the BRCA-1 gene have a 40 to 80 per cent chance of developing breast cancer, a 10 to 60 per cent chance of developing ovarian cancer, and there is an increased risk of prostate cancer in males with this genetic abnormality. The BRCA-2 gene causes a similar increased risk of breast and ovarian cancer in women and an increased risk (up to 10 per cent) of prostate, male breast, and pancreatic cancers (NBCC 2002). (Remember, these gene changes are also carried by males.)

Tumour Suppressor Gene (Tp53) is another rarer (1 in 10 000) genetic mutation that can cause an increased risk of breast, bone and soft tissue cancers.

Genetic testing for breast cancer genes

Genetic testing is currently available in Australia for determining changes in the BRCA-1 and BRCA-2 genes. (Tp53 testing is also possible.) It is only offered to high-risk women. It is inappropriate for low-risk individuals as it is very unlikely to provide any helpful information and is also likely to give false reassurance. In a high-risk family, the individual first tested is almost always the one who has had breast cancer. Initial testing is seldom offered to unaffected individuals.

It is important to realise that genetic testing is not perfect. A significant number of people possessing BRCA-1 or BRCA-2 changes will be missed and there may well be other inherited genes responsible for breast cancer that are as yet unknown and cannot be tested for. Thus, an important limitation of these genetic tests is that a test that does not find an abnormality may be giving false reassurance to the tested person and other family members.

Genetic testing should only be done after thorough counselling that includes discussion of all management options and the consequences for the woman and other members of her family if there is a diagnosis of a harmful genetic abnormality. Such problems include fear and anxiety for themselves and their children, family planning issues, and disruption of immediate and broader family relationships. For the above reasons, genetic testing should be organised through Family Cancer Clinics. You can ask your GP for a referral. A list of clinics is available through the National Breast Cancer Centre (details of which are provided at the end of this chapter).

Breast cancer risk

A number of factors can increase your risk of developing breast cancer. Some of these you will not be able to alter. They include increasing age, a family history of breast cancer, and a previous personal history of breast cancer. Never having a child or having your first child after the age of 35 years also increases your risk slightly. Those risks that can be altered include an alcohol intake of over 20 grams per day and obesity. They both significantly increase your risk by increasing oestrogen levels.

An increased lifetime exposure to the naturally occurring hormone oestrogen increases the risk of breast cancer. This occurs when menstrual periods are commenced early (before teens) or are finished late (in late 50s) or when women go on hormone replacement therapy at menopause. (The increase in breast cancer incidence with hormone replacement therapy is quite small.) The reverse is also true, with reduced oestrogen exposure reducing the risk of breast cancer. Thus, late menarche (16 years) reduces the breast cancer risk to about half the normal incidence and early menopause (at 42 instead of 52 years) reduces the risk to about 66 per cent of the normal incidence. Also, women who have their first child by the age of 18 reduce their oestrogen exposure and have half the risk of women that have no children. Asian women living in Asia have lower oestrogen levels and thus have lower breast cancer rates—only 10 to 20 per cent the risk of Western women.

Breast cancer prevention

Preventing breast cancer requires both minimising exposure to risk factors and early cancer detection. Breast cancer may exist for long periods as a non-spreading or locally spreading tumor before becoming malignant (i.e. spreading to other parts of the body). This delay allows time for early detection and curative treatment. There is a 90 per cent survival rate at five years after diagnosis when the cancer is contained within the breast at diagnosis compared with an 18 per cent rate at five years when the disease has spread beyond the breast (Zobias 2000).

Detection of early breast cancers can be done by several methods including breast self-examination, yearly medical examinations and mammograms. Annual breast examinations by your doctor can find some cancers that are missed by mammogram. While its benefit as a screening technique is still uncertain, it should certainly be part of a routine yearly medical from at least the age of 40.

Factors that can reduce your risk include maintaining a normal weight and keeping alcohol consumption to a maximum of two standard drinks a day. As stated above, hormone replacement therapy may increase your risk slightly but in most women its other benefits outweigh this increased risk.

Recognising cancerous changes in the breast

Reporting changes in a breast as soon as they are evident is vital for the early diagnosis of breast cancer. Any of the symptoms listed below can by itself indicate that breast cancer is present and need immediate investigation.

- Any lump, lumpiness or thickening.
- Nipple discharge, especially if it is only on one side or from a single duct, occurs spontaneously or contains blood or mucous.
- Nipple change, such as ulceration, inversion, redness, change in shape or crusting.
- Changes in the skin over the breast, such as puckering, dimpling, change in colour or unusual redness. (Remember that your breast tissue extends almost to your armpit.)
- Pain in your breast, especially if on one side or if it does not improve after your menstrual periods.

The most common change observed is a lump, but a lump does not have to be felt for cancer to be present. All women should ensure they know what their breasts feel and look like and should report any change they find immediately to their doctor. Breast self-examination has for a long time been part of this process and, although it is not certain that it reduces breast cancer deaths, it is a worthwhile adjunct to continually monitoring your breasts for changes. (About 30 per cent of women do regular breast self-examination.)

Once you have reported your symptom, it is important it is investigated quickly and thoroughly. This should always involve appraisal by your doctor (i.e. taking a history and performing an examination) and, if necessary, investigation by imaging (mammogram and/or ultrasound) and aspiration/biopsy of the lesion with a fine needle. Many women with a breast lump will want an accurate diagnosis for reassurance and this requires a biopsy of the lesion.

As with all potentially serious medical conditions, it is important for your peace of mind that you are happy with the management your breast problem receives. If for any reason you are unhappy, make sure you tell your doctor. You can always ask for a referral to a specialist for a second opinion.

The National Breast Cancer Centre has recently published a hand-out regarding breast changes and how they should be managed called 'Do you have a breast change?' It is available at www.nbcc.org.au/pages/info/resources/nbccpubs.htm—look in the section on consumer booklets, audio etc—or it can be sourced from the National Breast Cancer Centre through your GP.

Why do women delay presenting with cancer symptoms found in their breasts?

Unfortunately many women with breast cancer symptoms still delay consulting their doctor about the symptom. This is a serious problem as early detection is the main method by which death from breast cancer can be reduced.

The main problem is a fear of finding out they have cancer combined with a belief the treatment will not help breast cancer anyway. Fear of disfigurement associated with surgical treatment is another important cause. (Many breast cancers can now be treated with removal of the lump only, especially if they are caught early.) Finally, some women lack sufficient knowledge about the symptoms, other than breast lumps, which are associated with cancer. Many women presenting with breast cancer have symptoms in addition to a lump alone. Other common presenting symptoms include nipple and skin changes.

But I'm too young to worry about breast cancer

This is unfortunately not the case. While the incidence of breast cancer increases with age, about 10 per cent of breast cancers occur in women under the age of 40. In 1997, women under the age of 30 made up 0.7 per cent of those diagnosed with breast cancer. No matter what your age, if you have a new breast symptom, particularly a lump, you need to see your doctor immediately to determine its cause. Most will not be cancer but you cannot afford to assume this will be the case.

Screening using mammograms

Mammograms are X-rays of the breast and they can be done for two different reasons. Firstly, they can be done as a screening test to help find abnormalities in breasts that look and feel normal (i.e. no lump or other abnormality has been previously found). This test is called a screening mammogram and is the type of mammogram we are referring to in this section. It is generally not performed by a doctor.

Mammograms can also help diagnose the nature of a lump that has already been found. This is called a diagnostic mammogram. It involves more X-rays and is interpreted by a doctor (a radiologist). All mammograms are X-rays, not ultrasounds.

Mammograms pick up about 85 per cent of breast cancers and, if all Australian women in the 50 to 70 year age group had regular screening mammograms, the breast cancer rate could be halved at least. Unfortunately, at present only about 50 to 60 per cent of Australian women in this important age group have screening mammograms and this explains why breast cancer mortality has to date only been reduced by 23 per cent. This is still a wonderful result but it can be improved!

Breast cancer is detected in about 0.5 per cent (5 in 1000) of those screened for the first time, with the incidence slightly less at subsequent screenings.

Screening mammograms are free of charge for all women over 40 years of age at BreastScreen. (Phone 13 20 50 anywhere in Australia.)

Mammograms in the 40s and over 70s—are they worth it?

Mass screening for women aged from 40 to 50 years at normal risk is not currently recommended in Australia. However, this is a controversial issue and there is evidence that it may be of benefit to these women. Your decision?

Screening women in their 40s will help prevent some deaths (about four deaths for every 10 000 women screened in this age group), with most of this benefit occurring in women in their late 40s.

On the other hand, there are several good reasons for you not to have mammograms if you are in the 40 to 50 year age group. Firstly, it increases the likelihood of you having an unnecessary investigation as there is a higher incidence of false positives in younger women. For women in their 40s, 96 per cent needing further investigation following a mammography won't have cancer. This compares with 92 per cent in their 50s and 88 per cent in their 60s. This higher incidence of false positive tests also causes extra unnecessary anxiety.

There is also an increased rate of false negative tests (i.e. missed cancers) in younger women as screening is less sensitive in pre-menopausal women due to their denser breast tissue. The inconvenience and discomfort of the procedure and the extra expense to the community are also issues to consider. Extra radiation exposure is minimal and not significant.

Mass screening of women over 70 years of age is not recommended at present. However, the benefit is about the same as screening the 40 to 49 year age group, so it is reasonable for women over 70 to continue their screening program if they wish to do so.

Breast implants and cancer screening

Breast cancer is no more common in women with breast implants and the prognosis is no worse. Mammograms are, however, not as effective in women with implants as some breast tissue can't be visualised.

Table 29 Suggested routine screening for breast cancer

Age group	*Self-examination and awareness of symptoms*	*Yearly medical examinations*	*Mammograms*
Before 40	Always	Yes	No
40 to 44	Always	Yes	Not usually considered necessary
45 to 49	Always	Yes	A reasonable option for women seeking optimum protection—discuss with your GP if this option is preferred and see section on mammography
50 +	Always	Yes	Yes, every two years until at least age 70

Further information

National Breast Cancer Centre
Website: www.nbcc.org.au.; Ph: (02) 9036 3030

BreastScreen Australia
For information regarding mammograms or to book a mammogram—Ph: 13 20 50; Website: www.breastscreen.info.au

NHMRC Breast Cancer Centre
For further advice regarding inherited breast cancer—Ph: (02) 9334 1700

Breast Health Link
Website: www.breasthealthlink.com

Cervical cancer

Cervical cancer is a disease that should not be underestimated. Prior to the introduction of Pap smear screening, cervical cancer was the most common gynaecological cancer in women and the most common cause of cancer deaths in women. (This is still the case in underdeveloped countries.) The introduction of Pap smears has had a dramatic effect on this disease and to date it has saved the lives of over 5000 Australian women.

In Australia, cervical cancer accounts for about 3.7 per cent of female cancers, with the vast majority (85 per cent) of these occurring in women who have not had a Pap smear or who have had inadequate smears in the past ten years. Women who have been sexually active at any time (including homosexual women) should have the test every second year. (Women with a history of abnormal smears will need to have them done more frequently.) Having a Pap smear once every two years can prevent over 90 per cent of cervical cancers. At present, only about 60 per cent of women have a Pap smear every two years and about 80 per cent have one every three years. This less than optimal Pap smear rate explains why cervical cancer still causes about 2.4 per cent of cancer deaths and the tragedy is, these deaths often occur in young women (see figure 24). Fifty per cent occur before the age of 50.

The problem is especially prevalent in remote indigenous communities, where lack of screening for cervical cancer has meant it is the most common cause of gynaecological cancer death. In white Australians the death rate per year is 2 in 100 000 women while in indigenous Australians the rate is about 14 times greater at 27 in 100 000. The overall Australian death rate per year is about 8 in 100 000.

What causes cervical cancer?

Almost all cervical cancers are due to exposure to the sexually transmitted human papilloma virus (HPV). Cervical cancers are rare in women who have not had sexual intercourse. In all there are about 35 types of HPV that affect the cervix, but only a few high-risk types are responsible for cervical cancer.

Most initial HPV cervical infections resolve by themselves, irrespective of whether the initial infection is due to a high- or low-risk type of HPV. By themselves, these initial infections cause only a mild abnormality on the Pap smear and, like the HPV infection that causes them, these mild Pap smear abnormalities usually go without treatment and do not progress to cancer.

The development of cervical cancer requires a high-risk type of virus to become incorporated into the genes of the cervical cell. For this to occur, it is thought that an additional cancer-causing factor must also be present, such as cigarette smoking.

Pap smears as prevention

All women who have been sexually active should have Pap smears. They should commence at the age of 18 or within two years after first sexual intercourse. Women can stop having pap smears at age 70 if they have had two normal smears in the previous five years and have had no other suspicious symptoms. A woman who has had a hysterectomy does not need Pap smears when all the following apply: there was no evidence of uterine or cervical cancer found at the hysterectomy; all previous smears were normal; she is not severely immunosuppressed; and she has had no symptoms.

At present Pap smears are done every two years. (The additional pick-up rate for doing them yearly is about 0.5 per cent and is not worthwhile economically.) If you are pre-menopausal, the best time to collect a specimen is midway between your periods. Contact bleeding with the procedure is relatively common and does not increase the likelihood that cancer is present.

Only about 60 per cent of women have Pap smears every second year, with compliance being worse in low socio–economic groups, in non-English-speaking women, and in country areas. Almost all deaths occur in women who do not have regular Pap smears and over 50 per cent of deaths occur in women who have never had a Pap smear. To help this situation there are now national and state programs to monitor women participating in Pap smear screening. They incorporate registries, recall systems and promotional schemes.

Having had a Pap smear, it is important you contact your doctor to find out the result. While doctors have a responsibility to notify patients of their results and most doctors have

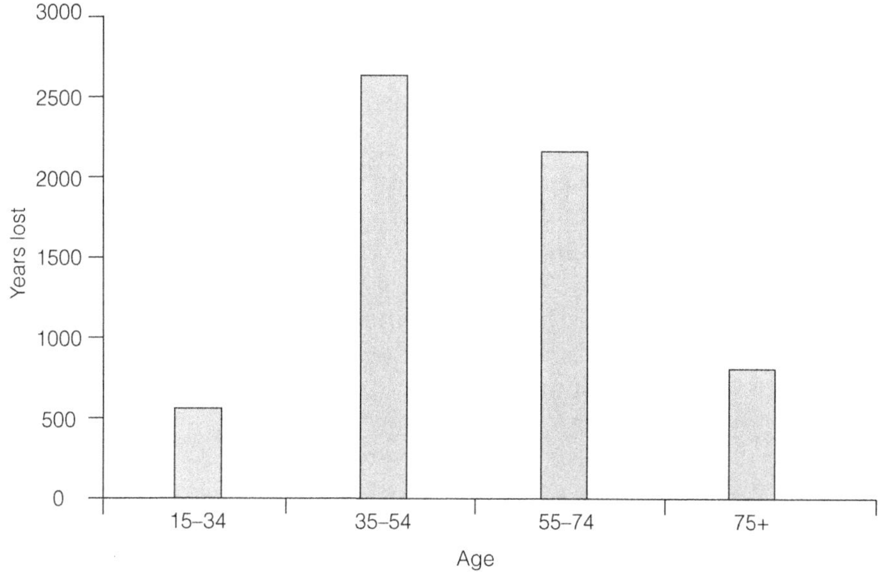

Source: Adapted from Australian Institute of Health and Welfare: Mathers, 1999.

Figure 24 Years lost due to disability and mortality (DALYs) from cervical cancer (1996)

very good systems in place to ensure abnormal tests are not missed, it doesn't hurt to play safe. It is your body; make sure you take an interest.

All states in Australia have Pap smear registers. These government-run registers act as reminder services for women who are overdue for their next Pap smear test. They also work with medical practitioners to ensure women with abnormalities have adequate follow-up care. You should ask to be registered with your state register the next time you have a Pap smear test.

The vast majority of male GPs, while being competent at performing Pap smears, understand that some women prefer a female doctor to perform their smears. Do not be afraid to ask for a female doctor in your practice to do your smear or see a female doctor in another practice.

WHAT DOES A NORMAL PAP SMEAR MEAN?

Pap smears are not perfect. Abnormalities can be missed and this is one of the reasons why Pap smears need to be done every two years. A normal Pap smear tells you that you have a very low risk of either having cancer or developing cancer in the next few years. It does not indicate you have no risk of developing cancer. If you have symptoms, such as bleeding after intercourse or bleeding between periods or after menopause, you cannot assume you have no cause for concern. You should consult your GP to make sure there is no sinister cause.

THE NEW 'VEDA-SCOPE'

The 'Veda-Scope' is a new device used to perform Pap smears. The smears themselves are performed in exactly the same manner as traditional smears and there is no difference in the quality of smears being taken. The difference is that the vagina is expanded by a flow of air, rather than the traditional speculum, and the cervix is seen under internal illumination and magnification of up to six times. The main advantage is that this system is reported to be more comfortable for the patient. There can, however, be occasional problems with increased air-drying of smears, which makes them unreadable. These smears cost about $8 more and this cost has to be borne by the patient.

Terms used to describe abnormal Pap smears

Cervical cancer occurs in cells called squamous cells. Pre-cancerous changes in these cells can be graded either low or high according to the likelihood they will progress on to actual cancer. In increasing order of severity they are:

1. Normal smear
2. Atypical squamous cells (possible low-grade squamous intraepithelial lesion)
3. Atypical squamous cells (possible high-grade squamous intraepithelial lesion)
4. Low-grade squamous intraepithelial lesion (HPV or CIN I)
5. High-grade squamous intraepithelial lesion (CIN 2 or CIN 3)
6. Squamous cell carcinoma (actual cancer)

This terminology is relatively new and may not yet be in general use.

NEW METHODS OF EXAMINING CERVICAL CELLS TAKEN DURING PAP SMEARS

Over the past few years, newer laboratory techniques aimed at more accurate diagnosis of cervical cancer have been developed. Before discussing these tests, it is important to emphasise that these tests are done in addition to the normal Pap smear test (i.e. the specimen is examined twice, once by the normal technique and once by the newer technique).

Retesting conventional smears by computer: These techniques use computer-assisted microscopes to look for abnormal cells. (The PAPNET and Autopap tests are examples of this type of test.) One recent study found that PAPNET could pick up about 7 per cent more abnormalities than manual screening. However, most of these were low-grade abnormalities (Heley 2001). As these tests are more expensive, they are mainly used for quality control by most laboratories.

Different slide preparation (The ThinPrep/Autocyte method): In this method, your doctor makes a conventional slide for the Pap smear and then places the remaining cells in a liquid medium. The slides prepared from this liquid medium enable the pathologist to have a clear view of just the cervical cells. This is an advantage over normal smears as normal smears are sometimes difficult to read due to the presence of thick mucous or blood. Problems with reading conventional smears means that about 1 to 2 per cent of conventional smears need to be repeated.

At present, there is no convincing evidence that these newer techniques are significantly better than conventional smears. This is because many of the extra lesions they detect are low grade and may not have needed further investigation. As stated before, many low-grade abnormalities regress and do not reappear. Finding these extra low-grade abnormalities usually just causes extra anxiety for patients.

With regard to high-grade abnormal smears, these newer techniques are able to diagnose a few more lesions—about 5 per cent more (Heley 2001). However, a proportion of these extra high-grade lesions are found due to the material being examined twice rather than the superiority of the newer techniques.

As these techniques add about $30 to the cost of a Pap smear, it is doubtful they are cost effective. All of this extra cost is at present paid by the patient.

The newer tests may, however, be useful when excessive mucous, blood or discharge makes a conventional smear difficult to read. The use of the test in this situation as a back-up may prevent the need to return for a second test. (These tests reduce the number of unsatisfactory tests that need to be repeated to about 0.4 per cent, compared with 2 per cent for conventional Pap smears.) They may also be useful in women who have needed past Pap smears repeated due to inflamatory changes or too few cells being present. Anxious women may also benefit from the reassurance of a second test.

It needs to be re-emphasised that 85 per cent of cervical cancers in Australia occur in women who do not have regular smears.

Screening techniques for detecting HPV

As stated previously, there are about 35 types of Human Papilloma Virus (HPV) that affect the cervix, with only a few high-risk types being responsible for cervical cancer. In women over 35, there is a strong association between persistent HPV infection (over six months) and high-grade cervical abnormalities. In these cases, testing for HPV may well be of benefit in predicting those likely to develop cancer. At present, this test is not recommended as a screening test by the National Health and Medical Research Council (NHMRC) because the test cannot tell which HPV infections are likely to cause cancer. There is also a high incidence of positive tests for HPV that are not causing cancerous lesions.

Testing should not be done in women under the age of 35 as the false-positive rate is far too high in this group. This is because women under 35 have a much higher incidence of recent HPV infection. A positive test for HPV in this group is unlikely to be significant as the test is indicating an acute infection that will clear up without causing any harm.

The test for HPV can be done on a cervical swab or on fluid from a ThinPrep or Autocyte test. However, at $80 per test (all paid for by the patient), it is expensive and, not surprisingly, rarely done.

Skin cancer prevention—melanomas

Australia unfortunately has the highest rate of skin cancer in the world. Approximately 66 per cent of people living in Australia will develop skin cancers, with about 1200 dying of these cancers each year. It is an unfortunate fact that almost all of these cancers, including melanomas, are either preventable in the first place or completely curable if caught early. Almost all skin cancers are the direct result of long-term exposure to ultra-violet radiation (UVR) from the sun. Sun beds and solariums also cause exposure to harmful UVR.

Types of skin cancer

Melanomas

Melanomas are pigmented skin cancers that can cause death by spreading throughout the body (a process termed metastasising). They are less common than the other main types of skin cancer, but are much more dangerous. They are responsible for most of Australia's skin cancer deaths. Australia has the highest rate of melanoma occurrence in the world, with the incidence and death rate being considerably higher for males.

Pigmented skin lesions (naevi) are the precursor (starting) lesions for these melanomas. Almost all of these lesions are acquired due to sun exposure, with fewer than 2 per cent of the population being born with pigmented lesions. Pigmented lesions tend to develop in the first 40 years of life, with few appearing after this time. Thus, while most of the burden of disease from melanomas occurs from middle age onwards (see figure 25), preventing melanomas relies on minimising exposure to damaging UVR in childhood and early adult life. Childhood protection is paramount in preventing melanomas!

The first sign of a melanoma is a new spot or a change in an existing spot. Existing pigmented spots that are irregular in outline and uneven in colour (called dysplastic naevi) are the lesions most likely to become melanomas. Melanomas can vary greatly in appearance. Commonly, they have an irregular edge and/or surface and they can be flat or raised. Their colour is usually uneven and may be any combination of black, brown, blue, red, white and light grey. They may bleed or itch. Any new mole in an adult should be suspected of being a melanoma.

Risk factors for the development of melanoma include having fair skin that tans poorly, a tendency to freckle easily, high sun exposure (especially if this occurred as a child), the presence of over 100 pigmented lesions on the body, and the presence of atypical or unusual pigmented lesions. People with depressed immune systems are also at greater risk. There is also a slightly increased risk if a first degree family member has had a melanoma.

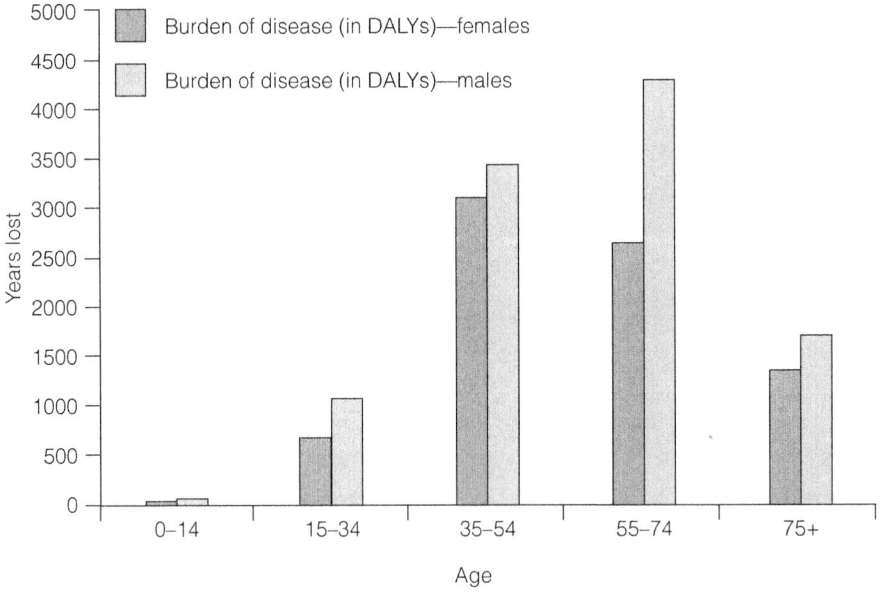

Source: Adapted from Australian Institute of Health and Welfare: Mathers, 1999.

Figure 25 Years lost due to disability and mortality (DALYs) from melanoma (1996)

Other important skin cancers

The two other main types of skin cancers are squamous cell carcinoma (SCC) and basal cell carcinoma (BCC). Both these cancers are also due to sun exposure. However, unlike melanomas, they usually do not spread. The main exception to this rule is squamous cell cancers on the face, especially the lips. BCC can cause considerable disfiguring local damage if not treated early.

Common precursor lesions for SCC are the solar keratoses that are regularly burnt or frozen off the bodies of almost all Australian adults from middle age onwards.

Preventing skin cancers

Almost all skin cancers are caused by the sun's ultra-violet radiation (UVR), which causes skin cancer cells to be formed through mutations to skin cell genes. It also weakens the skin's immune system. (The immune system helps detect and destroy cancer cells that have been produced.) UVR also damages the deeper parts of the skin called the connective tissues. This damage is responsible for the early ageing that occurs in sun-damaged skin. There are two types of ultra-violet radiation, UVA and UVB, and exposure to both types should be reduced. This is important when choosing your sunscreen.

In Australia, avoiding UVR means a life-long ritual of reducing time spent in the sun, wearing adequate protective clothing, and the use of sunscreens. Fortunately, there are early signs that this improved sun protection is having an effect, with evidence from some states showing the incidence of melanoma is starting to fall in younger adults.

Reducing time spent exposed to UVR

You should stay out of the sun whenever possible, especially during the middle of the day (from 11 a.m. until 3 p.m. during the daylight saving months and from 10 a.m. until 2 p.m. during other times). UVR levels can be quite high even on cloudy days and it is important to keep in the shade whenever possible. When heading outdoors, take shade with you in the form of hats, umbrellas etc., and try to provide as many shady areas around your home as possible, especially near/over pools and children's play areas.

UVR is also present during winter and is especially a problem in the snow country, where up to 88 per cent of UVR is reflected onto your face. At higher altitudes there is also significantly more UVR present. For example, at a height of 2000 metres the UVR levels are about 30 per cent higher than those at sea level.

Wearing appropriate protective clothing

You should start with a good hat that has a tight weave and a broad brim (8 to 10 centimetres for adults and 6 centimetres for children). When wearing a hard hat at work or while riding a bike, a brim and neck flap should be attached. Baseball-type caps are not as good a choice as they do not protect your ears, neck or much of your face—all of which are common sites for skin cancers. Whichever hat you choose, sunscreens are still needed for the head and neck to protect against UVR reflected from the ground.

Your clothes should cover your limbs and neck (i.e. have collars) and be made of a fabric that has a fairly close weave. Try to avoid sleeveless tops with no collars. Rash vests offer good protection for both adults and children when in the water. Long sleeves are best but, remember, their UVR protection does decrease as the garment ages.

Apply a good sunscreen and do it properly

When about to be exposed to UVR, it is important to apply a broad spectrum SPF 30+ sunscreen which protects against UVB and UVA and gives immunoprotection from sunlight. An eight-minute exposure to sunlight can reduce the skin's immune protection by up to 35 per cent. The sunscreen should also be water resistant if you are swimming or likely to sweat a lot.

Sunscreens need to be applied 20 minutes before exposure. This is because rubbing in the cream breaks down the sunscreen's 'water-in-oil emulsion' barrier to UV light. This takes about 20 minutes to reform. Sunscreens should be reapplied every two hours or more frequently if the cream is likely to have been rubbed, sweated, or washed off while swimming or exercising. (Sunscreen is often rubbed quickly off the face, especially around the eyes, when swimming and needs to be reapplied every 30 minutes or so.) The cream should be applied evenly to the skin and, as mentioned previously, should also be water resistant if you are swimming or likely to sweat a lot.

Before using a new sunscreen, try a small patch test on your arm overnight to identify any allergy or irritation. As a general rule, creams and lotions are less likely to cause skin problems than alcohol-based products.

It is important to understand that sunscreens cannot filter out all UVR. A SPF 30+ preparation applied properly can be expected to cut out 97 per cent of UVR. Thus if you were going to get sunburnt in ten minutes with no sunscreen, you will still get sunburnt in about 300 minutes with properly applied SPF 30+ cream; and a lot sooner if it is not properly applied initially or reapplied regularly. SPF 15+ sunscreens give only half the protection of SPF 30+ sunscreens and should be avoided unless a SPF 30+ product is not available. Sunscreens do deteriorate with age and it is important to check the expiry date of the cream you are using.

What's in sunscreens?

Active ingredients—these may act by either absorbing or reflecting UVR:

- UVA and UVB protective—titanium dioxide, oxybenzone, zinc oxide
- UVA protective only—homosalate, butyl methoxydibenzoylmethane
- UVB protective only—octyl methoxycinnamate, octyl salicylate, padimate O, octocrylene.

Stabilisers—these act to stop the active ingredients being broken down by UV light:
- Preservatives.
- Perfumes.

(Quayle 2001)

DO SUNSCREENS HELP PREVENT SKIN CANCERS? YES!

Sunscreens have been proven to prevent longer-term skin damage and reduce the development of pigmented lesions. These are the known causes of melanomas and other skin cancers and it is therefore extremely likely that long-term regular sunscreen use will greatly reduce the future incidence of skin cancers in Australia. At present there are numerous studies being conducted to confirm the ability of sunscreens to stop skin cancers developing. To date, these studies have shown that adults who apply sunscreens regularly do have a reduced incidence of SCCs.

While melanomas and BCCs both appear from middle age onwards, both are likely to be initiated by sun exposure much earlier in life. Thus, it is necessary to study the use of sunscreens in children and younger adults to prove that sunscreens do in fact reduce the incidence of these cancers. As such studies take a long time to perform, there have to date been no completed studies to confirm protection against melanomas and BCCs. However, early results have been encouraging and, as sunscreens have been shown to stop solar UVR from causing the skin damage and pigmented skin lesions that cause these cancers, it is extremely likely they will be shown to prevent melanomas and BBCs.

It is important to emphasise once again that preventing melanomas requires the protection of children's skin.

UVR sun cancers and solariums

The use of sun beds and solariums causes exposure to UVR, which results in skin damage and adds to the risk of developing skin cancers. Do not believe any reassurances you might be given—they are not safe.

Screening for melanomas (and other skin cancers)

Finding and treating melanomas early should ensure that the vast majority of people with the cancer can be cured. For this reason, all people at increased risk of melanoma should be screened at least annually from their early teenage years. This involves looking at all skin areas, as melanomas can occur anywhere, including under nails, on the soles of feet, and even inside the eye. Those at increased risk include:

- People with multiple pigmented lesions.
- People with a previous history of melanoma or lesions that are more likely to turn into melanomas. (These are called dysplastic naevi and are pigmented lesions that are irregular in shape and uneven in colour.)
- People with a family history of melanoma or pre-melanoma lesions (dysplastic naevi) in a primary relative (parent or sibling).
- People with freckles or who burn easily rather than tan.
- People with a past history of non-melanoma skin cancer.
- People with light/red hair colour.
- People with high levels of sun exposure, especially if this occurred as a child. (Significant episodes of sunburn in childhood are thought to be a causal factor and should be especially avoided.)

In addition, as part of routine medicals, everybody should be checked regularly (preferably each year) for skin cancers. Any skin lesion that you are concerned about should be seen immediately by your GP and not left to increase in size. (Do not wait until your next routine visit.) This applies especially to pigmented lesions and any lesions on the face or ears as these can be much more difficult to treat. Dysplastic lesions need careful observation. The signs to be concerned about include any new lesion, spots etc. that change size, shape or colour, sores that don't heal, and anything else that worries you.

It is also very important for people at increased risk of melanomas to regularly (monthly) examine themselves for new skin lesions or changes in existing skin lesions and to have these reviewed by their GP. (Areas such as the back and head need to be examined by another family member or friend.)

UV light and sunglasses

Numerous eye problems are related to sun damage. These include:

- BCCs and SCCs on the skin around the eye. SCCs can also occur on the conjunctiva (the white part of the eye).

- Melanomas on the skin surrounding the eye, on the conjunctiva, on the iris (the coloured part of the eye) and in the eye itself. About 180 eye melanomas occur in Australia yearly.
- Pterygiums, which are non-cancerous growths that occur across the cornea.
- Cataracts (opacities in the lens of the eye). These are mostly caused by chronic exposure to UVB radiation.

To give adequate protection, your sunglasses should fit close to your face and wrap around your eyes. They should also meet with the Australian Standard 1067.2 specifications for sunglasses, which should be shown on the tag attached to the glasses. Such glasses protect against 99 per cent of UVR. Neither the colour of the glass nor the cost of the glasses influence the degree of protection given.

Modern prescription glasses have adequate filters for UV light already built in so tinting is not needed.

Prostate cancer

Prostate cancer is the most common cancer in males, with about 13 per cent being affected during their lifetime. However, it occurs mostly late in life and many men with the disease die of another condition before it can have a fatal effect. Only about 3 per cent of males die from prostate cancer.

The disease is inherited in about 9 per cent of cases. However, this rate is much greater in young men. Forty-three per cent of cases occurring in males under the age of 55 are inherited. A male with a first-degree relative (father or sibling) with the disease has twice the risk of developing the disease.

While screening of patients without prostate symptoms is of questionable benefit, it is important to emphasise that males with prostate symptoms should see their doctor for investigation. These symptoms include poor or decreasing urine flow, increased frequency of passing urine with smaller amounts, needing to pass urine at night, pain with passing urine, or passing blood in the urine.

Examination of the prostate is done by a digital (by finger) rectal examination. This examination is not performed often as part of a routine medical check-up and is usually done only if a patient's symptoms suggest bowel or prostate problems.

Diet and prostate cancer

There is some evidence that the consumption of fish, especially fatty fish such as salmon, herring and mackerel, reduces the risk of prostate cancer (Terry 2001). This is probably due to the effects of omega-3 fatty acids contained in these fish. These omega-3 fatty acids also offer significant protection against vascular disease, such as coronary artery disease.

There is evidence that a diet high in vegetables (especially tomatoes due to their lycopenes) helps in reducing prostate cancer incidence (Saxalby 1999) and that lack of exercise and excessive dietary fat may increase its incidence.

Screening for prostate cancer by Prostatic Specific Antigen testing

Screening for prostate cancer involves the measurement of Prostatic Specific Antigen (PSA) in men with no prostate symptoms. PSA is a chemical (a glycoprotein) secreted by the prostate (mostly into the semen but also into the blood). Its rate of production is actually decreased in men with prostate cancer. However, a larger percentage is secreted into the blood and this causes the PSA level in the blood to rise in many patients with prostate cancer. PSA exists in the blood in a bonded and a free form and both of these can be measured. The total PSA is the measurement of both forms together.

The total PSA test is used for prostate cancer screening. It can be raised by reasons other than cancer, including examination of the prostate, ultrasound examination of the prostate, prostatitis (i.e. prostate infection) and recent ejaculation. Thus, testing should not be done soon after these events.

At present, there is still considerable debate regarding the use of PSA testing in screening healthy men for prostate cancer.

The case against PSA screening

Unfortunately, as can be seen from the points below, the PSA test is quite inaccurate, producing many false positive and negative results. Results are classified as follows (Stricker 2001):

- *Normal range* (PSA of 0.0 to 3.9ng/mL)—25 per cent of men with prostate cancer have a PSA in the normal range and are missed by the test.
- *Suspicious range* (PSA of 4.0 to 10.0ng/mL)—only 25 per cent of men in this range will actually have prostate cancer. Thus, many are unnecessarily investigated.
- *Suggestive of cancer* (PSA over 10.0ng/mL)—50 per cent of the men in this group that have prostate cancer will be incurable.

If PSA screening is to disclose the majority of curable cases of prostate cancer, it is necessary to investigate those with PSA levels in the inaccurate middle or 'suspicious' range. The accuracy of the PSA test in predicting prostate cancer in the suspicious range can be improved by calculating the free to total PSA ratio. (A ratio below 15 to 25 per cent indicates an increased chance of cancer being present.) Using age-related upper limits of normal for (total) PSA can also reduce the rate of false positive tests. (The upper level of normal for PSA also varies according to age.)

The position of the Cancer Council of NSW and Cancer Council Australia is not to recommend for or against PSA screening in men with no symptoms of prostate disease. They feel the man involved should make his own informed decision based on the arguments for and against screening.

The case against screening is based on the following facts:

- There is no conclusive evidence that screening for prostate cancer increases your life expectancy and early detection does not guarantee you a cure.
- Doctors cannot tell which cancers are going to spread further, so if you have a cancer that is in the prostate only, it is not clear whether you will benefit from treatment.
- Treatments and investigations have significant side effects that may adversely affect your quality of life. For example, surgical treatment by radical prostatectomy causes minor incontinence in about 20 per cent of men and impotence problems in about 70 per cent.
- Screening for cancer using PSA readings is inaccurate with many false-positive results. If you have a false-positive test, you will suffer unnecessary anxiety and endure unnecessary investigations. Only 1.5 per cent of men tested will have a significant cancer and at least 66 per cent of these men will die of another disease.

The case for limited PSA screening

Some well-respected doctors and medical organisations actively support limited prostate cancer screening for men once they have been fully informed of the limitations of both the test and available prostate cancer treatments and have decided they would like to have the test done. Their view is based on the belief that screening is the best way to minimize illness from this common cancer and that the fall in prostate cancer death rates may be due to increased screening levels. Screening is suggested for all men without prostate symptoms between the ages of 50 and 70 (unless they have a life expectancy of less than 10 years), especially if there is a family history of prostate cancer. A younger starting age of 40 is suggested by some for men with a family history. Even for those men with a family history of the disease, the NSW Cancer Council's position is still neither for nor against screening. Men over 70 should not be screened because most diagnosed with prostate cancer would die of another disease.

All screenings should be done as a combination of a PSA test and a digital (finger) examination of the prostate via the anus, and, to be of maximum benefit, should really be done each year.

Several large studies into screening for prostate cancer are being undertaken at present and hopefully they will help clarify this issue. Information from these studies is still, unfortunately, some years away.

As stated before, men with prostate symptoms need these symptoms investigated by their doctor and this would normally include a PSA.

What to do if your PSA is abnormal?

Firstly, do not panic. It may well be that your result was elevated due to another cause, such as recent sexual activity, recent examination of the prostate, or a prostate or other urinary tract infection. If the examination of your urine suggests infection, then the infection should be treated. It can take three to six months for a PSA level to drop to normal after treatment of a prostate infection.

If your initial test was abnormal, whether due to the above causes or not, it should be repeated and this repeat test should include a free to total PSA ratio. If your test is still abnormal, then you should be referred to a specialist urologist for further investigation. This will normally require a biopsy of your prostate. Ultrasound investigation of the prostate is of no benefit as it does not assist in the diagnosis of cancer. Most men with a persistently raised PSA have a benign enlargement of the prostate, not prostate cancer.

Finally, a negative biopsy following a positive PSA test may not be the end of the story. Biopsies are not perfect and your raised PSA will require further follow-up to ensure a cancer has not been missed. (About 15 per cent if men with a raised PSA and a negative biopsy will have cancer found at a subsequent biopsy.

Further information

Australian Prostate Cancer Collaboration
Website: www.prostatehealth.org.au

Part 7

Other preventative health issues for women

Preparation for pregnancy and screening in pregnancy

The decision to become pregnant

Pregnancy is one of the most important periods in any relationship. It is a time of huge change that is unavoidably associated with increased stress. To ensure each pregnancy is the happy and fulfilling experience that it should be, it is very important to prepare for the event properly. This can best be achieved if the couple make an active decision to become pregnant and discuss the many issues involved before the event.

With the above in mind, it is an unfortunate fact that approximately 50 per cent of pregnancies are not planned. Some of these pregnancies are 'accidental', with alcohol often being a contributing factor. However, many also occur because an active decision to become pregnant is such a momentous one that many women and men are happier to just let it happen. This causes several problems, including losing the opportunity to share in this decision, less than optimal timing with respect to jobs, finances etc., which can unnecessarily increase stress on the couple, and less than optimal medical preparation for the pregnancy.

A pre-pregnancy check-up is a good way to start your pregnancy planning process and this should be done as soon as you or your partner has any thought about wishing to start a family. It should be done before contraception has ceased.

Prior to starting a family, you will probably have needed to see a doctor only occasionally. This all changes with pregnancy and the raising of children and it is important you find a good family doctor. Hopefully you will already have a long-standing relationship with a GP. If not, it is important to get to know your GP well before becoming pregnant. Make sure you are comfortable with his/her attitudes and manner as it is very likely you will be relying on your GP's judgment often from now on.

The pre-pregnancy consultation

There are numerous medical topics you will need to address in the pre-pregnancy consultation. They include:

- General information regarding pregnancy and any concerns you may have.
- Genetic problems, especially if you have specific problems relating to you or your partner's family or ethnic group.
- Your attitude to testing for Down syndrome—you should make informed decisions regarding this issue before pregnancy.
- Medications that are safe or unsafe to take during the pregnancy.
- The effect of alcohol and smoking during pregnancy.
- Your need for iron or vitamin supplements, including specific advice regarding folate supplements.
- Your options regarding public versus private care during the pregnancy and delivery and the hospitals that are available—this will affect who delivers your baby.
- How to avoid potentially harmful infections during pregnancy.
- Issues you might have regarding social problems in your family, such as domestic violence, alcohol, family support, and relationships with other family members.
- Advice regarding the prevention and recognition of depression during the pregnancy. This is a very common problem that can occur at any time during the pregnancy, not just in the post-natal period.
- How to prevent incontinence associated with pregnancy—any woman who has a pregnancy that lasts past 20 weeks has an increased risk of developing a problem with incontinence.
- Tests that need to be carried out before becoming pregnant.

Routine tests at the pre-pregnancy check-up

Rubella titre: Up to 10 per cent of all pregnant women are not immune to rubella. (This figure is higher in some immigrant groups where immunisation levels are low.) Thus, rubella titre needs to be checked in all women and immunisation given if needed. Remember, it is not possible to vaccinate against rubella during pregnancy as there is a slight risk the baby will be affected by the vaccine. Should you accidentally be immunised while pregnant, please contact your doctor immediately. There is, however, some recent evidence that most babies born to women who were accidentally immunised when pregnant were born quite normal (Woodhead 2001).

Full blood count: It is important to ensure anaemia is not a problem. (A full blood count can help identify low iron status and the possibility of thalassaemia.)

Chickenpox (or varicella): All women who have not had or who are uncertain about whether they have had chicken pox in the past should have their immunity checked. Those found not to have immunity should be offered vaccination before they become pregnant (but not if they have problems with their immune system). About 5 per cent of women who state they have had chicken pox are not immune. For this reason, it has been suggested by some doctors that all women should be checked for immunity to chicken pox. This is not accepted practice at present because very high levels of immunity in the adult community make it unlikely these women will contract the disease.

Thalassaemia tests: This is discussed below.

Pap smear: if not done in past 12 months.

Blood sugar test: for women at increased risk of gestational diabetes. (See the chapter on Diabetes.)

Tests for HIV and Hepatitis B and C

Foetal genetic abnormalities

Down syndrome

One in every 700 live births in Australia has Down syndrome and the proportion of cases will increase as the age of mothers increases in our society (see table 30). Most cases (over 97 per cent) of Down syndrome are due to an additional chromosome 21 (Classical Trisomy 21). This occurs as a sporadic event and is not inherited.

The other cause is a translocation abnormality of chromosome 21. This can run in families and sufferers of Down syndrome need to be checked for this abnormality so that other family members can be advised if they are at increased risk of having a Down syndrome child. This risk can be as high as 10 per cent.

Decisions about whether to test a foetus for Down syndrome are best made prior to becoming pregnant. There are two main types of tests, screening and diagnostic.

Table 30 Risk of Down syndrome

Maternal age	*Risk at 12 weeks gestation*	*Risk at 20 weeks gestation*
20	1 in 1068	1 in 1295
25	1 in 946	1 in 1147
30	1 in 626	1 in 759
32	1 in 461	1 in 559
34	1 in 312	1 in 378
36	1 in 196	1 in 238
38	1 in 117	1 in 142
40	1 in 68	1 in 82
42	1 in 38	1 in 46
44	1 in 21	1 in 26

Source: Royal Australian College of General Practitioners, CHECK PROGRAM—Genetics, March 2001.

SCREENING TESTS

These tests do not diagnose the disease; rather, they categorise women into low risk (one in more than 250 to 300) or high risk (one in less than 250 to 300) of having a Down syndrome baby. Women found to be at high risk need further investigation with a diagnostic test.

Screening tests are available to all women and are especially useful for women who are either at a low risk of having a Down syndrome child (i.e. healthy young mothers) but would like some extra reassurance without having to endure an invasive procedure or who do not wish to risk a miscarriage with diagnostic tests. (Amniocentesis carries a miscarriage rate in addition to normal of about 1 in 200 and chorionic villus sampling carries an extra miscarriage rate of 1 in 100.)

There are two disadvantages of these tests. Firstly, some Down syndrome pregnancies show as being at low risk and thus not all Down syndrome cases will be diagnosed. The pick-up rate is about 70 to 80 per cent by the second trimester, so about 20 to 30 per cent of Down syndrome cases are missed by screening tests. Secondly, women who have a false-positive result will be unduly alarmed and can go through unnecessary invasive diagnostic tests that will result in occasional, unnecessary miscarriages.

There are two types of screening test that are equally effective. (These tests will also pick up most cases of Trisomy 18, another type of genetic abnormality, and neural tube defects.)

Triple or quadrupal screening tests: These are blood tests taken from the mother early in the second trimester. (The triple test checks for alpha fetoprotein, oestriol, and beta-HCG.)

Ultrasound of the foetus (nuchal translucency measurement): This checks the fluid content of the foetal neck skin folds. It can also be abnormal in foetuses with heart and kidney problems. The test must be performed by a specially trained ultrasonographer.

DIAGNOSTIC TESTS

Diagnostic tests are invasive and involve taking either a sample of amniotic fluid (amniocentesis) or a sample of the placenta (chorionic villus sampling [CVS]). CVS can be done earlier (at 11 weeks) than amniocentesis. As stated above, they are associated with an increased risk of miscarriage.

These tests actually sample foetal cells to check them for the chromosomal abnormality associated with Down syndrome. Therefore, unlike screening tests, they actually diagnose the condition with 100 per cent accuracy.

Diagnostc tests are generally available only to women who are at high risk, usually because of their age (over 35 years is the usual criterion) or because they have a high-risk result from their screening test.

Testing for beta-thalassaemia status

Beta-thalassaemia is the most common human gene disorder in the world. It is estimated that 1 in 100 Australians carry the beta-thalassaemia trait and it is more common in people of Italian, Greek, Turkish, Cypriot, Lebanese, Maltese or Southeast Asian descent. If you belong to one of these groups, you should definitely have this test done. (It is reasonable for you to request the test irrespective of your racial group.)

Tests that can show whether a person carries the thalassaemia trait are a full blood count, haemoglobin electrophoresis and a serum ferritin. (DNA testing may be needed to confirm the diagnosis.) If your test is positive then your partner should be tested for the abnormality as this disease is a significant problem only if the gene is passed to the child from both parents.

Family genetic problems

If you have a family history of a genetic disease specific tests may be required. It is important to discuss any family genetic disorders with your GP before becoming pregnant. (Such conditions include haemochromatosis, cystic fibrosis, thalassaemia, neurofibromatosis and muscular dystrophy.)

As well as known family problems, any family history of birth defects, multiple miscarriages or intellectual disability may indicate you have inherited genetic problems and you should also mention the presence of any of these problems.

Table 31 Genetic conditions of ethnic groups

Ethnic group	*Disease*	*Carrier frequency*
Italian, Greek, Lebanese, Indonesian	Beta-thalassaemia	1 in 7 to 1 in 20
Anglo-Scottish	Cystic fibrosis	1 in 20
Ashkenasi Jews	Tay-Sachs disease	1 in 20
African	Sickle cell disease	1 in 30
South east Asian	Alpha-thalassaemia	1 in 10

Source: Royal Australian College of General Practitioners, CHECK PROGRAM—Genetics, March 2001.

Some genetic abnormalities have a significantly higher incidence in certain ethnic groups (see table 31). Members of these groups need to discuss with their doctor potential problems relating to diseases in their racial group and carefully research any family history of the disease.

Other preventative health issues

Folate supplements

Increasing folate intake prior to becoming pregnant is the best way to reduce the risk of spina bifida and anencephaly (both are types of neural tube defects). There is also some preliminary evidence that folate supplements may protect against other diseases such as oral cleft palates and heart and kidney malformations (Hernandez-Diaz 2001) and even early childhood cancers such as leukaemia (Thompson 2001). (These later benefits are definitely not established yet.)

Protection against neural tube defects is achieved by taking a folate supplement of 0.5 milligrams per day, commencing at least two months before becoming pregnant and continuing for three months into the pregnancy. This should be in addition to a diet rich in folate. Women with a family history of neural tube defects should increase their dose to 5.0 milligrams per day. (Discuss this with your doctor.)

While most Australian women are aware of the benefits of folate supplements, only about 50 per cent are taking such supplements at the time they conceive their child. An important reason for this is that, as stated before, about 50 per cent of pregnancies, irrespective of the socio–economic status of the parents, are unplanned. If you are a woman of child-bearing age, you should ensure you have a diet high in folate and, if there is any chance of you becoming pregnant, you should take folate supplements. Foods rich in folate include cabbage, peas, wholegrain cereals, Brussels sprouts, lentils and lettuce. Mandatory folate supplementation of flour has been conducted in the USA since 1998. It has resulted in a rise in blood folate levels in women aged 15–44 and in a 19 per cent reduction in neural tube defects (Rouse 2003). Mandatory food supplementation is being considered in Australia.

Alcohol, smoking, social drugs and other harmful medications

Women who need to take routine medications should discuss their best options with their medical practitioner before becoming pregnant. All social drugs should be avoided during pregnancy, especially in the first trimester. This includes alcohol, tobacco and illicit drugs. Alcohol and smoking are both causes of low-birth-weight babies.

Maternal infections

TOXOPLASMOSIS

This is an infection that generally causes no symptoms when contracted by healthy people after birth, however, it can be transmitted from the mother to the foetus. Infected babies are well at birth but can develop many symptoms later, including eye problems, epilepsy and retardation. Infection occurs mostly from eating undercooked meats or raw unwashed vegetables, or from contact with infected soil. It can occur from cats' litter boxes but rarely from direct cat contact. Diagnosis is usually made by blood tests. Prevention is best achieved by washing hands well before eating any food, ensuring all meats are well cooked and all fruits and vegetables are thoroughly washed before being consumed, and by avoiding handling cat litter boxes.

LISTERIA INFECTION

Listeria is a bacterial infection that can cause still births, premature labour, and illness in the newborn. Pregnant women who contract the disease (from food) usually have only minor, non-specific viral-like symptoms and so, like toxoplasmosis, it is difficult to diagnose early. Prevention is best achieved by thoroughly cooking food from animal sources, avoiding unpasteurised milk and milk products, washing raw vegetables well before being eaten, washing hands and implements after handling uncooked meats and raw vegetables (including cutting boards), separating prepared food from uncooked meats and unwashed vegetables, avoiding soft cheeses such as brie, camembert and blue-veined, and avoiding takeaway foods containing meat (or cooking them again at home). Care also needs to be taken with delicatessen foods.

PARVOVIRUS

This disease (also known as Erythema infectosum/fifth disease/slapped face disease) is usually a disease of children that occurs in epidemics that often last several years. Exposure in pregnant women is via their school-aged children or when in contact with children through their work. It presents in children with a rash (especially on the face), and fever and joint pains. In adult women there are often no symptoms. In the foetus, it is mainly a problem in the first 20 weeks of a pregnancy. Only about 40 per cent of women are susceptible, the rest being immune from previous infections. Of those susceptible, only about half will get the disease, and only in half of these will the foetus become infected (Gilbert 2001).

While prevention of the disease is difficult, it needs to be emphasised that even when a foetus is infected, the disease is usually benign. However, in some cases, anaemia develops and this can lead to death of the foetus. (The rate is about 10 per cent in those women infected in the first 20 weeks of their pregnancy.) Management depends on evidence of infection and the stage of the pregnancy.

RUBELLA

Refer to 'Routine tests at the pre-pregnancy check-up' section.

Older mothers

In recent times there has been an increasing tendency for women to commence their families later in life. Most women have very good reasons for making this decision and older mothers may well be able to cope better with the mental and financial stresses associated with having children. However, you should be aware that a decision to delay having children does, unfortunately, increase the risk to the child and the pregnancy.

A significant proportion of women who choose to leave having children into their mid to late thirties will have problems falling pregnant due to reduced fertility. The changes of menopause actually start about 10 to 12 years before menopause occurs, with the reduction in egg (follicle) numbers accelerating from the age of 36. So don't leave it too late.

Some congenital abnormalities also increase with maternal age, such as Down syndrome and low birth-weight. Many foetuses with more severe congenital abnormalities will miscarry and this fact may partly explain why the foetal death rate (due to miscarriages, still births and ectopic pregnancies), increases with increasing maternal age; especially after the age of 35. The rate at a maternal age of 22 is 9 per cent while the rates at 35 and 42 years of age are 20 and 50 per cent respectively (Anderson 2000).

Urinary incontinence in women

Urinary incontinence is a very common problem that causes significant social and hygiene problems for many women. It occurs at all ages but increases with age. Studies have shown prevalence rates in women varying from 30 to 50 per cent, with the higher levels being more indicative of the true incidence. About 66 per cent of those suffering do not seek help. Overall, about 14 per cent of women have incontinence severe enough to wear pads regularly, with the incidence increasing with age to about 42 per cent in the elderly. (Men also suffer from incontinence, mainly in old age due to prostate problems.)

Part of the underlying problem is that mild incontinence is seen as a normal part of ageing and something that just has to be put up with. In other words, a small amount of leaking is normal. This is not the case. Incontinence is not normal and many women can be cured or significantly improved with treatment. For example, up to 80 per cent of stress incontinence, the commonest type of incontinence, can be cured with pelvic floor exercises alone. So mention it to your GP if you have any incontinence!

There are several types of incontinence and these are summarised in table 32. Stress incontinence is by far the most common cause, and luckily the most easily treated. Before any treatment is commenced, it is important you consult your GP regarding the cause of your problem. Your GP can assist by making an accurate assessment of the type of incontinence problem and its severity, and order appropriate investigations or referrals to specialists to assist with diagnosis. The use of voiding charts is often of great benefit in sorting out the type of incontinence present. (These charts record the time of voiding and amount of urine passed on each occasion for two to three days. Any leakage episode is also recorded.)

Table 32 Types of Incontinence

Type	*Causes*	*Features*
Stress	A weakness in the valve at the base of the bladder that controls flow. Weak pelvic floor muscles due to childbirth, menopause, surgery etc. Pelvic organ prolapse may be present. Spinal injury (neurogenic bladder).	Most common type of incontinence. Involuntary loss of (usually) small amounts of urine with coughing, laughing, exercise or lifting. There is usually a feeling of pressure.
Urge	Bladder wall muscle instability causing the bladder to suddenly contract (overactive bladder). Occassionally caused by neurological disease.	Involuntary leakage of large amounts of urine at unexpected times. Associated with a strong desire to void (urgency).
Mixed	Combination of stress and urge incontinence.	Common problem with one symptom predominating.
Overflow	Blockage, due to tumours or strictures, to outflow from the bladder. (Very common in older men due to prostate enlargement.)	Involuntary leakage of small amounts of urine from a full bladder. May present as dribbling or like the symptoms of stress or urge incontinence.

Risk factors for incontinence

The numerous factors that increase the risk of developing incontinence are:

- Pregnancy with vaginal delivery/episiotomy—in fact, any pregnancy that successfully progresses past 20 weeks increases the risk. (About 66 per cent of women experience incontinence during pregnancy.)
- Hysterectomy—women who have had a hysterectomy initially have up to a 40 per cent increase in the incidence of incontinence; this may increase up to about 60 per cent by age 60 (Saunders 2000).
- Pelvic floor weakness.
- Oestrogen deficiency (menopause).
- Significant obesity.
- Chronic cough, especially in smokers and asthmatics.
- Chronic constipation with straining.
- High-impact physical activities.
- Low fluid intake.
- Diabetes.

- Medications, such as fluid tablets and drugs that impair bladder muscle emptying funtion. These include tricyclic antidepressants, sedatives and calcium channel blockers.
- Caffeine—interferes with bladder muscle stability and a high intake can double the risk of incontinence (Lily 2000).
- Being elderly, confused or immobile or having had a stroke.

Physical activity and incontinence

Participation in sport is an important risk factor for incontinence, with around 50 per cent of those regularly participating experiencing some incontinence and up to 20 per cent stopping specific activities due to the problem (Kron 2000). It occurs mostly with running, track and field, high-impact sports such as aerobics, gymnastics and basketball, horseback riding, and tennis. It is a problem for both women who have been pregnant and those who have not. Low-risk sports include swimming, rowing, walking, bicycling, yoga and Tai Chi.

Prevention and treatment of incontinence

Treatment of stress incontinence

Bladder retraining and pelvic floor exercises and stimulation are the main options for the treatment of stress incontinence. Biofeedback and topical or oral oestrogen can also be beneficial. There is usually not much success with drug treatment and surgery is only an option when all else fails.

Treatment of urge incontinence

As with stress incontinence, pelvic floor muscle training and bladder training are important treatments, together with fluid management and topical oestrogen. Drugs to help reduce bladder overactivity, such as anticholinergic drugs and tricyclic antidepressants are useful, although tricyclics have problems with side effects. Smooth muscle relaxants (e.g. hyoscyamide) are widely used but there is little evidence to show they are very effective. Caffeine intake should be reduced. Once again surgery is an option only when all else fails.

Pelvic floor exercises

The pelvic floor is made up of layers of muscle that stretch, like a hammock, from the pubic bone in the front to the tail bone at the back. It acts to support the contents of the abdomen, especially the lower abdominal organs lying directly above, which include the bowel, bladder and uterus. The outlets for these three organs (the vagina, the urethra or front passage and the rectum or back passage) all pass through the pelvic floor.

The pelvic floor muscles play an important role in supporting the organs in the abdomen and in controlling bladder and bowel function. It is therefore important you keep your pelvic floor muscles strong. This is especially the case with older women, where menopausal hormonal changes can weaken the pelvic floor muscles, and in pregnant women, where the pelvic floor muscles have to support the extra weight of the pregnancy. A healthy, strong pelvic floor prior to pregnancy will recover quicker and better following pregnancy.

Pelvic floor muscles should be assessed before treatment, either by digital examination or by physiotherapists using special pressure measuring instruments. Strengthening pelvic floor muscles helps incontinence by strengthening the muscles surrounding the bladder and vaginal outlets. This technique can improve or cure 80 per cent of patients with mild to moderate incontinence.

Factors weakening the pelvic floor are as follow (where possible, they should be avoided or treated):

- menopause
- coughing/sneezing (stopping smoking and treatment for hay fever, asthma and bronchitis are important)
- heavy lifting
- straining from constipation (Adopting from good posture while defecating helps reduce this problem. You should lean forward with a straight back and have your legs apart and wait until your perineal muscles have relaxed before defecating. After defecation or voiding, you should do your pelvic floor exercises.)
- pelvic surgery, especially hysterectomy
- excessive weight
- excessive exercise
- pregnancy, especially with a vaginal delivery.

CONCEPTS RELATED TO TREATMENT WITH PELVIC FLOOR EXERCISES

It is important to identify the muscles that comprise the pelvic floor before starting an exercise program to strengthen them. This is best achieved by tightening the ring of muscle around your back passage. You should not feel like you are squeezing your buttocks. It should be done while relaxed in a lying or sitting position, such as when on the toilet, and should be repeated until you are sure the correct muscles are being tightened.

Another method of identifying the correct muscles involves trying to stop the flow of urine when voiding and then restarting. This can be done weekly to check progress in muscle strengthening. It should not be done more regularly as it interferes with normal bladder emptying.

The pelvic floor muscles stretch between the pubic bone at the front and the sacrum at the back. They act as a sling to support the organs of the pelvis. Strong pelvic floor muscles give good support to these organs, allowing the bladder to function properly. Weak, saggy muscles do the opposite and result in reduced control of bladder emptying.

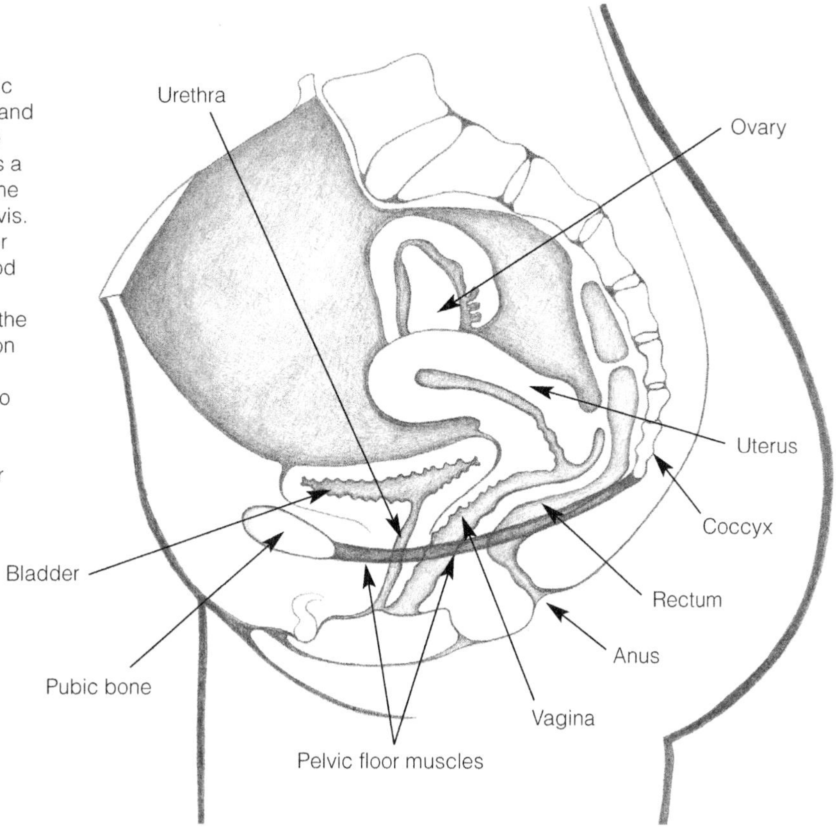

Figure 26 Cross section of female pelvis

If you are not confident you have identified your pelvic floor or you are not able to slow urine flow during voiding, then medical help is required.

It is important you do pelvic floor exercises about five times a day every day of your life. For this reason, it is best to incorporate them into your daily routine. Appropriate times include after going to the toilet and when waking or going to bed. As many women perform pelvic floor exercises incorrectly and get little or no benefit, it is wise to consult your GP or physiotherapist for advice before commencing. One or two visits is usually enough to give adequate tuition. Good results take some time to occur.

If you already have incontinence, you should see your GP for proper assessment of the problem and then have an individual program of pelvic floor exercises worked out. This generally requires about four to six sessions in the first month and then monthly sessions for about six months. Remember, good results take some time (several months) to occur but initial benefits should be evident in a few weeks.

A SIMPLE PELVIC FLOOR EXERCISE ROUTINE

Whether you have incontinence or not, you need to do pelvic floor exercises on a daily basis! They take very little time. The routine below is recommended by the Continence Foundation of Australia.

The exercise: Tighten and draw up the muscles around your anus, vagina and urethra all at once. Try to maintain this contraction strongly for at least five seconds and then release. There should be a definite feeling of letting go. (You can hold longer, up to ten seconds, if you are able.) This exercise should be repeated up to eight to ten times per session. You need to rest for about 10 seconds between each contraction. This should then be followed by five to ten short fast strong contractions.

What not to do: When doing pelvic floor exercises, it is important not to hold your breath, not to push down instead of squeezing and lifting up, and not to tighten you abdomen, buttocks or thighs.

The whole program should be repeated four to five times per day. Try to find routine times for doing the exercises. Progress can be monitored by your ability to stop your urine flow while voiding but remember to do this about once a week only. Significant improvement should be noticed in a few weeks. If you are uncertain about how to do pelvic floor exercises, ask your doctor!

If you are not making progress, then you may need additional types of pelvic floor exercises. These are best provided by a doctor or physiotherapist with training in this field.

Bladder training

Bladder training is useful for stress incontinence and especially urge incontinence. Its aim is to increase bladder capacity and therefore the time needed between voiding. The program includes progressively increasing the time between voiding and trying to delay voiding once the urge to void is present. To perform this training, patients must be mentally and physically able and must be highly motivated.

Prior to starting and during bladder training, a bladder diary should be kept to indicate progress. (It should record times and amounts of urine at voiding and the occurrence of any leaking.)

As part of bladder training, it is important to avoid social voiding (i.e. going to the toilet when it is not needed) or going 'just in case' you might need to later. Try to void only when your bladder is full.

Other aspects of treatment

Avoid bladder irritants: Substances that irritate the bladder muscle make incontinence worse by making the bladder more likely to contract involuntarily. They include coffee, tea and artificial sweeteners, such as aspartate.

Fluid management: A fluid intake of between 1500 millilitres and 2000 millilitres a day is needed to avoid constipation. (Other diseases, such as kidney or heart disease, may have an overriding influence on fluid intake.) Diuretics, such as caffeine, should be avoided.

Elevating devices: The use of a tampon to assist in elevating the pelvic floor is beneficial if you need temporary relief from symptoms (e.g. during exercise).

HRT: Hormone replacement therapy is useful in preventing or reducing incontinence in post-menopausal women. It is equally effective when taken as topical vaginal cream or when taken as tablets, patches or implants. (Topical creams do not have the side effects or additional benefits of the other forms.)

Drug and surgical treatments of incontinence are beyond the scope of this preventatively orientated book.

Further information

National Continence Help Line
Ph: 1800 330 066; website: www.contfound.org.au

Menopause and hormone replacement therapy (HRT)

Women often find the changes to their body that accompany menopause distressing. Menopausal changes occur due to the normal reduction in the production of the hormone oestrogen (from your ovaries). This process usually occurs gradually over a period of several years. Menopause happens at the time your periods cease (i.e. you don't have a period for the next 12 months) and this reflects an almost complete cessation of hormone production by your ovaries. Symptoms including menstrual (period) irregularities usually commence several years prior to the actual menopause and occur for about four to six years. On average the menopause occurs at 51 years, but the normal range is between 45 and 55 years. Hormone replacement therapy (HRT) is simply the replacement of this naturally occurring oestrogen with administered oestrogen supplements.

Replacement oestrogen is given every day, either as tablets, patches applied to the skin or pellets implanted under the skin. (The pellets last for about six months.) Oestrogen can also be applied locally in the vagina to relieve the vaginal symptoms of menopause, such as dryness, which may lead to painful sexual intercourse. When used in this manner alone, the oestrogen affects only the vaginal area and does not assist in reducing other menopausal symptoms or osteoporosis.

In women with a uterus, oestrogen should always be given with a progestin. This is because if oestrogen is taken alone there is an increased risk of cancer of the uterus. This also applies to women who have had an endometrial ablation operation. It needs to be emphasised that when oestrogen and progestin are taken together, there is no increased risk of uterine cancer.

The progestin is usually taken in the form of a tablet or skin patch and can be taken either for 10 to 14 days per month (usually in women who are within a year or two of the onset of their menopause) or continually (usually in women one or two years past their menopause).

Who needs HRT?

HRT should be offered to any woman who suffers significant symptoms due to reduced oestrogen, as long as there are no medical problems with its use. There are, however, two problems in quantifying the significance of menopausal symptoms. Firstly, symptoms affect women differently and, secondly, menopausal symptoms are often vague, therefore women may not attribute them to menopause.

To help overcome these problems, a list of 20 symptoms typically experienced by oestrogen-deficient women has been included in table 33. Each symptom is rated from 0 to 3 depending on the severity felt (0 for no symptom up to 3 for a severe problem). The scores for all 20 symptoms are then added, giving a range of scores from 0 to 60.

If you scored over 15, it indicates you probably have a significant oestrogen deficiency and your symptoms are likely to improve with the use of HRT. There are three questions you need to consider before you commence HRT, though.

- Would HRT significantly benefit my menopause symptoms?
- Does HRT provide other health benefits for me?
- Does HRT pose any health risks for me?

Additional health benefits of HRT

Protection against osteoporosis: HRT gives significant protection against osteoporosis, reducing the risk of fractures by 50 per cent. This benefit continues right through into old age as long as HRT is continued, but reduces quickly when HRT is ceased.

Reduced skin ageing: There is evidence that HRT may reduce changes to the skin through ageing.

Disadvantages/health risks of HRT

A slight increase in the incidence of breast cancer: HRT causes a very slight increase in the risk of breast cancer. It is thus appropriate for all women taking HRT to be aware of ways to minimise their risk of breast cancer, including self-breast examination and having

Table 33 Menopausal symptom checklist

Symptom	*Score**
Hot flushes	
Light headedness/dizziness	
Headaches	
Feeling of crawling under the skin	
Sleeplessness/altered sleep pattern	
Irritability	
Depression	
Feeling of being unloved/unappreciated	
Anxiety	
Mood changes	
Backache	
Joint pains	
Muscle pains	
New facial hair	
Dry skin	
Unusual tiredness	
Reduced sexual feeling	
Uncomfortable intercourse	
Dry vagina	
Passing urine more often	
Total score	

* Each of the above symptoms is rated from 0 to 3, depending on the severity felt by the woman (0 for no symptom up to 3 for a severe problem). The scores for all 20 symptoms are then added. A score of over 15 indicates significant menopausal symptoms.

Source: Royal Australian College of General Practitioners, CHECK PROGRAM—HRT, September 1998.

mammograms. The use of HRT in women who have had breast cancer needs to be discussed with your GP. It is also worth noting that *excessive* alcohol consumption is likely to increase breast cancer just as much as HRT and should be avoided in all women, especially those on HRT.

Cardiovascular disease: At present there is considerable controversy about any possible reduction in cardiovascular disease and HRT. In women with established coronary artery disease, there is some evidence that it may actually make coronary artery disease slightly worse. (The probable reason for this is that HRT increases, very slightly, the risk of clots forming.) Thus, it is presently recommended that HRT should not be used in women with established coronary artery disease.

The situation in women without coronary artery disease is yet to be determined. It has for some years been felt that lower blood cholesterol that occurs with taking HRT should cause a significant reduction in the incidence of coronary artery disease. There have, however, been no completed studies to show this effect and one that suggests a slight detrimental effect. In view of these findings, it is probably best not to assume any cardiovascular disease benefit from HRT and perhaps assume a slight detrimental cardiovascular effect from HRT.

Having said this, there is at present no cardiovascular reason that should prevent well, young women without cardiovascular disease from taking HRT as a treatment for their menopausal symptoms. Views relating to this topic are changing quickly and no doubt will have altered by the time this book has been published. For this reason, you will need to discuss this issue with your general practitioner. (You can also source information from the Australasian Menopause Society website—see the end of this section.)

Slight 'period' bleeding: In women with a uterus, oestrogen replacement will usually cause light periods. These will vary according to your age and the dose of progesterone given (as well as individual variation). In the time around menopause, oestrogen is given continuously (every day) with a course of progesterone being added for 10 to 14 days each month. Initially this will be associated with a slight withdrawal bleed that lasts for a few days and occurs a few days after each course of progesterone is ceased. This will hopefully reduce with time.

Once you have been on HRT for about two years, your uterus is less hormone sensitive and the program can be changed to taking both oestrogen and progesterone every day. Slight break-through bleeding often occurs in the first six months of this combination and then bleeding usually ceases. If it continues, you need to consult your doctor. (Unfortunately, if this combination is given around menopause, it leads to more significant and inconvenient irregular break-through bleeding.)

Slight increase in the incidence of deep venous thrombosis: The incidence of deep venous thrombosis is increased to about two times the normal. (The most common form of this disease is clots in the legs.)

Oestrogen side effects: Oestrogen symptoms include breast discomfort and enlargement, headaches, abdominal bloating, pelvic discomfort and nausea. These can usually be reduced or prevented by adjusting the dose of oestrogen given. Older women commencing HRT who are well past their menopause need to start on a very low dose as they are particularly sensitive to these symptoms. Their doses can then be increased very gradually.

Other minor disadvantages: These may include a slightly increased risk of developing gallstones, dry eyes and a worsening of migraines and autoimmune diseases if you already have these problems. HRT is not effective as a form of contraception.

There are several conditions that have been incorrectly attributed to HRT. HRT does not cause an increase in blood pressure, an increased risk of diabetes, an increased risk of uterine cancer (as long as it is given with progestin), or an increase in weight. If any weight gain does occur, it is no more than the normal average for the age group.

Potential contra-indications to HRT

Women who have had or have an increased risk of the following medical problems need to discuss these issues with their doctor before commencing HRT:

- breast cancer
- cardiovascular disease
- deep venous thrombosis (clots)
- autoimmune diseases, migraines
- uterine (endometrial) cancer.

Many women with the above conditions may still be able to take HRT.

When should you stop HRT?

The length of time you take HRT will depend on the reason that you are taking it. Women who are using it solely for the relief of menopausal symptoms should review its use after about two years. They should also start on a small dose and increase it gradually until symptoms are relieved. In this way they will ensure they are taking the minimum dose possible.

Women who take HRT to reduce their risk of osteoporosis need to take it for considerably longer. To gain significant benefit with respect to osteoporosis prevention, healthy women with no increased risk of breast cancer, cardiovascular disease or clotting would need to continue treatment for at least five and probably ten years.

While HRT use does decrease the incidence of osteoporosis, there is considerable debate as to whether there is any overall health benefit for women who take HRT for longer than a couple of years. This is especially the case in women who are at increased risk of breast cancer, deep venous thrombosis (clots) or vascular disease (heart attack and stroke). Opinion regarding the use of HRT for osteoporosis is changing quickly, so you will need to discuss this matter with your medical practitioner. There are other treatments available for osteoporosis as well as HRT, but few other preventative options.

Much of this controversy has been brought about by the findings of the WHI (Women's Health Initiative) study relating to a slight increase in breast cancer and cardiovascular disease in study participants who took HRT. The reporting of this study was, unfortunately, misleading. Firstly, the increase in these conditions was very slight and the overall risk for women using HRT was still very small. Secondly, the average age of women in the study was 63 and a significant number had risk factors for vascular disease. Such women are not normally prescribed HRT in Australia and the findings are thus less relevant to the use of HRT by most Australian women. Also the study only looked at one type and one dose of HRT and there are other perhaps more suitable alternatives that may not have caused the above effects.

Other treatments for menopause

There are several other treatments for menopausal symptoms for those women who cannot take HRT or do not wish to do so.

Tibolone

Once in the body, tibolone breaks down into three separate active compounds that have effects similar to that of traditional HRT on various body tissues. They are as effective in preventing bone loss as oestrogen-based HRT, thus they should be equally effective in preventing fractures, although there is little data to confirm this. Also they reduce menopausal symptoms including hot flushes, night sweats, dizziness, fatigue, sleeplessness, irritability, mood problems and vaginal symptoms such as dryness. Tibolone also has the advantage of not having oestrogen-like effects on the uterus and breasts. This provides several benefits over conventional HRT, including no breast soreness and allows most women to be 'bleed free' after three months of treatment. As with the oestrogen/progesterone HRT, there is no increased risk of uterine cancer.

This medication does have a slight 'male hormone' (androgenic) effect. While this may benefit mood and libido, it may also cause a reduction in 'HDL cholesterol', increasing vascular disease risk. At present, this medication is not on the medical benefits schedule and patients must pay the full cost of the medication. There is little data regarding cardiovascular, breast cancer, or thrombosis (clotting) risk with this drug.

Raloxifene

Raloxifene is a selective oestrogen receptor modulator. Like tibolone, it causes less vaginal bleeding and breast symptoms than HRT but is less effective with regard to hot flushes. Raloxifene (about $90 per month) is much more expensive than tibolone (about $35 per month), and neither are on the Pharmaceutical Benefits Scheme.

Phytoestrogens

While there is some evidence that phytoestrogens are of benefit in reducing symptoms associated with menopause, they are nowhere near as good as HRT. A recent report (Glazier 2001) looked at 74 studies on phytoestrogens and menopause. It found that they did reduce some menopausal symptoms, but that this effect was quite small and often not of great benefit, especially when compared to traditional HRT. (The benefit is about the same as taking a placebo.) There was also some evidence that some of them could reduce cholesterol and that some reduce osteoporosis.

A significant problem with phytoestrogens is that there are numerous types and there is not enough evidence to sort out which ones are most beneficial. Also, there is little information regarding appropriate dosages or the side effects of taking larger doses than those contained in our normal diets. Soy-derived isoflavones are an often-promoted source of phytoestrogens.

Further information

Australasian Menopause Society
Website: www.menopause.org.au

International Menopause Society
Website: www.imsociety.org

North American Menopause Society
Website: www.menopause.org

Part 8

Osteoporosis, injuries, asthma and other preventative health issues

Osteoporosis

Osteoporosis occurs when bone becomes more porous than normal—that is, the density of bone is less. The bone that is present is normal in structure. As calcium is the main constituent of bone, accounting for 67 per cent of your bone mass, osteoporotic bone has a reduced-calcium density. This reduced bone density makes the bones weaker and increases the risk of fractures.

Scientifically, osteoporosis is defined as a bone mineral density (BMD) at any site in the skeleton that is 2.5 standard deviations (or 25 per cent) below the 'normal' mean (i.e. the norm for a young, healthy person). Bone density is usually measured by an X-ray technique called dual X-ray absorptiometry (DXA).

It is important to realise your bones do not stay the same as you age. They are continually changing, with new bone being added and old bone being resorbed. In osteoporosis, this balance tilts in favour of bone and calcium removal. The most common cause of this altered balance in women is the lowering of the hormone oestrogen that occurs with menopause. Peak bone density is reached in early adulthood and unless there is some medical problem, this level does not change greatly until menopause in women and about 50 years of age in men.

Figure 27 shows the bone loss that occurs in males and untreated women with age and indicates the likely age osteoporosis will occur—65 years in untreated women and 75 years in men. Osteoporosis is a normal, although unfortunate, ageing process. While appropriate diet and exercise will help minimise the problem, you cannot assume it will definitely prevent it. Many women (and men) will suffer the fractures that result from this problem unless they receive treatment with medication.

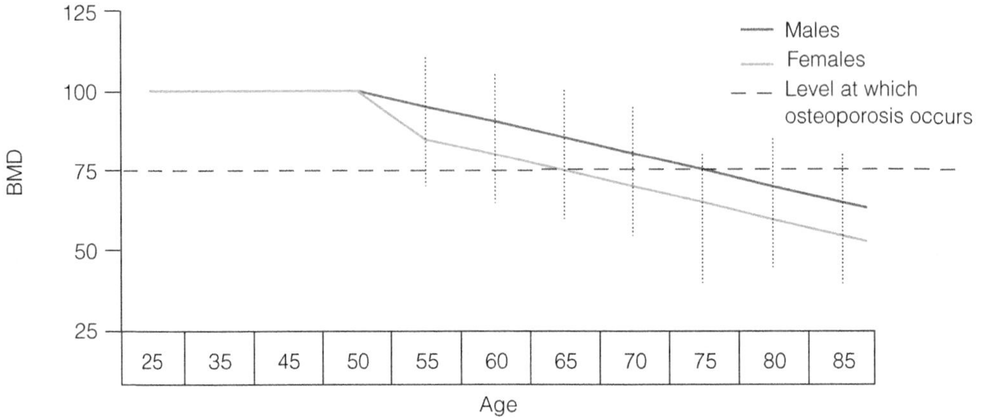

Figure 27 Bone mineral density change through life

In women, bone loss occurs quickly once menopause starts unless hormone replacement medication is taken. Five years after menopause, 15 per cent of bone mass has been lost, with most occurring in the first couple of years. (Five per cent in first year after menopause, 4 per cent in the second, 3 per cent in the third, 2 per cent in the fourth and 1 per cent in the fifth.) This may seem like a small amount, but by the age of 70, women will have lost 30 per cent of the bone mass they had at 50 years of age.

As a general guide, the risk of fractures doubles with each 10 per cent loss of bone mass and with each ten years of age. Table 35 gives an indication of how these age changes affect the likelihood of fractures. By the age of 70, a woman not treated for osteoporosis is 32 times more likely to have a fracture than she was at 50 years of age. The use of oestrogen replacement reduces these risk levels by 50 per cent.

Bone mineral density (BMD) also steadily decreases in men after the age of 50, although the initial rate is slower than that of women. (Men lose about 0.5 to 1 per cent of bone mass per year after reaching 50.) Approximately 30 per cent of males over 60 years of age will also experience a fracture due to osteoporosis during their lifetime. However, due to lack of awareness of osteoporosis as a causal factor, as few as 5 per cent of these men receive treatment for their osteoporosis. For this reason, any male over 50 who has a fracture with minimal trauma should be investigated for osteoporosis. Underlying medical causes for osteoporosis are more common in men. Sixty per cent of males with a fracture due to osteoporosis have an underlying medical cause, the most common being male hormone abnormalities, excess alcohol intake, chronic diseases, and the use of prescribed steroid medications.

Facts about osteoporosis

- Osteoporosis is much more common in women than men and occurs principally after menopause due to reduced oestrogen levels.
- Sixty per cent of women suffer bone fractures due to osteoporosis at some time during their lives.
- Twenty-six per cent of those suffering with these fractures do not regain independence and remain in nursing homes for the rest of their lives.
- Three per cent of women with fractures die of complications resulting from the fractures (especially hip fractures).
- About 30 per cent of men suffer an osteoporotic bone fracture at some time during their lives, although they occur later than in women. (The fracture incidence in men would be close to that in women if men lived as long.)
- The spine is the most common site for osteoporotic fractures and about 65 per cent of these fractures occur without symptoms. These need to be diagnosed by X-ray, with a loss of height greater than 20 per cent in any part of the vertebral body signifying a fracture.

Table 34 Risk of fracture in untreated women compared to risk at age 50 years*

Age	*Risk of fracture due to age*	*Risk of fracture from bone loss (% bone loss)*	*Total risk of fracture compared to a woman aged 50*	
			with no HRT	*with continuous HRT*
50	1 time	1 time (0%)	1 time	1 time
60	2 times	4 times (20%)	8 times	4 times
70	4 times	8 times (30%)	32 times	16 times

* Assumes menopause starts at age 50

Source: Royal Australian College of General Practitioners CHECK PROGRAM—HRT, September 1998.

Osteoporosis risk factors

Numerous factors and diseases cause an increased risk of osteoporosis. The most important risk factors are:

- Menopause in women when HRT is not being used
- History of fracture after 40 years of age

- Family history of osteoporosis or likely osteoporotic fractures
- Smoking
- Low bodyweight, especially with eating disorders such as anorexia. This can also occur in people who over-exercise, such as elite athletes.

Other important risk factors include:

- Low calcium intake.
- Immobilisation—people confined to wheelchairs or bed.
- Lifestyle factors—excess alcohol consumption, smoking and lack of exercise all increase bone calcium loss.
- Predisposing medical conditions, including conditions causing excess glucocorticoid (steriod) secretion, chronic renal or liver disease, Turner's syndrome, male hypogonadism, rheumatoid disorders, malabsorption disorders and primary hyperparathyroidism.
- Medications. An important cause is prolonged use of medical steroid therapy. All people, male or female, on more than 7.5 mg per day of the drug prednisone or 2000 mg per day of beclomethasone (a steroid spray used for asthma) for three months or more should be investigated for osteoporosis. Excess thyroxine, some epilepsy medications (especially phenytoin) and loop diuretics such as frusemide (Lasix) also cause increased bone resorption. A calcium-retaining thiazide diuretic would be a better choice that frusemide.

For women, it is important that the above risk factors are considered before as well as at menopause as they need to be identified and avoided or treated as early as possible.

Osteoporosis Australia's one-minute risk test

The risk of osteoporosis can be assessed by using Osteoporosis Australia's 'One Minute Risk Test'. If you answer 'yes' to any of the following questions, you have an increased risk of osteoporosis and a consultation with your GP is advisable.

1. Have either of your parents broken a bone after a minor bump or fall?
2. Have you broken a bone after a minor bump or fall?
3. For women after menopause, did you undergo menopause before the age of 45?
4. For women before menopause, have your periods stopped for 12 months or more (other than with pregnancy)?
5. For men, have you ever suffered from impotence, lack of libido or other symptoms associated with low testosterone?
6. Have you ever taken corticosteroid (prednisone, cortisone) tablets or used large doses of steroid puffers for respiratory diseases such as asthma?

7. Have you lost more than 5 centimetres of height?
8. Do you regularly drink heavily (above the safe driving limits)?
9. Do you suffer frequently from diarrhoea?

Diagnosing osteoporosis

Osteoporosis is diagnosed by measuring your BMD. It is recommended for those women who are at significant risk of developing osteoporosis. This includes the following:

- all postmenopausal women over 60 who are not taking HRT
- women who have suffered a fracture with minimal trauma after the age of 40
- postmenopausal women not on HRT who have other significant risk factors including smoking, low body weight and a family history of osteoporosis.

Even without the presence of an increased risk, some women may choose, quite reasonably, to have their bone density measured around menopause as a precaution. After menopause your bone loss will accelerate rapidly and any existing osteoporosis is best diagnosed before this time so that preventative measures can be taken to minimise further loss. BMD measurement is only eligible for a Medicare rebate in a few circumstances, such as when an osteoporotic fracture is present. You will need to check with your GP as to whether you fall into one of these categories. Women choosing to have BMD measured as a precaution have to pay all the costs involved.

The most common method of measuring BMD is dual X-ray absorptiometry. The measurement of BMD at any site in the body is a good predictor of the bone density at all sites in the body. Initial assessment is usually done at the femoral neck (the hip) with further monitoring at the wrist. Measurements taken are the most consistent (i.e. reproducible) at the wrist and least reliable at the spine, with the hip in the middle. For this reason, a change in BMD of 1 to 2 per cent in the wrist may be significant but the same change may only be normal result variability in the spine.

The 'T' score measures the variation of BMD above or below what is normal for a young, healthy woman (or man). The units of measurement are standard deviations, with each standard variation equalling a 10 per cent change from the above normal score. As a general rule, the risk of fracture doubles with each standard deviation below the normal mean. A 'T' score of negative one indicates a bone density 10 per cent below the average and that you have twice the risk of having a bone fracture due to bone loss as a young, healthy person. A 'T' score of negative three, 30 per cent below the average, increases the risk of fracture to eight (i.e. 2 × 2 × 2) times.

Table 35 'T' scores for bone mineral density (BMD)

Score	*Risk of fracture due to osteoporosis*
A positive score	Above normal BMD and a risk of fractures below that of a young, normal person.
0	The same level of risk as a young, healthy person.
Negative 1 to negative 2.5 (i.e. 1 to 2.5 standard deviations below normal)	A bone density 10 to 25% below that of a young, healthy person. A slightly increased risk of fractures
Less than negative 2.5 (i.e. over 2.5 standard deviations below normal)	A bone density greater than 25% below that of a young, healthy person. Osteoporosis present. A significantly increased risk of fractures.

The 'Z' score also measures BMD, but instead of comparing your result with the reading for a young person, it compares your result with the result for what is considered normal for your age group. Thus, the 'Z' score gives an indication of how your BMD compares with the normal for your age group. If the 'Z' score is less than negative two (i.e. more than 20 per cent below the normal for a healthy person of the same age), it is an indication that, in addition to bone loss from normal ageing, there is bone loss due to an additional medical problem.

While bone ultrasound testing done with good equipment and a competent operator is also reliable in determining bone density and in predicting the likelihood of future fractures, X-ray is still the preferred investigation. Ultrasound heel testing, usually offered in shopping centres, is less accurate and any positive test needs to be repeated with a proper X-ray. (It can sometimes give false positive and false negative tests; that is, it indicates that some people without osteoporosis have the problem and vice versa.)

Prevention and treatment of osteoporosis

Most women and men feel that lifestyle measures, including diet and exercise, will provide adequate protection against osteoporosis. Unfortunately, as figure 27 showed, this is not the case. Many people will need to use medication as well. Prevention can be divided into four areas:

- lifestyle
- treating any medical causes, including prescribed medications
- using medications that will slow or reverse bone loss
- and fall prevention measures.

Lifestyle measures

Successful prevention of osteoporosis relies on attaining maximum BMD levels in childhood and maintaining these levels as much as possible during adult life. The lifestyle factors that contribute to maximising BMD are:

- maintaining an adequate calcium intake throughout life
- maintaining adequate weight-bearing exercise to increase bone calcium levels and to help maintain adequate levels of fitness and agility to reduce the risk of fractures
- reducing alcohol consumption to two drinks per day (the maximum beneficial level)—alcohol increases bone resorption and can reduce calcium absorption from the bowel
- ceasing tobacco use, as smoking increases bone resorption
- maintaining adequate vitamin D levels.

ADEQUATE CALCIUM INTAKE

A recent study of 1000 women in Australia (Pasco 2000) found that 76 per cent had calcium intakes less than that recommended by the National Health and Medical Research Council. It also found 14 per cent had a severely low intake level of less than 300 mg per day. Table 36 shows the recommended calcium intake for men and women.

As well as being the best source of dietary calcium, dairy products also provide calcium that is the most easily absorbed from the intestine. To achieve adequate calcium intake from diet alone, you need dairy products of some sort. The best way to achieve this is with two 250 ml glasses of calcium-enriched low-fat milk. These milks have no fat and about 400 mg

Table 36 Daily recommended calcium intakes

Person	*Recommended calcium intake (mg per day)*
Males	
up to 11 years	800
12–15 years	1200
16–18 years	1000
19 years and over	800
Females	
up to 7 years	800
8–11 years	900
12–15 years	1000
16–54 years	800
Post-menopausal	1000
Pregnant—First two trimesters	1100
Pregnant—Last trimester and lactating	1200

of calcium per 250 ml serving (or 160 mg per 100 ml). Other low-fat dairy products, such as low-fat yoghurts, can also be used but be careful with reduced-fat cheeses as they still have a considerable fat content and much of it is saturated fat. Soy products with added calcium are a good alternative if you can't consume dairy products.

Post-menopausal women require 1000 mg of calcium per day and, as can be seen from the above figures, many women find this difficult to achieve from diet. For women who can't get adequate calcium from their diet, calcium supplements will need to be used. When using these supplements, be careful not to confuse the weight of the calcium contained in each tablet with the total weight of calcium carbonate in each tablet. It is the weight of the calcium that you need to know. Depending on the tablet, this can vary from 20 to 600 mg of calcium per tablet. Therefore, you must check when purchasing or when your doctor prescribes calcium tablets.

Calcium absorption can be affected by the foods you eat. Substances that can decrease absorption include tannins in tea, iron, caffeine, excess alcohol, the phosphate in soft drinks and phylates, which are present in fibre. Calcium carbonate is best absorbed with food but does interfere with iron absorption. Calcium lactate, citrate and gluconate can be taken at any time. Salt, caffeine and an excess intake of protein foods can also increase calcium loss in your urine.

Vitamin D helps increase calcium absorption from the bowel and helps in depositing calcium in the bone. It can be sourced from oily fish, eggs and milk products. The best source, however, is sunlight, which allows your body to produce its own vitamin D. Lack of vitamin D is mainly a problem for those with a poor diet or who have limited sunlight exposure—mostly house-bound elderly people. For these people, vitamin D supplements should be considered, whether osteoporosis is present or not.

EXERCISE

Exercise in people without osteoporosis: Daily exercise helps keep your bones strong and aids in the prevention of injury. Exercise during childhood and adolescence is particularly important for increasing bone mass and strength, while adult exercise is important in maintaining the levels achieved. To be beneficial, your osteoporosis exercise needs to be done regularly, at least three times a week, every week throughout your life. The benefits of exercise quickly reverse once you stop.

Only the bones placed under stress during exercise benefit, so it is very important to perform a wide variety of exercises that affect the bones in your arms, legs and trunk. There are two main types of exercise that are beneficial for osteoporosis: weight-bearing and strengthening (resistance) exercise.

Weight-bearing exercise involves being in an upright position, allowing gravity to have an effect. It includes walking, jogging, netball, gymnastics, tennis, dancing and golf. Resistance or strength training usually involves the use of weights on your arms and legs while doing an exercise routine, and it can be done on land or in the water. Gradually increasing the size of the weights used will increase the benefit. One to three sets of eight to twelve repetitions at least three times a week is recommended. High-impact sports that involve activities such as jumping are also beneficial, as are balance and co-ordination exercises. Arthritis and the risk of injury makes participation in high impact sports difficult as people age and such activities should be replaced by resistance exercises in association with balance training in this age group.

To avoid injury, all exercise programs need to be introduced gradually. A consultation with your GP is recommended before starting, especially if you are over 45, have an existing medical problem, or have not been exercising regularly.

Exercise in people with osteoporosis and older people: While similar principles apply to those mentioned above, this group is at increased risk of injury from exercising and should definitely consult their GP before starting. Certain exercise limitations and precautions are also needed including:

- avoiding jarring, high-impact, twisting or abrupt movements
- avoiding abdominal curl-up type exercises
- avoiding forward bending from the waist, especially if carrying any weight
- avoiding heavy lifting
- weight-bearing exercise may also not be appropriate for those with established osteoporosis.

In people with osteoporosis, it is more appropriate to aim at achieving improved muscle strength, balance and stability, and co-ordination, as all these attributes can help prevent falls. A strengthening exercise program and a falls prevention program are better at achieving these aims. Water exercises may be of benefit for frail people or in those recovering from a fracture. Tai Chi is also advocated for some people.

It is best to have an individual program designed for you by a physiotherapist. Their supervision can also help you reduce the risk of falls and they can give advice regarding the relief of acute and chronic pain that may be associated with your osteoporosis.

Fall prevention is an important area of health prevention, especially if you have osteoporosis or are elderly and this is discussed below. Also, special pads can be worn to protect the hips. These pads reduce the risk of hip fractures from falls by about 50 per cent.

How much exercise: Exercises should be introduced gradually until you achieve about 30 to 40 minutes a day, four days a week. This does not have to be done continuously. It can be broken up into several smaller amounts during the day. Pain is usually a sign you are over-exercising or that something is wrong and you should consult your doctor if this occurs.

Finally, over-exercising can be as bad as under-exercising. Young female athletes and dancers are two groups likely to over-exercise. You should not allow exercise to reduce your weight below a body mass index of 20, and should definitely not allow it to affect your menstruation, as this will actually cause bone loss, not gain. You need to see your doctor if you stop menstruating due to weight loss.

Adjusting medication that exacerbates osteoporosis

Several medications can exacerbate osteoporosis and should be avoided where possible in elderly people or those with established osteoporosis. These are mentioned in the section on causes of osteoporosis. Drugs that increase the risk of falls should also be ceased where possible. (See fall prevention section.)

Medications to reduce osteoporosis progression

OESTROGEN (HORMONE REPLACEMENT) THERAPY

Oestrogen therapy is the most effective treatment for preventing osteoporosis in post-menopausal women. This oestrogen needs to be given continuously with no monthly break and is normally given with a progesterone hormone.

You will need to take hormone replacement therapy (HRT) for a prolonged period (10 years at least) to gain a significant benefit for osteoporosis prevention. There is, however, considerable debate at present as to whether the adverse effects of HRT outweigh the benefits of osteoporosis prevention (see pages 319–22).Views regarding this matter are changing quickly and you will need to discuss the subject with your GP.

OTHER MEDICATIONS

Bisphosphonates reduce bone breakdown and may increase bone density and are commonly used for osteoporosis. Side effects include nausea, heartburn and stomach pains. Tibolone and raloxifene can also be used and were discussed on page 323. The naturally occurring hormone calcitonin increases bone density in the spine and is occasionally employed. These medications are usually utilised for the treatment of osteoporosis rather than its prevention.

Fall prevention

Falls are a huge problem for elderly Australians with one in three Australians over the age of 65 falling each year (and one in two over the age of 80). While luckily only a few of these falls are serious, resulting in fractures, they still have very significant consequences. A fall reduces the confidence of an elderly person, making them less likely to engage in physical activity in the future. This leads to less physical competence and an increased likelihood of falling again. Fifty per cent of those who have fallen once will fall again. Falls are the sixth most common cause of death in the elderly and the most common cause of a person's placement in a nursing home.

What to do

Preventing falls requires an overall assessment of the person and their environment by doctors, physiotherapists and social workers. Physical impairments, such as low blood pressure, lower limb arthritis, gait and balance problems, and visual and hearing abnormalities, need to be assessed and, where necessary, medication adjusted. Drugs associated with a high risk of falls include anti-hypertension medications and drugs for the treatment of mental health problems, such as depression, anxiety and schizophrenia. The risk of falling can also be reduced by physical activity programs to improve gait and balance, and by creating a safer home environment, both internally and externally.

If you have already had a fall or lack confidence in your physical activity capabilities, proper assessment can help prevent you falling in the future. You should also be assessed if you have any of the following risk factors for falls or fractures:

- osteoporosis
- giddiness, feeling faint
- arthritis
- weakness or walking abnormalities, such as unsteadiness—these can be caused by neurological conditions or numerous other chronic medical problems
- being on multiple medications (four or more)
- acute illness or recent hospital discharge
- visual and hearing impairment
- postural hypotension (dizziness from low blood pressure that occurs when rising from a lying position)
- depression.

Altogether, those requiring assessment include at least 25 per cent of those over 70 years of age. However, anyone who wishes to reduce their risk of falls should seek assessment.

Postural hypotension is dizziness due to a fall in blood pressure that occurs when getting into an upright position. Assuming there is no correctable cause for this problem (especially medications), people who get dizzy getting out of bed need to assess how long it takes their blood pressure to adjust to an upright position. This can vary from half a minute to ten to 20 minutes. During this time you need to remain seated on the edge of the bed.

Physical activity and home assessment programs

Being physically active is one of the best ways to minimise the risk of falls. It is important that your physical activity program is designed specifically for you, as different people have different physical and medical problems. You should not start without seeing your GP and physiotherapist first. Programs organised by a physiotherapist should aim to achieve balance, mobility and strength and include strategies to improve confidence in mobility.

Education concerning minimising the risk of falls and assessment regarding home hazards, illness, medications, and the need for a walking aid should all be part of the program.

Tips to avoid falls outdoors

Most outdoor falls happen on uneven surfaces, wet floors, and curbs and steps, and commonly occur when bending or turning or in the dark. The following practical tips are useful in minimising these dangers.

Use glasses if you need them and, on sunny days, sunglasses and a hat to reduce glare. Ensure stairs and pathways are well lit and avoid walking in the dark at night or carry a torch when you do. Allow your eyes to adjust to a darkened environment before proceeding.

Avoid slippery or uneven surfaces and be aware of curbs, gutters, steps, and broken paving stones. Look ahead to help anticipate problems/obstacles and slow down when approaching them. Keep pathways swept and clear of obstacles, such as garden tools, toys, pets and children. Wear low-heeled, well-fitting shoes with a good tread.

Consider installing stair rails and use walking aids if needed.

(Adapted from publications from the National Ageing Research Group.)

Tips to avoid falls indoors

All flooring needs to be dry and not heavily waxed or slippery. Ensure there is no loose carpet and fix rugs with non-skid backing. Avoid dim lighting in the home and you can also install movement sensitive lights near stairs and in the bathroom.

Ensure stairs are in good repair, place non-slip, easily-seen adhesive strips on all treads, and ensure stairs are lit with switches at the top and bottom. In the bathroom, use rubber mats on the floor and in the shower and the bath. Avoid door locks in bathrooms/toilets and place a seat in the bathroom if needed. Medicine cabinets should be well lit with drugs clearly labelled.

In the kitchen, place a rubber mat near the sink and wear rubber soled shoes. Store frequently used objects at waist height to avoid bending. Avoid tripod or pedestal style tables.

Around the house, be aware of any children's toys, shoes left on the ground, and grandchildren or pets playing. Avoid moving furniture into positions that may cause obstructions. The pathway to the toilet should be unobstructed. All furniture should be in good repair. An ideal chair should allow your feet to reach the floor with knees at a 90 degree angle. Avoid chairs with wheels.

(Adapted from publications from the National Ageing Research Group.)

Further information

Osteoporosis Australia
An accident and falls prevention video is available by ringing 1800 242 141 from anywhere in Australia. Also provided are books on fall prevention and information on falls clinics and programs. Website: *www.osteoporosis.org.au*

National Ageing Research Centre
Ph: (03) 8387 2148; Website: www.nari.unimelb.edu.au

The Osteoporosis Society of NSW
Ph: (02) 9683 1622

Accidents and injuries

Disability and death through preventable accidents are a major problem in our society. Falls, road accidents, poisoning, drowning and workplace injuries are almost all preventable and account for over 5 per cent of the total burden of disease in the overall population. They are even more important in children.

Childhood accidents and injuries

Injury is a leading cause of child death and disability in Australia, being responsible for 12 and 9 per cent of the total burden of disease in boys and girls respectively. Boys are considerably more likely to be injured than girls in all types of injuries, with bicycle and pedestrian injuries and drowning being particular problems. In boys, the highest rate of hospitalisation was in the 1 to 4 and 10 to 14 year age groups. In girls, it occurred in the 1 to 4 age group. Over 50 per cent of injuries occur in the home, with another 25 per cent occurring at school or associated with sport.

Injury is more common in rural and, especially, remote areas. Compared to metropolitan areas, death from injury was 1.6 times more common in rural areas and 2.9 times more common in remote areas. Children on farms also suffer different types of injury, with drowning and injury involving farm equipment often being involved. Injury is more common in poorer communities, especially by motor vehicle accidents and drowning.

In decreasing order of importance, the incidence of childhood injuries in 1996 was:

- Motor vehicle accidents—the provision of adequate child restraints and their use until the child is large enough to safely use adult seat belts is a major issue.
- Falls, which are common in all age groups, especially after infants start walking.
- Drowning, which occurs mostly in the 1 to 4 year age group—the incidence in boys is three times that of girls. Thirty-three per cent of drownings occur in swimming pools.
- Burns/scalds, which occur mostly in children 4 years of age or under.
- Bicycle and other transport-related accidents, especially boys aged between 10 and 14. Pedestrian accidents are important in children with the maximum incidence occurring in the 1 to 4 year age group and then decreasing with age.
- Suffocation by foreign bodies, which mainly affects the 0 to 4 year age group.
- Intentional injury (assault), which occurs mostly in children under 1 and in boys aged 10 to 14.

In addition to those mentioned above, there are other less-well recognised preventable causes of injury including poisonous plants, insect/animal bites and stings, dog bites, horse riding accidents, sudden infant death syndrome, and dangers associated with child furniture/equipment, such as bunk beds, cots, mattresses, chairs, strollers, ceiling fans, toys etc.

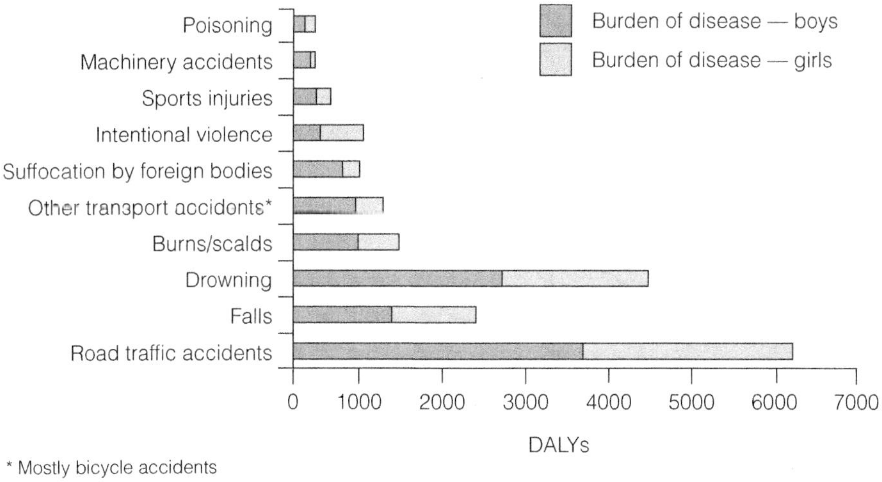

Source: Adapted from Australian Institute of Health and Welfare: Mathers, 1999.

Figure 28 Total burden of disease from injury and poisoning in boys and girls age 0 to 14 years in 1996

There is insufficient space in this book to cover all these topics. However, an excellent information source for all the above topics and many more is the website of The Children's Hospital at Westmead, a major paediatric hospital in Sydney, www.chw.edu.au/parents. Of special importance is their home safety check list. This can be accessed on www.chw.edu.au/parents/factsheets

Child protection in motor vehicles

The use of properly fitted approved child restraints is of paramount importance in protecting children in the car. These restraints must be fitted properly and children should not be moved out of their restraints before they are large enough to use the next sized restraint safely.

Infants should be kept in rear-facing restraints until they physically won't fit and should be able to sit and hold their head upright before moving into a forward-facing child seat. The child should stay in this seat until he or she is too big for it as it provides better protection than booster seats. An older child should not be moved into a booster seat because the child seat is needed for the next child. Booster seats should be rigid with side-wings and a sash guide to keep the belt in place. Remember, it is the size of the child, not their age, which determines when they can move up to the next size of restraint. It is never safe for someone to hold children in the car while driving.

For further information about child restraints, including their fitting, contact your state roads and traffic authority or your motorist organisation. The NSW RTA also tests and rates child restraints and produces a buyers guide with its recommendations. It is obtainable from the RTA website: www.rta.nsw.gov.au (look in: safety > road safety information > child restraints).

Children should never be left in a car alone. Parked cars can become hot very quickly, with the temperature inside reaching a level much greater than that outside. Most of this temperature rise occurs in the first five minutes and leaving the window open slightly makes little difference. Other risks include choking and even abduction of the child.

Fall prevention for children

Falls are the second most important cause of injury after motor vehicle accidents and they occur in all age groups. In the under five age group, most falls result from furniture, nursery equipment, stairs, and bicycles. Prevention includes the use of door gates and stair barriers, and always using harnesses in prams, strollers and high chairs. Avoid using baby walkers and never leave children alone on change tables or in supermarket trolleys.

Important issues with older children include ensuring play areas have soft fall surfaces (such as sand) that are at least 300 mm in depth under all play equipment, helmets are always worn when riding horses, bikes or skateboards, and elbow and knee pads are worn when using skateboards, scooters, roller blades or roller skates.

For all children, ensure bunk beds have guard rails and fixed ladders and don't allow wheeled riding toys on uneven surfaces. Try to have non-slip surfaces around the house where possible.

Drowning

Drowning is a major preventable health issue for Australian children and accounts for about 21 per cent of childhood deaths due to injury. About 750 children died from drowning in the period from 1991 to 2000. It is three times more common in boys and most prevalent in the one to four year age group.

As an Australian, you should ensure all members of your family can swim well and are adequately educated with regard to swimming safely in the surf. AUSTSWIM is Australia's national organisation for the teaching of swimming. The possession of an AUSTSWIM certificate is the industry standard for swimming teachers. Your local council or pool should be able to provide a list of accredited teachers or visit the AUSTSWIM website at www.austswim.com.au

Over 11 800 people were rescued from Australian beaches by lifesavers in 2001. To get more information regarding 'surf education', you can visit your local surf life saving club on any Sunday and enquire about the programs provided in your area. (Programs are also run through some schools.) You can also access the Surf Life Saving Australia website on www.slsa.asn.au And remember, swim between the flags! Other important issues in preventing childhood drowning include the following.

ADEQUATE SUPERVISION

It is essential adequate adult supervision is provided at all times when children are near water. It is also imperative the supervising adult does not consume any alcohol. When away from home, there is usually a delegated driver who can fill this role. The supervising adult should concentrate on this task and not be interrupted by numerous other activities. For example, it is not possible to prepare food at a picnic and watch children swim.

SAFE HOME ENVIRONMENT

Your home should be 'water safe'. Remember a child can drown in 5 centimetres of water. About a third of all childhood drownings occur in swimming pools, mostly in the one to four year age group. Adequate pool safety requires pool fencing with gates and locks that are well maintained, competent supervision of children at all times and the display of a CPR (cardiopulmonary resuscitation) chart (available from your local council). There should be no objects close to gates that might be used by children to climb on and open the gate lock.

Do not consider flotation aids as life-saving devices. They are no substitute for supervision. Spas should be emptied when not in use. In rural areas, dams, lakes, rivers etc. need to be checked for hidden dangers and access may need to be restricted to these swimming spots. This may require fencing in your home. Supervision of all water activities is essential.

Outside, open drains or garden ponds should be covered with a grill. Inside, children should never be left unsupervised in the bath. When very young children are about, all buckets filled with water, such as nappy buckets, should be covered and the lid should be kept on the toilet.

Finally, learning cardiopulmonary resuscitation (CRP) can help save the lives of your family and friends. Courses are available from St John's Ambulance www.stjohnnsw.com.au, The Royal Life Saving Society of Australia www.rlssa.org.au or the Red Cross of Australia www.redcross.org.au

Burn and scald prevention

Burns and scalds can occur from numerous sources, including scalding from hot water, contact burns, and flame burns. They are responsible for about 7 per cent of illness due to accidental injury and occur mostly around the home and in children under the age of five years. Contact burns occur most commonly from touching heaters, BBQs, ovens, irons and cigarettes. Preventative measures include the following:

- Place suitably-sized guards made of a heat-resistant or low-conducting metal around fires. These should be able to be secured to the floor or walls.
- Doorway barriers to keep children out of the kitchen when cooking and oven guards to prevent children touching hot oven doors and stove elements should be used. These also protect children from pulling pots and saucepans containing hot fluids over themselves.
- Keep children away from smoking adults and keep cigarettes, ashtrays and matches out of reach.
- Keep children away from BBQs, camp fires (which should be put out with water, not sand or dirt), hot exhausts from motor bikes, and hot tools such as soldering irons. Even lamps and the inside of a hot car can cause burns.

As well as being kept away from radiators and fires, children should wear night clothing that has a low fire danger. Well fitting clothes, such as track suits, are a good choice. All child night clothes sold in Australia must have a label stating the fire danger of the garment. Category one garments are the safest, being made from materials that are slow to burn. Category two garments are styled to reduce fire danger (like track suits) but are made of more flammable materials, and category three garments have a high fire danger.

Hot water is a very common source of burns. These occur mostly in the bathroom due to tap water that is too hot. Water at a temperature of 60°C can cause severe burns in one second, whereas water at 50°C takes five minutes. It is important to reduce the maximum temperature of bath tap water and this is best achieved by installing temperature controlling devices or by reducing the temperature setting of your hot water system. Other preventative measures include child-proof taps or taps that have a hot water limiter. It is also important to practise safe bathroom habits, such as keeping the bathroom door closed when not in use and not leaving the bath unattended once it has started being filled. (Taking the phone off the hook will help avoid interruptions.) Never run a hot tap by itself, test the water before putting the child in, and turn off taps tightly.

House fires are often started by children with matches. Lighters and matches should be kept away from children and child-resistant cigarette lighters should be used. It is important to install smoke detectors in your house and have two planned escape routes that the whole family knows well in case of fire.

If a child's clothing has caught alight, stop them from running, drop them to the floor, and roll them until the flames are extinguished. A blanket is helpful for this purpose. Remove clothing unless it is stuck to the skin and apply cold water to the burnt area for 30 minutes. Do not use ice and do not put anything else on the burn, such as creams. The child should be kept warm and medical help should be sought.

Choking on food

Young children cannot grind and chew properly and are therefore more likely to inhale larger pieces of food. For this reason, they should not be given small hard foods, such as nuts, popcorn, hard lollies or corn chips, or foods that can break off into hard pieces, such as raw carrots and pieces of apple. Hard foods need to be grated, cooked or mashed and meat and sausages should be cut into small pieces and have any hard skin removed.

Inhalation of food is more likely if children are moving about while eating, so ensure they sit quietly and an adult is present while they eat. Forcing your children to eat can increase the risk of choking.

Poisoning

Most poisonings occur in the home and involve children under the age of six years. The main causes of poisoning include:

- inappropriate storage of drugs and chemicals in the home
- product mislabelling, label misreading and putting chemicals or drugs into unlabelled containers
- excessive dosage of pharmaceutical drugs due to dosing errors and inappropriate prescribing
- recreational drug use.

In your home you should have a child-proof cabinet where medications, alcohol, and other drugs and dangerous household products, such as caustic detergents, automotive products, cleaning products etc., can be kept. Products should be returned to their safe storage place immediately after use. Children should not self-administer any medication, including paracetamol.

Out-of-date or unwanted medicines or chemicals should be disposed of promptly. A check should be made every three months. Purchase household products in child-resistant containers. Check your garden does not have poisonous plants.

All chemicals and medications should be kept in their original, properly labelled containers, and never put chemicals into a container that may be or was used for drink or food.

Adult accidents and injuries

Adult drowning

Alcohol is involved in about half of all adult drownings so you should not consume any alcohol or other intoxicating drugs before or while swimming. If you have a medical problem that compromises your swimming ability, you should either not swim at all or do so with others very close at hand if this is a safe option. Education regarding safe swimming in the surf is also important for adults.

Road safety

Road traffic accidents cause 2.2 per cent of disease burden in Australia and no discussion on accident avoidance would be complete without mentioning road safety. Campaigns to reduce road trauma are continually being run by governments, with the following issues being of paramount importance.

DRUGS AND DRIVING

Alcohol continues to be a major cause of motor vehicle accidents and to ensure your safety in the car, you must ensure the person driving has not consumed excess alcohol. You may find this difficult if the person is a family member or friend. However, if you expect your children to demonstrate this type of responsible behaviour, you should certainly do no less yourself. Remember, it only takes one accident. Excess alcohol should also not be consumed the night before a long day of driving.

As with alcohol, you should avoid illegal drugs when driving. Cannabis use is common in young people and it is also a major cause of motor vehicle accidents.

When purchasing any legal medication, be sure to ask whether it will have an effect on driving capability.

DRIVER FATIGUE

To ensure you do not suffer from driver fatigue, you should rest at least every two hours and avoid driving long distances after a long day at work or at night (especially in the early hours of the morning). Power napping will help you prevent driver fatigue if you have sleep deprivation and sharing the driving load can be a great help. You should be wary about driving when unwell.

Death rates from motor vehicle accidents are three times more common in country areas, so take special care. Contributing factors in addition to driver fatigue include poorer roads, speeding, and greater distances travelled per person. Make sure that, when undertaking long trips, your motor vehicle is fully roadworthy, as it should always be.

TEENAGE DRIVER EDUCATION

Driving when young can be a dangerous activity. Death rates from motor vehicle accidents in the 15 to 24 year age group are three times that of the general population and males of this age account for 20 per cent of hospitalisations due to road accidents (see figure 29). Thankfully obtaining a driver's licence is much more difficult than it used to be, with learners having to accumulate a considerable amount of on road experience. Make sure you assist your children by sharing your time and knowledge.

You should also be aware that novice teenage drivers (aged 17) have an increased risk of accidents of up to four times when they are driving with others under the age of 20 in the car. As a parent, you should consider advising your newly-licensed adolescent not to drive with other young people in the car until he/she has had more on-road experience. Similarly, your teenager should probably not be driven by other unexperience drivers where there is no accompanying adult.

DRIVING AND THE AGED

When approaching the end of your driving career, please do so gracefully and stop before you are made to do so. Be aware of your own limitations and take heed of any concerns expressed by family members, friends or your doctor. Injury to one's loved ones or others in the community is very hard to live with, especially if you were already aware of the problem that caused it. Likewise, if you have older family members that should not be driving, don't be afraid to express your concerns to them.

Workplace injuries

Workplace injuries are far too common in Australia. Most jobs are associated with some kind of risk, whether it be from working with machinery, working at heights, excessive tiredness from long hours etc. It is not always possible to reduce this risk level to zero, however the risk should always be minimised. This is the responsibility of all employees from top management down. Everyone is important and no accident is acceptable. The information provided in this section is by necessity a very general outline of the issues involved in workplace safety.

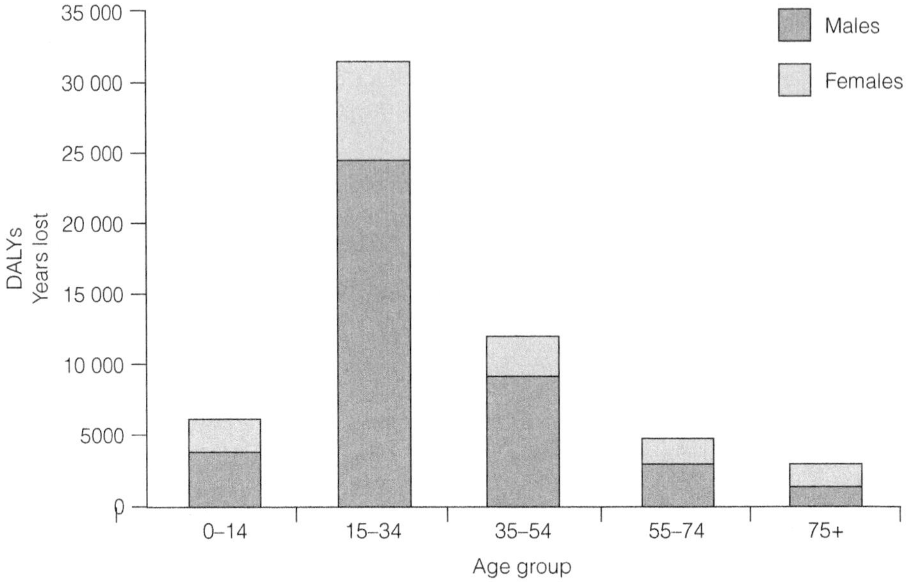

Source: Adapted from Australian Institute of Health and Welfare: Mathers, 1999.

Figure 29 Age related loss of years due to disability and death from motor vehicle accidents (1996)

The causes of workplace injury are numerous. They include unsafe attitudes, ignoring proper procedures, lack of knowledge regarding safe work practices, unsafe working equipment, a substandard working environment due to factors such as poor lighting, excess noise and moist floors, and distorted thinking due to fatigue, drug use, personal problems etc.

WAYS OF REDUCING WORKPLACE RISK

- Establish a workplace Occupational Health and Safety Committee at your workplace. These committees are of great benefit in reducing injury and are compulsory in businesses employing more than 20 people where the majority of employees request such a committee be formed. Workcover can advise on how to form such a committee.
- Determine what can be done to reduce risk. There are numerous people and organisations that can help provide this information, including an occupational health representative at your workplace, your union representative at work or the union you belong to, your employer, employer associations, Workcover in NSW (www.workcover.nsw.gov.au), Worksafe Australia—National Occupational Health and Safety Commission

(www.nohsc.gov.au), or private occupational health and safety consultants. (A directory is published by Workcover.) It is important those directly responsible for worker safety and the workers themselves be kept informed with up-to-date information about worker safety. This means the continued education about safety issues. There should also be written safety instructions for each job, if necessary in several languages, which are updated as needed.

- Provide safety equipment. The employer needs to provide and keep up-to-date all equipment needed to keep a safe working environment and to ensure that it is maintained in good condition.
- Provide adequate supervision by management to ensure worker compliance with safety procedures.
- Install effective systems to report hazards noticed by workers.
- Ensure there are effective ways of dealing with safety hazards.
- Create effective systems for checking the workplace for hazards.
- Have regular (at least annually) reviews of the health and safety program.
- Have an effective accident reporting system.
- Ensure the workplace is a drug-free environment, especially with regard to alcohol.

HEARING LOSS AND THE WORKPLACE

While adult-onset hearing loss is not a major cause of mortality, it is a major cause of disability in Australia. It is significantly more common in males and is a major workplace injury that receives insufficient attention, mainly because it usually develops slowly over a long period. Be aware of this fact and make sure that proper hearing protection is provided and used in your workplace (and at home).

Further information

Surf Life Saving Australia
Website: www.slsa.asn.au

Austswim
Website: www.austswim.com.au

Respiratory diseases

Asthma

Australia has one of the highest rates of asthma in the world, with about two million people being affected (about 20 per cent of children and 10 per cent of adults). Thus, it is not surprising that asthma is our ninth most important cause of disease burden.

Asthma is often considered a disease of the young and, indeed, most of the cases are diagnosed before the age of 15. However, the fact that asthma is a long-term condition means most asthmatics are actually adults and two-thirds of asthma disability occurs in people over the age of 15.

Prevention of asthma

Genetic predisposition makes the prevention of asthma difficult in most cases. Providing information about the prevention of asthma in infants is difficult because the issues involved are complicated and the knowledge base inadequate. However, there are a few points worth noting. Please remember that these relate to the prevention of developing asthma, not reducing its occurrence in those with the disease already.

- Prevention is only worthwhile considering in those children who are at high risk of developing the disease because they have a strong family history of asthma or other allergic conditions such as eczema. It has not been shown to benefit other children.

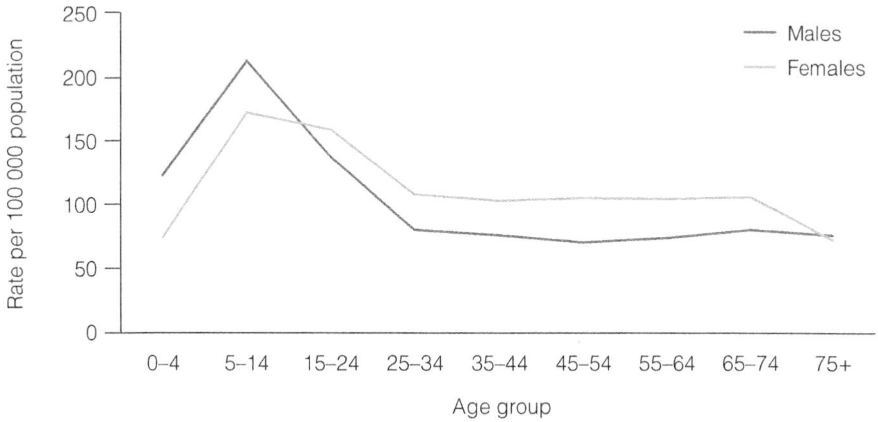

Source: Australian Institute of Health and Welfare, 2000.

Figure 30 Prevalence of asthma in Australia

- Avoiding cigarette smoke from both active and passive smoking definitely helps prevent asthma. This should start during the pregnancy and continue throughout life. This also helps avoid sudden infant death syndrome.
- While breastfeeding exclusively for the first six months of life has been shown in some studies to prevent asthma and other allergies in the long term, this benefit is not definite. There is also evidence that delaying the introduction of solids does not influence asthma. (Delaying solids till six months and allergenic foods, such as peanuts, milk, egg and tree nuts, until at least 12 months may help reduce eczema [Joshi 2002].) There is no advantage in dietary restrictions to prevent asthma or other allergic diseases in older children as sensitisation to these foods has occurred already.
- Avoiding the consumption of allergenic foods, such as cow's milk, peanuts, eggs, and fish, by the mother while breastfeeding is unlikely to reduce asthma incidence in the child, although it may give some protection against eczema in young high-risk infants. This benefit ceases after the first few years of life.
- Avoiding specific allergenic foods during pregnancy has no beneficial effect and may adversely influence maternal nutrition.
- Reducing exposure to house dust mites may be helpful in reducing sensitisation and thus asthma. Such measures need to continue throughout life and should begin during pregnancy. Thus, prevention measures need to be adopted in both the parents' and child's bedrooms. To date, such measures have been shown to provide benefits in the first few years of life. However, such preventative benefits seem to cease by the age of four (Joshi 2002).

- There is no clear evidence that preventing exposure to pets, including cats, helps prevent developing asthma or other allergies, although it may exacerbate the problem if already present.

Reduction/prevention of asthma attacks in people with asthma

The numerous risk factors detailed below can, if minimised, reduce asthma symptoms in many sufferers. Most people with asthma are sensitive to only a few of the triggers mentioned and restricting them all is unnecessary. You should see your doctor about identifying those that are of particular concern to you. All families with a history of asthma should strive to have a low-allergy home.

It is essential for all asthmatics to see their GP regularly to monitor their disease, have a management plan for exacerbations, and identify and minimise exposure to risk factors that help cause these exacerbations.

HOUSE DUST MITES

House dust mites are a significant trigger for asthma attacks. They occur commonly in temperate moist coastal climates, such as the east coast of Australia, and are encouraged by carpeted flooring, mattresses and feathered doonas/pillows. They are also in soft toys. Sensitivity to house dust mite needs to be diagnosed as early as possible because chronic exposure leads to increasingly severe reactions to the mite and these more severe asthma (and eczema) symptoms are difficult to treat. Reducing exposure in the first place is your best treatment option. (See boxed section below.)

House dust mite prevention

- Air your baby's bedding, including the mattress, in the sunlight regularly. This drying-out process reduces dust mites.
- Encase parent's and children's mattresses, doonas and pillows in good quality, impermeable mattress/pillow covers.
- Avoid sheep skins and soft toys in the cot, prams, and car capsules as they contain large numbers of dust mites.
- Wash all your baby's sheets and soft toys at least once a week.
- Putting your child's favourite toys in the freezer regularly kills mites.

- Keep your home dry and well aired, as this will reduce both moulds and house dust mites. Use extractor fans in the bathroom, kitchen and laundry, and keep windows open where possible.
- Areas commonly used by your children, such as playrooms and bedrooms, should not be carpeted as vacuum cleaners cannot adequately remove dust and dust mites from carpets.
- Clean your house regularly with damp dusting, damp mopping and vacuuming. The best vacuum cleaners have strong suction, a good filter system (HEPA, triple or electrostatic types) and double filter bags. Windows should be left open while vacuuming and for 20 minutes after vacuuming to help evacuate dust disturbed by vacuuming.

SMOKING

Both active and passive smoking increase the incidence of asthma and all homes should be free from cigarette smoke.

POLLENS

Most pollens do not travel far unless it is windy. You can usually avoid developing plant allergies by making sure you do not place plants that commonly cause allergies close to the house. In general, choose plants that are not heavily scented and are pollinated by birds and insects rather than by the wind. Avoid being in the garden on windy days, and hot still days. Compost heaps should also be avoided. Choose grasses that produce little pollen and don't need too much mowing, such as buffalo, and wear a protective mask when mowing. It is especially important to avoid allergenic grasses, such as Ryegrass and Timothy grass.

ANIMALS

Family pets are an area of controversy at present. In the past it was thought that exposure to pets, especially cats, increased the incidence of asthma in many sufferers. However, there is now some evidence this is not the case and that even the opposite may be true. Until there is more conclusive evidence one way or another, probably the best course to take is to live with the animals you have while your child is young. They should also probably not be allowed to sleep with children. Having said this, domestic animals, especially cats, do exacerbate asthma in some people. It is flakes of cat skin, not fur, that are mostly responsible for the cat-allergy problem. They can remain airborne for hours and are very difficult to get rid of, even if the cat has left the home for good. When animals are a problem, exposure needs to be avoided to minimise sensitisation. Animals should be kept outdoors whenever possible but this is difficult with cats as they tend to roam and attack native animals and birds. The decision to keep your pet will depend on the balance between symptoms and emotional attachment.

MOULDS

Sensitivity to moulds can cause significant asthma and reducing mould exposure in the house may help. This can be achieved by drying clothes outside, reducing home humidity by using exhaust fans or portable dehumidifiers, emptying kitchen garbage bins regularly and scrubbing bathroom crevices.

FOODS

Food is not a common trigger for asthma, with less than 2 per cent of adults and 11 per cent of children being affected. Symptoms usually occur within minutes of taking the food and include mouth swelling, vomiting, cramps, diarrhoea and skin rashes as well as asthma. Allergies to food are clear-cut and only foods that have been properly diagnosed by a specialist doctor as a trigger need to be excluded. Most people will be allergic to only one kind of food, the common ones being peanuts, shellfish and eggs. Contrary to popular belief, dairy products are an uncommon cause of asthma and should be part of your normal diet (especially low-fat varieties) unless you have a definitely diagnosed allergy. Food-induced asthma should be tested by blood or skin prick tests and then confirmed by your doctor with a well-supervised challenge test.

FOOD ADDITIVES

Sulphite preservatives (additive numbers 220 to 232 on food labels) used in wine making, preserving fruit, fruit juices, dried fruits, processed meats, canned fish, salads and pickled vegetables can make asthma worse. Colouring dyes such as tartrazine (additive number 102) are rarely a cause of asthma. Preservative-free products are available.

SIGNIFICANT AIR POLLUTION

If this is a problem, you will need to be careful about where you choose to live.

WORKPLACE IRRITANTS

Numerous allergens are found in the workplace including wood dust (especially western red cedar and oak), flour and grains, castor bean and green coffee bean, laboratory animals (especially rats), biologic enzymes (e.g. laundry detergents), metal salts (platinum, chrome, nickel) and industrial chemicals and plastics such as epoxy resins, isocyanates, toluene diisocyanate, persulfates, ethylenediamine, p-phenyl-enediamine, and trimellitic anhydride.

DRUGS

A number of drugs can cause or exacerbate asthma including aspirin, non-steroidal anti-inflammatory drugs used for arthritis, beta-blockers and some herbal preparations.

EXERCISE

A vital part of a good asthma plan is keeping fit and healthy. Exercising can, however, make your asthma worse. This occurs because you breathe more quickly through your mouth and the air that reaches your lungs does not get time to be warmed and moistened by passing slowly through your nose. This cooler, drier air causes your airways to become narrower. Your doctor can help you manage this problem so you can be active and play sport. This management usually involves using puffers five to ten minutes before you warm up and perhaps longer-term preventative medication. You should always warm up for 15 to 20 minutes before exercising and cool down afterwards. Always have your reliever medication with you while exercising. If you get symptoms, you should stop and use the medication. Scuba diving should not be done by asthmatics.

EMOTIONAL STRESS

People who find stressful situations a problem for their asthma should take preventative measures before such stress occurs. They should also carry medication.

RESPIRATORY TRACT INFECTIONS

Such infections commonly exacerbate asthma. Preventative asthma medication needs to be increased while the infection is present.

POLYUNSATURATED FATS

Omega-3 fats have anti-inflammatory qualities that theoretically might reduce the incidence of asthma. It has been suggested that one reason for the increase in asthma over recent years might have been the increase in the intake of omega-6 polyunsaturated fats, mainly as margarines, which has led to an imbalance in the ratio of omega-6 fats and omega-3 fats. There is, however, no hard evidence this has caused an increase in asthma, and, in any event, this imbalance is becoming less of a problem due to the increasing use of monounsaturated fats in margarines in preference to polyunsaturated omega-6 fats. Increasing the proportion of omega-3 fats in the total fat intake is worthwhile in everyone's diet as it also is protective against coronary artery disease and perhaps arthritis.

Smoking and chronic obstructive lung disease

After lung cancer, most deaths due to respiratory diseases are from chronic obstructive lung disease (chronic bronchitis and emphysema). By far the main cause of these diseases is smoking, with some contribution from exposure to other substances, such as coal dust and silica, in the workplace. Such exposure is more common in males.

It is important to note that the majority of people with chronic bronchitis remain undiagnosed as most just feel their breathing problems, including being a bit short of breath and coughing, are part of the normal ageing process. They therefore do not seek help and do not receive treatment. If you are a smoker and over the age of 35, ask to have your lung function assessed by your GP at your next visit. Many symptoms of chronic bronchitis can be improved to a degree with treatment and ceasing smoking will halt the progress of the disease.

Smoking was discussed in detail in Part 6 in the section on 'Prevention of lung and other smoking-related cancers'.

Asbestos and other work-related causes of lung disease

The association between asbestos and lung disease has been recognised for many years. It causes two forms of lung disease.

Mesothelioma

This is a very deadly form of cancer that arises from the outside lining of the lung and, once diagnosed, the patient is usually dead within two years. The cancer is always caused by exposure to asbestos and it is important to understand the cancer can be caused by relatively minor exposures to this substance. Thus, all exposure to asbestos needs to be eliminated. This especially applies to the building industry where contact with asbestos in older dwellings is relatively common.

Asbestosis

Chronic exposure to asbestos can cause permanent damage to the lung tissue that resembles the changes of chronic bronchitis in smokers. This can lead to long-term disability and even death, especially if associated with cigarette smoking.

Further information

A good source information about making your house and garden 'low allergenic' with lists of low allergenic plants and plants you should avoid—

The Asthma Association of NSW
The association's website has numerous good downloadable articles on many asthma topics. Specific information about making your house and garden low allergenic can be found on www.asthmansw.org.au/peopleinfo/lowallergenhouse.htm and www.asthmansw.org.au/peopleinfo/lowallergengarden.htm, which includes lists of low allergenic plants and plants you should avoid.
Website: www.asthmansw.org.au

Asthma Australia
Website: www.asthmaaustralia.org.au

National Asthma Council
Website: www.nationalasthma.org.au

Renal disease

Kidney disease often goes undiagnosed in Australia, with an estimated 500 000 Australians having undiagnosed, and therefore untreated, early kidney failure. Diseases that exclusively affect the kidneys account for only a small percentage of disability and death in Australia. However, the kidneys are affected by numerous more common problems, such as diabetes and hypertension, and these diseases are responsible for most kidney damage and kidney failure.

Testing for abnormalities in the urine is done for three reasons: it helps detect diseases originating in the urinary tract, including the kidney, bladder etc.; it helps detect diseases originating outside the urinary tract that affect the kidneys; and, finally, it detects excess excretion of substances in the urine that indicate an abnormality in the body. For example, patients that are jaundiced through liver disease excrete abnormal amounts of bilirubin in the urine.

Screening for kidney disease

There are six groups of people who have significant increased risk of kidney disease and these individuals need regular screening of their urine. These groups are:

- anyone over 50 years of age
- Aborigines and Torres Strait Islanders
- those with a family history of kidney disease
- smokers

- those with high blood pressure
- people with diabetes. (It is worthwhile remembering that almost half the diabetics in Australia are undiagnosed. Those at increased risk of developing diabetes should also be screened for kidney disease.)

A screening program for all these at-risk people would allow early detection and early treatment of the majority of kidney disease. This in turn would prevent about one-third of all cases of end-stage kidney failure, which requires dialysis treatment. Renal failure requiring dialysis is a particularly debilitating condition that is definitely best avoided!

If you belong to one of the above groups, you should have your urine checked each year for blood, protein, glucose (sugar) and nitrites. Such routine urine screening tests can be done easily when you present to your GP for a check-up. While screening is necessary if you are included in the at-risk groups listed above, all people should really have a urine test every time they have a check-up. Urine testing has always been an integral part of routine medicals and as such has saved many lives. Any persistent abnormality found on testing your urine will require further investigation to determine the actual disease affecting your kidneys.

Protein in the urine and other disease

Protein in the urine is often associated with diabetes, however, there is increasing evidence (Gerstein 2001) that indicates the presence of albumin (protein) in the urine is a strong predictor of increased risk for several other diseases, including heart failure (risk increased up to three times) and heart attacks (risk increased up to two times). The overall death rate is also higher in people with protein in their urine.

The degree of increased risk is related to the amount of protein in the urine. This is measured by the albumin/creatinine ratio. However, even those with low ratio levels are at increased risk. The measurement of protein in the urine is performed via an easy 'dip-stick' test and should be done at all check-ups.

Determining kidney function

It is important to understand that while testing the urine is very good at identifying the presence of kidney disease, it does not give any indication of how much damage has been done to the affected kidney. All urine tests can do is say that something is wrong. Determining how much damage a particular disease has done to the kidneys requires taking a blood test and often a 24-hour sample of urine.

A blood test, called a serum creatinine level, can help determine the amount of kidney tissue that is working normally. When looked at by itself, the serum creatinine only starts to become abnormal when at least half the overall function of both kidneys is lost. This is too late. However, the serum creatinine can be used to determine the GFR (Glomerular Filtration Rate). The measurement of GFR is the main way to accurately measure your kidney function and the extent of kidney disease. Doing repeated GFR tests is also the best way of knowing if your kidney disease is getting worse. Measuring blood urea levels can also help assess the extent of kidney damage.

An abnormal GFR indicates the kidneys have been damaged. People with an abnormal GFR need to be referred to a kidney specialist (a renal physician) to help determine the cause and implement a management plan to minimise further damage. Many people are referred too late, reducing their chance of avoiding kidney failure.

Hearing and sight

Adult-onset hearing impairment

After dental caries, adult-onset hearing loss is Australia's most common health problem. It is also a serious problem, and is one of the top 16 causes of total burden of disease, especially in males in the 45 to 65 year age group. It is a problem that worsens as you get older and particularly affects males from 45 years onwards. While only about 3 per cent of 40 year olds have hearing impairment, by the time you reach 60 your chances of being affected are 50 per cent.

People with impaired hearing have difficulties with conversations and, even when they concentrate, they can still miss half of what is said. This causes frustration and can lead to social isolation, which is already a significant problem for many elderly people. The risk of accidents on the road and at work is greater because hearing may be impaired enough so that 'warning' sounds are missed. Having the car radio turned up too loudly does not help matters. The everyday sounds that surround you are one of life's great joys. Being unable to hear music is a real loss.

The cause of adult-onset hearing loss

There are numerous causes of adult-onset hearing loss, but by far the main cause is long-term exposure to loud noise. This occurs so gradually that you are very unlikely to even notice it. Chronic exposure to loud noise damages or even breaks the very delicate hair-like structures which detect sound in the cochlear part of the inner ear. The parts of the ear that conduct high-pitched sounds are affected first.

Noise does not have to be painfully loud to cause this damage. Long-term exposure to noises, such as those made by a ride-on mower, is enough. To prevent hearing loss, the World Health Organisation recommends you should not be exposed to noise levels of 85dB(A) for more than eight hours a day. This is about the level of heavy traffic noise. Figure 31 gives an indication of the time you can listen to a sound without damage to your hearing.

Young people's exposure to loud music is a considerable area of concern. Young males tend to be exposed to more noise of this kind than young women and are also exposed to

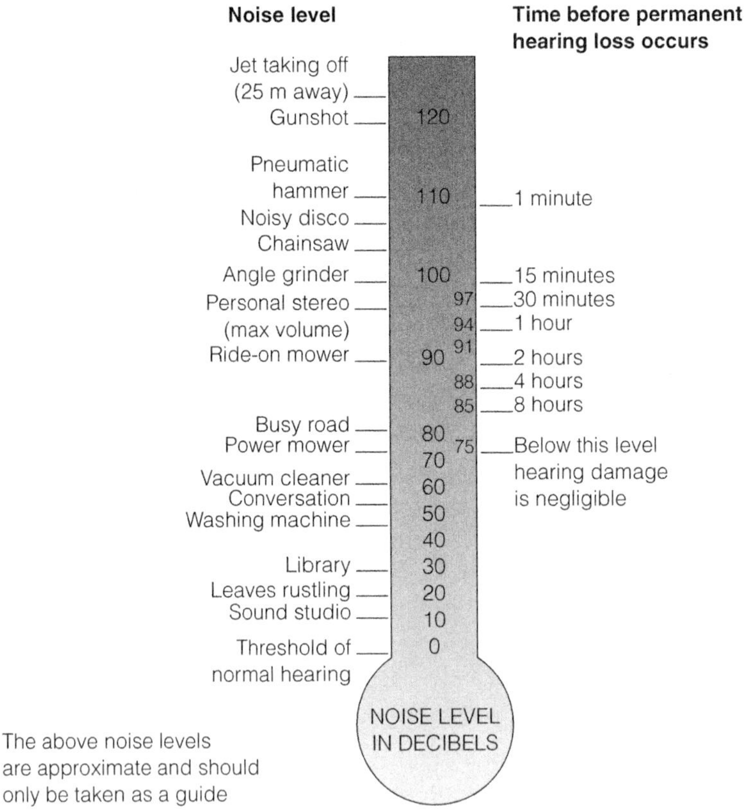

Source: Reproduced with permission of Australian Hearing.

Figure 31 Time taken to cause permanent hearing loss at different noise levels more noise at work. For this reason, they can expect to encounter deafness about ten years earlier.

Our modern urban environments are generally much noisier than in times past and it is likely that this will lead to hearing loss as early as 40 years of age.

Preventing hearing loss

The most important thing to do is to protect your hearing from loud noises. This should start from early in life and should be especially encouraged in teenagers and young people. In general, sudden, very loud noises are worse than continuous loud noise. Some practical tips (from Australian Hearing) include:

- Use headphones rather than turning the volume up when listening to personal stereos.
- Avoid long periods of loud noise, such as a loud concert.
- Wear proper protective earplugs or earmuffs when working in a noisy environment or doing loud household chores, such as lawn mowing. Earplugs can also be used at loud concerts.
- Make your work environment as quiet as possible.
- Give your ears rest periods when continuously exposed to noise (see figure 31).

Continuous exposure to excess noise at work is a problem for many people, especially males. This can be reduced by locating noisy equipment in isolated or sound-proofed areas, purchasing less-noisy equipment, ensuring workers are only exposed to higher noise levels for short periods (i.e. they are given noise rests), and enforcing the mandatory use of protective earplugs or earmuffs. People exposed to loud noises at work should have their hearing checked regularly to identify hearing loss as early as possible.

It is also important to protect your ears by treating ear infections early and never putting objects into your ear canal as this is a common cause of ear damage.

Diagnosis and treatment of hearing loss

As stated before, hearing loss is often so gradual that it usually goes unnoticed. Many of those that do notice it deny they have a problem, preferring to believe people are not speaking properly etc. This is partly due to a belief there is nothing that can be done about their hearing loss. This of course is not true.

The above facts mean the diagnosis of hearing loss is often delayed. Here are some questions compiled by Australian Hearing that will help identify whether you have a hearing loss problem.

- Do you have difficulty understanding people unless they are facing you?
- Do you find it hard to understand conversations in a noisy room?

- Do you fail to hear the doorbell or telephone ring?
- Do people complain that you turn the TV or radio up too loud?
- Do you often ask people to speak up or repeat themselves?
- Do you have difficulties understanding telephone conversations?
- Do people complain that you do not hear them?
- Do you sometimes have ringing or buzzing in the ear?

If you answered yes to any of these questions, you need your hearing checked. This can be arranged through your GP and should be done by a qualified audiologist.

In addition to better communication, improvement in hearing can enhance mood, socialisation and thinking. Hearing aids are often necessary to treat significant hearing loss and assist by making the sounds you hear louder. Unfortunately, they do not always improve sound clarity. All hearing aids are not the same and treatment needs to be co-ordinated by a qualified audiologist who can design a suitable individual aid for you. The use of hearing aids in both ears (if needed) is sometimes preferable as it can give a more natural sound and helps with determining which direction the sound is coming from.

Tips for talking to people with hearing loss

- Face the person directly, preferably at their eye level.
- Make sure they can see your face by keeping your hands away from your face and ensuring bright lights are not shining into their eyes.
- Do not shout.
- Keep background noise to a minimum by turning off the TV and radio.
- Find a different way of saying something if you are not being understood.

Chronic glaucoma—a silent cause of blindness

Chronic glaucoma is a condition where the pressure in your eyes gradually increases. This increased pressure causes damage to the nerves at the back of the eyes, leading to irreversible loss of vision and, in the end, blindness. In most people it does not start to be a problem until the age of 60.

It is estimated that 300 000 people in Australia have this problem. However, only about 50 per cent of these people know they have the disease because the gradual nature of the visual loss means it is not noticed until significant loss of vision has occurred. It unfortunately usually involves both eyes.

Luckily, the condition is easily treatable and is also easily diagnosed by a very simple test that measures the pressure in your eyes. This should always be done in conjunction with an examination of the visual fields and a measuring of the cup-to-disc ratio in the retina as some people with damage have pressure readings in the normal range. Such testing is usually done by an opthalmologist or an optometrist.

If you have no risk factors for chronic glaucoma (see below), then you should start having screening eye pressure checks at about the age of 60 (some recommend 50) and then one every second year until you reach 70 years of age. After 70 it should be done yearly. The frequency of this testing will also depend on the pressure level found in the first test. If you wear glasses, your renewal consultations are ideal times to have your eye pressure checked.

This disease should not be confused with acute glaucoma. While both diseases cause an increase in eye pressure, in acute glaucoma the pressure build-up is fairly sudden. This causes acute severe pain that hopefully leads to quick diagnosis and treatment. Chronic glaucoma causes no such pain.

Risk factors for chronic glaucoma

There are three risk factors for chronic glaucoma:

- a history of increased pressure found in either eye
- increasing age
- a family history of glaucoma.

People with a first-degree relative with chronic glaucoma have a 16 per cent chance of developing the disease (Loane 2000). If you have such a family history, you should be tested every second year from the age of 40 until you reach 70, then yearly.

Further information

Australian Hearing
Website: www.hearing.com.au

Infectious diseases

Immunisation

All Australians need to ensure their vaccinations are up-to-date. This means you need to update your immunisations if you have missed any and ensure you have future vaccinations at the appropriate time. This includes adults. Exceeding the recommended time interval between doses, including missing doses, does not mean the course needs to be restarted or that supplementary doses need to be given. All that needs to be done is for the missed doses to be administered, although some doses can be omitted depending on the age of the person when they are receiving 'catch-up doses'. You should seek your GP's advice on the doses you need to 'catch-up'. Vaccinations should not be postponed by minor illnesses such as upper respiratory tract infections. It is pleasing to note that the level of fully immunised babies (one year olds) has been steadily increasing and is now over 91 per cent. In 1997, the figure was only 75 per cent.

The current vaccination schedule appears on page 368 and you should check this to see whether your immunisations are up-to-date. Please remember that vaccination schedules change reasonably regularly so you should check your immunisation protection with your GP at each visit. As an example, many adults will not be immunised against Hepatitis B.

Influenza

A common vaccination given to adults is the influenza vaccination, which is now recommended for everyone over the age of 65 and earlier in people at increased risk. It is provided free to these people by the Australian Government. By preventing influenza and its debilitating symptoms, this vaccine also reduces hospital admissions and death rates. At-risk groups include Aborigines and Torres Strait Islanders and those with significant other illnesses, such as heart disease. It is also recommended for adults travelling in large groups. Those allergic to egg or egg protein should not be given this vaccine.

Notes on vaccination in general

1. Vaccinations should not be postponed by minor illnesses such as upper respiratory tract infections.
2. Exceeding the recommended time interval between doses does not mean the course needs to be restarted or that supplementary doses need to be given. All that needs to be done is for the missed doses to be administered, although some doses can be omitted depending on the age of the person when they are receiving 'catch-up doses'. You should seek your GP's advice on the doses you need to catch up. (The exception to this is Hib vaccination. No Hib vaccination needs to be administered after the age of five years unless the person has no spleen.)
3. Immunisation levels should be checked in adults and missed doses administered.
4. Questions regarding the need to immunise are addressed in Commonwealth Government websites mentioned on page 374.

Pneumococcal vaccination in children

Some children need to be given the pneumococcal vaccination. These children include:

- those under five years with significant medical problems that increase their risk of pneumococcal infection
- all Aborigines and Torres Strait Islander children and all children from Central Australia under two years of age
- Aboriginal children aged two to five living in Central Australia or other areas with a similarly high incidence of pneumococcal infection
- those with a depressed immune system
- children with any one of a few specific anatomical abnormalities, such as a proven or suspected cerebrospinal fluid leak, or with cardiovascular disease associated with cyanosis or cardiac failure.

If appropriate, you will need to discuss this matter with your GP.

The Australian Standard Vaccination Schedule 2000–2002

Age		*Vaccination*	
Birth		Hep B	
		*Path 1**	*Path 2**
2 months		DTPa–Hep B and Hib and OPV	DTPa** and Hib (PRP–OMP)–Hep B and OPV
4 months		DTPa–Hep B and Hib and OPV	DTPa** and Hib (PRP–OMP)–Hep B and OPV
6 months		DTPa–Hep B and Hib and OPV	DTPa** and Hib (PRP–OMP)–Hep B and OPV
12 months		MMR and Hib and meningococcal group C***	MMR and Hib (PRP–OMP)–Hep B and meningococcal group C
18 months		DTPa	
4 years		DTPa and MMR and OPV	
10–13 years 1 month later 5 months after second dose	Hep B Hep B Hep B	Note: These Hepatitis B vaccinations are not necessary if the child has received 3 Hepatitis B doses previously.	
15 years***		Meningococcal group C	
14–19 years		Td	
Non-immune women who are post partum or of child-bearing age		MMR	
50 years	Td	Not necessary if the person has had a tetanus booster in the previous 10 years.	
50 years and over for indigenous Australians		Pneumococcal vaccine (every 5 years) Influenza vaccine (every year)	
65 years and over		Pneumococcal vaccine (every 5 years) Influenza vaccine (every year)	

* Different Australian states take different paths.

Notes:

DTPa **: Diphtheria Tetanus and Pertussus (whooping cough). (Try to give same brand for 2, 4 and 6 month vaccinations.)
DTPa–Hep B: Diphtheria Tetanus and Pertussus (whooping cough) and Hepatitis B
Hib: Haemophilus influenzae type B
Hib (PRP–OMP)–Hep B: Haemophilus influenza type B and Hepatitis B
OPV: Oral polio vaccination
MMR: Measles, mumps, rubella (German measles)
Hep B: Hepatitis B (first dose should be given at birth)
Td: Tetanus

*** Meningococcal group C vaccination will start early in 2003. In the first year it will also be offered to 15 to 17 year olds and in subsequent years to 15 year olds.

Likely additions to the above vaccination schedule in 2003

1. Pneumococcal vaccination for infants at two months, four months and six months of age. (This has been added because the bacteria *Streptococcus pneumoniae* is a major cause of meningitis in the under-five year age group. It is also likely to significantly reduce the occurrence of middle ear infections and the subsequent need for grommet tubes in young children.)
2. Vaccination against chickenpox (varicella) at 18 months, with a catch-up dose at age 10 to 13 years.
3. Meningococcal C vaccination at age 12 months (and as above in unimmunised adolescents).
4. A new two-dose Hepatitis B vaccination (Hep-B-VaxII) for unimmunised adolescents.

Sexually transmitted diseases

Most sexually transmitted diseases (STD) can be prevented by commonsense and a responsible attitude to sex. This, unfortunately, is not always the done thing and unsafe sexual practices are responsible for about 1 per cent of all burden of disease. The list of serious sexually transmitted diseases is large and includes HIV/AIDS, hepatitis B, genital herpes, chlamydia, syphilis, genital warts and gonorrhoea. Cervical cancer from Human Papilloma Virus could also be added to this list and the trauma of an unwanted pregnancy should not be forgotten.

STDs are most common in young people. (The average age of infection with chlamydia in Australia is 15 to 24 years in women and 20 to 35 years in men.) Young people are more vulnerable because they are less likely to be in a long-term relationship, are more likely to have multiple partners, and are more likely to take risks such as participating in intercourse without condoms.

Preventative measures were partly covered in the section on the preventing teenage pregnancy and that section is worth reading again. Prevention should include:

- *Anticipation.* If you are sexually active or soon likely to be, it is important that you see your doctor to obtain adequate contraception and advice about protection from STDs. Unfortunately, about 50 per cent of first time intercourse occurs without contraception. This is a topic that parents need to discuss with their daughters and sons early in their teens as feeling uneasy about approaching the family doctor is a major reason teenage girls (and boys) fail to address this issue.
- *Use condoms.* Unless you have decided to have one regular sexual partner for a prolonged period (not just a few months), you need to use condoms every time you have intercourse. This applies to both heterosexual and male homosexual relationships. To be useful, condoms need to be carried with you! You should never rely on your present partner's version of his or her previous sex life (or lack thereof) in deciding on the need to use condoms, especially if it is early on in your relationship. Practice has shown that such stories are often not factually based. If you have made the decision to become monogamous, then both partners probably need to be checked by a doctor first for sexually transmissible diseases. If either of you think this is too much hassle, then you should think again about your long-term commitment. Would you really want to be transmitting a serious disease to a potential lifetime partner who you love?

  Some sexually transmitted diseases such as genital herpes and genital warts can be present on areas that condoms do not cover. Thus, you should always ask your partner about such conditions. Having a look first is a good idea as well. (When putting on condoms is a good opportunity for women.) It is definitely too late after the event. However, seeing nothing abnormal does not mean you are safe and can forget the condoms.

While condoms are certainly better than nothing, they are not the most effective form of contraception and using the oral contraceptive pill as well is by far the best option.

- *Oral sex can also be involved in the transmission of STDs.* The most common STD resulting from oral sex is a genital infection that results from contact with an oral herpes simplex (cold sore) lesion. You should ask your partner about a past history of cold sores (and have a look) if this is relevant to you.
- *Discuss sexually transmitted diseases with your partner.* As stated, people are not always completely honest when it comes to discussing sexually transmitted diseases. However, any information that your partner does reveal about past or present STDs can only help and it does provide an opportunity for extra trust to develop in your relationship. This does not mean that you need not use condoms if your partner says all is OK. Many people are not aware they have STDs, especially chlamydia, genital warts and even more serious diseases such as HIV/AIDS.
- *Try to avoid excessive alcohol, especially 'loading doses'.* Excess alcohol will reduce your inhibitions and make you far more likely to take risks that you may later regret.
- *Learn refusal skills and skills to avoid date rape.* Further information regarding this topic can be gained from one of the excellent texts and references mentioned below.

If you are worried that you have a sexually transmitted disease, do not be apprehensive about seeing your doctor. They realise that such consultations are often difficult for patients and will be sympathetic and helpful. Additional information sources regarding STDs are mentioned on page 374.

HIV/AIDS

HIV is a viral infection that is mainly transmitted through sexual intercourse, with anal intercourse being the easiest method of spread. In Australia it mainly occurs in homosexual men. In Africa and other developing countries, vaginal intercourse is the more common method of spread. Transmission associated with intravenous drug use accounts for only about 4 per cent of cases in Australia but is a more common method of spread in Europe, Asia and the USA. Transmission by accidental needle stick injury only occurs in about 0.3 per cent of exposures to needles used by infected individuals and transmission by blood transfusion is exceedingly rare. Perinatal transmission from an infected mother to her baby occurs in about 20 to 45 per cent of cases unless preventative measures are taken. Such preventative measures can reduce this rate to about 5 per cent and include antiviral drug treatment during the pregnancy, the labour and after delivery; birth by caesarean section; and avoidance of breast feeding.

Preventing HIV/AIDS infection

- Unless both partners are in a monogamous, long-term relationship and do not have any sexually transmissible diseases, safe sex (condom use) needs to be practiced with every sexual encounter, whether vaginal or anal. Homosexual men need to be especially cautious. Safe sex is discussed in more detail in the section on sexually transmitted diseases. It is important to recognise that unsafe sexual practices are more common after illicit drugs or excess alcohol has been consumed.
- People who use intravenous drugs need to ensure that they do not share needles, swabs or any other materials that may be contaminated with blood.
- Needle stick injuries need to be minimised by adequate training of health professionals in the safe use and disposal of needles.
- Needle exchange programs need to be expanded throughout Australia so that all those at risk have access to safe injecting materials. All people infected with HIV need to be especially careful when disposing of blood contaminated materials.
- Infection can also occur with cosmetic procedures that involve piercing the skin, such as tattooing or having studs etc. inserted. It is best to make sure that such procedures are done professionally using instruments that have been properly sterilised (using an autoclave).
- Preventing the infection of babies requires that infected mothers be identified early in their pregnancy. All prospective mothers need to be questioned about whether they are likely to be infected with HIV and should be tested if there is any risk. If positive, they then need to be given careful counselling regarding the best options for reducing the risk of transmitting their infection.

Prevention of hepatitis B

Hepatitis B is a viral infection that affects the liver, with some chronic infections causing liver damage and liver cancer. About 25 to 40 per cent of people with chronic infections die from the disease. Whether infected individuals eradicate the illness or develop a long-term chronic infection depends on the age at which they are infected. People who develop the disease in early childhood have 90 per cent chance of being chronically infected. Only about 5 per cent of those infected as adults develop chronic disease.

Most cases in countries with a high incidence of the disease, such as China, Southeast Asia and the Pacific nations, occur due to infection from mother to baby at birth. In adults, transmission is mostly through sexual contact or injecting drug use. There are thought to be about 200 000 carriers of the disease in Australia. Transmission by needle stick injury occurs in only about 3 to 30 per cent of exposures from needles used by infected individuals. (Transmission depends on the state of the hepatitis B infection.)

Preventing hepatitis B infection

- Hepatitis B infection can be prevented by immunisation. This immunisation is part of the immunisation schedule in Australia. Some older children and adults will not have been immunised and if you are unsure of your immunity status for hepatitis B, you should discuss the matter with your GP.
- Methods for preventing infection through sexual contact or injecting drug use are similar to those described for HIV/AIDS.
- Infection of newborns can be prevented by immunisation and the administration of hepatitis B immunoglobin. It is therefore imperative that all mothers who are carriers of the disease are detected early in their pregnancy. (This involves testing those at risk of having hepatitis B and those who have not been immunised against hepatitis B.)

Prevention of hepatitis C

Hepatitis C is another viral infection that predominantly affects the liver. It is primarily transmitted by blood-to-blood contact, with 90 per cent of the new cases in Australia occurring in association with injecting drug use. (A very large percentage of injecting drug users have the disease.) There were about 11 000 new cases in 2000 and the spread of the disease is increasing quickly. In 1997 there were thought to be about 200 000 people with hepatitis C in Australia. About 75 per cent of infected people become infected chronically with about 20 per cent developing liver cirrhosis and 5 per cent liver cancer. The rate of transmission with sexual intercourse is thought to be very low, although the presence of menstrual blood may increase the risk. Transmission at birth is thought to be about 5 per cent and there is no established way to stop this transmission, although caesarean section may be of some help.

Preventing hepatitis C infection

- Prevention in injecting drug users is similar to those measures taken for hepatitis B and HIV. However, it should be noted that this infection is very easily spread, with only a minute amount blood being required. Infected individuals need to dispose of blood contaminated materials carefully.
- Unfortunately there is no immunisation for hepatitis C.

Dental caries

Dental caries is the most common disease known to man. It is due to acid, produced by bacteria in the mouth, that slowly destroys the hard tissues of the tooth and can occur as soon as teeth are present in the mouth (i.e. in young children). Over the past few decades, its incidence has decreased dramatically in communities where artificial fluoridation of the water supply is practiced. In most cases, dental caries can be avoided by good health prevention that includes:

- Regular visits (at least yearly) to the dentist from the age of three. Your dentist can help with preventative advice, applying fluoride, removing solids that accumulate on your teeth and arresting the progression of existing disease.
- Regular brushing of the teeth at least twice a day. In the morning after breakfast and before going to bed are the best times. It takes about two minutes to brush your teeth adequately. Good technique is essential and can be learned from your dentist. The use of dental floss to remove food from between your teeth aids greatly in this cleaning process and should be done each time you brush. Toothpicks and the like are not useful and can harm your gums.
- If your water supply is not fluoridated, then you should purchase supplements to add to your water. This principally applies to people who use tank water or bottled water for drinking. Fluoride used in recommended quantities causes no health problems.
- Eat wisely. Try to eat regular, larger meals and avoid snacks. Continually grazing on food, especially sweet foods, provides ideal growing conditions for the bacteria that cause dental caries. Carbonated soft drinks and new 'energy drinks', including the 'diet' varieties, are a significant cause of tooth decay as most are slightly acidic and this extra acid makes decay occur more quickly. This is especially important in children. Fruit juices are also generally acidic and *excessive* amounts, especially if they have added

sugar, can cause accelerate tooth decay. Letting an infant continually suck on a bottle filled with sweetened juice is a particular problem. Wine is also acidic but is generally only consumed occasionally and usually with food. (It can be a problem for wine tasters.)

Further information

On immunisation

Commonwealth Department of Health and Ageing

Immunisations: myths and realities answers questions commonly asked by people worried about or questioning the need for vaccination. Website: www.health.gov.au/pubhlth/immunise/publications

A supplement to this publication dealing with recent issues surrounding the MMR vaccine and inflammatory bowel disease and autism is also available at Website: www.health.gov.au/pubhlth/immunise/myth_measles.pdf

On sexually transmitted disease

Sexwise by Dr Janet Hall, Random House Australia

What every young person and parent should know about sex. Dr Hall empowers her readers by telling them the facts—and giving it to them straight.

Unzipped by Bronwyn Donaghy, HarperCollins

A book that deals frankly and sympathetically with the crucial role that love and emotions play in every aspect of adolescent sexuality.

The Children's Hospital at Westmead

Further titles regarding puberty and adolescent sexuality are available on website: *www.chw.edu.au/parents/books.*

Both the above books are mentioned on this web site and are recommended by staff at the hospital.

The Resource Centre for Adolescent Pregnancy Prevention

A good USA website that provides information and skills for both adolescents and for educators about preventing unwanted teenage pregnancies. Unfortunately it is not free.

Website: www.etr.org/recapp

Appendices

Quantifying the effects of illness—the 'burden of illness'

Appendix 1

The figures used in this book to grade the death and disability caused by each illness are derived from information gathered and interpreted by the Australian Institute of Health and Welfare (AIHW). In interpreting its information, the AIHW has recognised that each illness impacts differently on individuals with respect to death and disability. For example, the death of a 20-year-old motorcyclist is more significant than a death due to prostate cancer of a patient at age 80. For this reason, the AIHW adjusts the data they receive so that the importance to society of each individual event can be taken into account. They use the following three categories to do this.

Years of life lost due to premature death (YLL) is used to express death in terms of premature mortality (i.e. the burden of premature mortality). It indicates the years of normal life expectancy that is lost by a person due to their death. For example, assuming a 20 year old man would live to 80, the death of a 20-year-old motorcyclist would be given a YLL of 60. On the other hand, a 76-year-old cancer victim would on average be expected to live another eight years having reached the age of 76. His death would have been allocated a YLL of 8. (These calculations have not included discounting. See p. 378.) The YLL for each death that occurs from a particular illness can be added to give an indication of the overall importance of that illness compared to other illnesses. This information can also be looked at according to age groups to determine at what age the illness being examined causes the most premature death.

Years of life lost due to disability (YLD) indicates the years of healthy life lost due to poor health or disability (i.e. the burden of disability). These figures are calculated by determining the number of new cases of a particular disability causing illness and then looking at both the length of time the person suffers the disability and the severity of the disability. The severity is rated between 0 (for no disability) and 1 (for death). Thus, an illness that on average caused ten years disability and had a disability rating of 0.5 would be given a YLD score of 5. In this way the YLD and YLL scores can be compared and added together to give an indication of the total disability years of life lost.

By adding the YLL and the YDL together, the total illness burden for a particular disease (i.e. the total burden of disease) can be calculated. It is expressed in terms of disability adjusted life years (DALYs). One DALY is equivalent to one year of 'healthy life' lost. The significance of diseases that predominantly cause disability, such as anxiety or hearing loss, is often underestimated by both society and government. This system permits a comparison of the illness levels caused by all diseases, allowing an accurate assessment of the significance of illness in our community.

To allow for other illnesses that the affected person may have incurred if they had lived longer (in the case of YLL) or will incur in the future (in the case of YLD), all the above figures have an annual discount rate (of 3 per cent) applied to the calculations. If discounting were not done, YLL and YLD figures would be excessively high as people with multiple conditions would be counted more than once.

Evidence-based medicine

Appendix 2

Recently, there has been a strong move in traditional medicine to base all medical opinions and treatments on well-founded evidence. Reliable evidence can be divided into two groups that look at events either prospectively (towards the future) or retrospectively (in the past).

Prospective studies

The best type of evidence is gained by looking forward at what happens to participants in a study. Studies that do this are called prospective studies. The reason these are better is that they can look at randomly selected normal populations, not populations that have been selected because they already have a particular disease. There are two types of prospective trials/studies.

Randomised controlled trials

These trials provide the best information. They randomly select a group of subjects and divide them into controlled and uncontrolled groups. The uncontrolled group continues as before. The controlled group has one factor changed and the two groups are observed over a period of time to see if there are significant differences. For example, a study could be designed to examine the effect of increased calcium intake on bowel cancer.

If the participants and the observers are unaware of which group they are in, then the trial is called a double blind trial. In the example above, this might mean all participants were given similar tablets with only some containing calcium. Double blind trials are best because, as the participants and observers do not know who is in each group, it is not possible for their behaviour to affect the outcome.

The problems with these studies are that they rely on participants performing the trial properly, i.e. take their tablets, and they are time consuming and thus expensive. Also, due to the expense involved, they are usually restricted in follow-up time and if the time allowed is inadequate, it may mean the effect being looked for has not had time to appear.

Cohort (or longitudinal) studies

In these studies, a random group of individuals is selected and then observed at regular intervals for changes that might occur. Taking the calcium and bowel cancer example again, this type of study would randomly select a group and at regular intervals ask them about their calcium intake and any incidence of bowel cancer. Any causal relationship could then be assessed.

These studies are easier to do because the group is not being asked to do any specific task. They are also cheaper and easier to assess and thus follow-up can be over a much longer period.

Interpreting the results, however, is more difficult because there are many variables that might affect the outcome being investigated. In our example, individuals who had high calcium intakes may have a lower incidence of bowel cancer but the group may also have had a healthier diet rich in fruit and vegetables. It may have been this and not the increased calcium that caused the reduced bowel cancer. For this reason, these studies need to be carefully planned so that other known associated factors are also examined in the study and allowed for in the results.

Retrospective studies

Studies that look at a group of people with a particular medical condition, such as bowel cancer, and then try to work out factors that might have caused the problem are called retrospective studies.

Results from such studies are not as reliable as prospective studies because they are not looking at a normal population. They are looking at a population that already has the problem being researched (such as bowel cancer). This can affect the findings of the study as it may turn out that the findings do not apply to a normal population.

Case-controlled studies

Case-controlled studies look at a group of people with a specific problem and try to compare them with a similar population in the hope of finding the differences that caused them to develop the problem. In our example, both groups could be asked about their previous calcium intake and the findings compared.

The problems with case-controlled studies are that memories are not always accurate (and may be subject to bias) and numbers in the group with the problem are often small, making the findings less accurate.

Epidemiological studies

These studies look at the incidence of diseases and possible causes in population groups. From this information, it is possible to look for associations between diseases and possible suspected causes. For example, Japanese people have a high incidence of stomach cancer and also eat large amounts of charred food. From this it could be implied, but not proven, that eating large amounts of charred food causes stomach cancer. This is the least reliable type of evidence commonly presented.

Assessing all the available information about a topic

Usually there will be numerous sources of information about a particular topic. Some will obviously be better than others and some may give conflicting findings. All this information must be assessed in order to come to a conclusion and there will be some topics where the conclusion is obvious and others where it is less certain. For this reason, conclusions made from the analysis of evidence regarding a particular topic and advice based on these conclusions are graded according to the quality of the evidence assessed (a number) and the strength of the conclusion that can be reached from that evidence (a letter) as follows.

Quality of evidence

Level I —Evidence gained from a review of all relevant randomised trials.
Level II —Evidence gained from at least one properly designed randomised trial.
Level III—Evidence obtained from any of the following:

- well-designed pseudo randomised controlled trials
- comparative studies with cohort trials, case-control study or interrupted time series with a control group
- comparative studies with historical control, two or more single arm studies, or interrupted time series without a parallel control group.

Level IV—Evidence gained from case series, either post-test, or pre-test and post-test.
Level V —Opinions of respected authorities, based on clinical experience, descriptive studies or reports of expert committees.

Strength of recommendation

A —There is good evidence to support the recommendation.
B —There is fair evidence to support the recommendation.
C—There is poor evidence regarding including or excluding the recommendation.
D—There is fair evidence against the recommendation.
E —There is good evidence against the recommendation.

Thus, a 'IA' recommendation indicates that the most accurate trials possible have provided very conclusive findings. A 'VC' recommendation is not much better than personal opinion.

Appendix 3

Major foods contributing to fat intake

On average, Australians consume about 35 to 40 per cent of their energy as fat. Ideally this should be more like 25 to 30 per cent. In most people this equates to between 40 and 60 grams of fat per day. Where does this come from? The table below shows the amount of fat (and fibre and energy) in a typical example of good foods that should be eaten each day as part of a healthy diet.

This total fat figure can be varied up or down by altering food choices. A reduction can be achieved by not using spreads on bread and by reducing the fat content of cereals. Increases

Food	*Total fat in grams*		*Fibre*		*Energy in kJ*	
Fruit (2 pieces)	**0.0**		**6.0**		**580**	
apple (1 medium)		0.0		3.0		310
banana (1 small)		0.0		3.0		270
Vegetables	**0.0**		**9.0**		**360**	
3 serves (excluding avocado)		0.0		6.0		270
Salad		0.0		3.0		90
Carbohydrates (4 serves)	**12.0**		**17.0**		**3405**	
Pasta—1 serve (dry 100 g)		1.5		5.0		1430
Cereal—1 serve (high fibre such as natural muesli—½ cup or 60 g)		6.5		6.0		835
Wholegrain bread—2 slices		2.0		3.0		600
Wholegrain roll (60 g)		2.0		3.0		540
Protein (one and a half serves)	**7.5**		**0.0**		**1030**	
Lamb fillet rump, lean with all fat removed (130 g)—grilled		8.5		0.0		685
Chicken breast, no skin (150 g)—grilled with no oil		4.5		0.0		780
Fish (150 g)—grilled		2.0		0.0		600
Dairy products (2 serves)	**0.6**		**0.0**		**1135**	
Low-fat milk (250 mL)—1 serve		0.3		0.0		505
Yoghurt, fruit, low fat—1 serve		0.5		0.0		630
Oils and spreads	**24.0**		**0.0**		**960**	
Margarine (monounsaturated) 1 tablespoon (20 g)		14.0		0.0		590
Olive oil (used in cooking meats etc. and in dressings) ½ tablespoon (10 g)		10.0		0.0		370
Total	**44.1**		**32**		**7470**	

can be caused by poorer food choices. An example would be using lamb chops without removing excess fat, which would add well over 20 grams of fat to the total or using full cream milk, which would add 9 grams of fat.

The table does not include sauces used with pasta or meat. Sauces or marinades based on low-fat ingredients, such as tomatoes, vegetables, wine and herbs, add little in the way of fat. Cream-based sauces on the other hand can add significantly to total fat intake. Remember, fat is added to foods to enhance flavour. This is not necessary if you choose flavoursome foods to begin with.

Nutritionally beneficial fat-containing foods—use daily in moderation to make up your fat allocation		
Avocado* Cheese** Chicken (lean, with skin) Dairy products (low-fat) Eggs (boiled or poached) Fish (not fried*) Hamburger (homemade, low-fat) Margarine (monounsaturated*)	Mayonnaise (low-fat) Meats (beef, lamb and pork, lean with all fat removed) Milk (whole—in children less than five years) Monounsaturated oils, especially olive oil* Muesli (toasted*)	Nuts* Peanut butter* Salmon (red, canned*) Soy beverage (low-fat—'So-good'*) Tuna (canned*) Yoghurt (low-fat)
Less beneficial fat-containing foods—avoid or use only occasionally as treats		
Apple pie (baked) Bacon (grilled—3 rashers) Beef (cuts that are not lean or have visible fat) Beef dripping Biscuits (fat content varies greatly) Butter and dairy blend spreads Cake (most types especially mud-cake and cheesecake) Cheesecake Chicken nuggets Chicken (with skin) Chocolates (75 g) Coconut products (oil and cream and fresh and desiccated coconut) Confectionery (Mars Bars etc.) Copha Cream	Curries (using coconut or cream-based sauces) Croissant (1½) Crisps (100 g—potato or corn) Doughnuts (1½) Fried foods (all types) Fish (battered) Fish (crumbed, fried) Fruit cake or pie Garlic bread Hamburger (takeaway) Ice cream (fat content varies) Lamb (any cuts that are not lean or have visible fat) Lard Meat pie Milk (whole—necessary for children under five years) Muffins Noodles (fried) Omelette	Palm oil Palm kernel oil Pastries Pate Pizza Potato chips (hot) Potato crisps (100 g) Rice (fried) Salad dressings Salads prepared away from home (these often have lots of unnecessary added fat) Sauces (cream, butter, cheese or coconut based) Sausages (all types except low-fat) Sausage roll Soy beverage ('So good')* Soup (cream) Takeaway foods (hamburgers, chicken products etc.) Veal schnitzel Yoghurt (regular)

* Mostly unsaturated fat (and thus beneficial when consumed in moderation).

** Most cheeses have a high-fat content and need to be consumed in small amounts only. Try adding small amount (10 g) of a highly flavoured cheese, such as Parmesan, to salads etc.

Fat content of spreads and oils

Fat content	Total fat per 100 g	Saturated fat per 100 g	Saturated fat %	Mono-unsaturated fat %	Poly-unsaturated fat %
Spreads:					
Avocado	22	5	23	64	13
Margarine (monounsaturated—canola or olive based)	72	12	17	58	25
Margarine (polyunsaturated)	80	16	20	33	47
Dairy blend	80	42	52	29	19
Butter	77	54	70	26	4
Oils:					
Olive oil*	100	12	12	76	12
Sunola	100	7	7	85	8
Canola oil	100	7	7	63	30
Peanut oil	100	19	19	46	35
Polyunsaturated oil (sunflower)	100	11	11	23	66
Linseed (or flaxseed) oil**	100	10	10	21	69
Palm oil	100	51	51	39	10
Palm kernel oil	100	84	84	14	2
Coconut oil	100	92	92	6	2

* Olive oil is preferred because of its higher monounsaturated oil content and high content of antioxidants.

** About 78 per cent of the polyunsaturated oil in linseed is the omega-3 polyunsaturated oil alpha-linolenic acid. Linseed oil is oxidised easily and this causes an unpleasant smell. For this reason, linseed oil is not often used. To minimise oxidation, store it in the fridge, buy small amounts at a time and use it quickly, and reduce exposure to air by sealing with a vacuum top similar to those used for sealing wine. (It is oxidation that causes wine to go off also.)

The table also doesn't include treats. Again choosing low-fat treats such as jams and sorbets are good choices. High-fat treats should be consumed only very occasionally, perhaps once or twice a week.

The major sources of fat in Australian diets are shown in the table on p. 383 and the regular addition of any of these to your diet will significantly increase fat consumption. Most important are fats consumed as additives to food, such as fast foods and takeaways, crisps, chips, biscuits, pastries, confectionery (chocolates etc.), cakes, and fried foods. It is very difficult to know how much fat has been added to meals that you do not prepare yourself. For example, pasta prepared in a restaurant will often have oil added to it to help separate the strands. Thus, it is best to prepare as many meals as possible at home. Other common sources of fat are meat products and dairy foods. Eggs contribute only about 2 per cent of our total fat intake and only 1 per cent of saturated fat.

The foods in the table on page 383 are divided into two groups. The first group consists of foods containing beneficial fats, such as monounsaturated fats and omega-3s, or which

Fat content of other unprocessed foods

	Total fat	Saturated fat		Mono-unsaturated fat	Poly-unsaturated fat
Fat content	*per 100g*	*per 100g*	*%*	*%*	*%*
Animal products:					
Beef	5–20	2–9	43	50	7
Lamb	6–25	3–13	50	35	15
Chicken	4–14	1–4	30	56	14
Pork	5–25	2–11	43	43	14
Fish (white)	1.3–20	0.3–?	25	25	50
Fish (salmon grilled)	5–8 (8)	1–2	25	58	42
Fish (salmon canned)	8	2	25	50	25
Fish (tuna grilled)	3	1	30	30	40
Prawns	0	0	0	0	0
Dairy products	Varies		70	25	5
Nuts:					
Walnuts	66	6	9	18	73
Macadamia nuts	74	11	15	82	3
Peanuts	43	8	19	49	32
Pecans	68	6	9	63	28
Pine nuts	66	5	8	30	62
Others:					
Copha	100	98	98	2	0
Soy beverage	2	0.3	20	20	60

The statistical information used in this appendix has been taken from Rosemary Stanton *Good Fats, Bad Fats.* Allen & Unwin

contain other nutrients such as vitamins, iron, calcium and antioxidants. The second group consists of those that contain high amounts of total fat or saturated fat (usually both) and whose nutrients can be provided by alternative foods with lower fat levels. They should be used only occasionally as treats or avoided.

Appendix 4

Developmental milestones in children

Age	*Gross motor*	*Vision and fine motor*	*Social and understanding*	*Hearing and speech*
Newborn	Prone:* Pelvis high, knees under abdomen, turns face to side	Can fix on visual object and follow it briefly horizontally		Variable response to sound
4 weeks	Lifts head briefly when held in ventral suspension**	Follows object through 90°	Quietens when picked up	Soft guttural noises when content
6 weeks	Head lag not complete when pulled to sit	Hands often open	Social smiling	Quiets in response to soft sound 15 cm from ear
3 months	Prone: Lifts chest off bed taking weight on forearms. Only slight head lag when pulled to sit	Holds rattle placed in hand. Starts to look at own hands	Pleasurable response to familiar, enjoyable situations (bottle, bath)	Turns head to soft sound at ear level
6 months	Spontaneously lifts head when supine.*** Prone: Lifts chest on extended arms	Hand regard goes. Transfers objects between hands. Palmar grasp	Shows fear of strangers. Can imitate (e.g. cough), laughs	Visually locates soft sounds at 40–50 cm on ear level
9 months	Crawls. Stands holding onto support. Sits unsupported for 10 minutes	Pincer grip developing	Looks for toy fallen out of sight. Can play peek-a-boo	Tries to communicate vocally. Locates soft sounds above and below ear level at 1 metre
12 months	Walks alone with one hand held	Throws objects on floor repeatedly. Less likely to take all objects to mouth	Knows and turns to own name. Drinks from cup.	Says two or three words with meaning
18 months	Jumps using both feet. Walks backwards	Spontaneous scribble. Tower of three or four blocks	Points to two or three parts of the body. Indicates toilet needs	5–20 recognisable words. Understands many more
2 years	Runs well. Kicks ball without overbalancing	Copies vertical and circular strokes. Tower of six to seven blocks	Develops negative behaviour. Fantasy play. Gives first name	Two and three word phrases
3 years	Rides tricycle. Stands on one foot momentarily	Copies circle. Nine block tower	Mainly dry at night. Competent with fork and spoon. Knows own sex	Gives full name. Uses plurals. 3–5 word sentences
4 years	Hops on one foot. Stands on one foot for three to five seconds	Copies cross. Draws person with three parts. Matches five primary colours	Very imaginative play	Asks many questions. Gives name and address. Names four primary colours
5 years	Can skip	Copies square. Draws person with six parts	Understands rules of play. Washes and dries face and hands.	Speech fluent, good articulation

*Prone indicates lying on stomach

**Ventral suspension means being held horizontally with face down

***Supine indicates lying on back

Note: Dr Goyen gratefully acknowledges The New Children's Hospital at Westmead for agreeing to the reproduction of Appendix 5 from 'Developmental milestones in children' as published in *The Hospital Handbook* (1999).

Major foods contributing to iron and zinc intake

Appendix 5

Foods high in iron (in deceasing order)	Foods high in zinc (in decreasing order)
Parsley	Oyster, raw
Branflakes	Beef and veal
Liver, lamb's fry	Crabmeat
Pasta, wholemeal	Lamb
Beef	Kidney
Lamb	Prawns
Pumpkin seeds	Lobster
Muesli	Sunflower seeds
Tofu	Pumpkin seeds
Baked beans	Soy beans
Raisins	Cashew
Lentils/chickpeas	Pine nuts
Beans	Almonds
Cashews	Tofu
Sweet corn	Bran, rice
Apricots	Pasta, wholemeal
Spinach	Rice, brown (or white)
Bran, rice	Peas
Dates	Lentils/chickpeas
Breakfast biscuit, wholewheat	Bulgur (cracked wheat)
Bulgur (cracked wheat)	Branflakes
Almonds	Peanuts/peanut butter
Pine nuts	Salmon/tuna, canned
Oysters and mussels	Fish, steamed
Soy beverages	Milk, whole
Fish, battered	Cheese
Rice, brown cooked	Yoghurt
Crabmeat	Rolled oats
Chicken	
Bread, wholemeal	
Rolled oats	
Egg, boiled	
Salmon/tuna, canned	

Source: Adapted from Rosemary Stanton's *Healthy Vegetarian Eating*.

Appendix 6

A list of low glycaemic index (GI) foods (also low fat)

The contribution of a food to the glycaemic load of a meal increases in proportion to the amount of carbohydrate it contains. The foods below are listed (approximately) in order of carbohydrate content, with foods having the highest content being at the top. Thus, foods near the top of the list are more important in reducing the glycaemic load than foods near the bottom. (This also means they contain more energy and this fact needs to be considered in dietary planning also.)

Breakfast		*Lunch/dinner*		*Morning/afternoon tea*	
Food	*GI*	*Food*	*GI*	*Food*	*GI*
Muesli, natural	49	Rice, Doongara (an Australian rice)	56	Apple muffin, low-fat**	44
All bran™ cereal	42	Noodles (low-fat)	47	Grapes	46
Porridge	46	Fettuccine	40	Banana	52
Special K™	54	Spaghetti, white	41	Pear	38
Fruit loaf	47	Spaghetti, wholemeal	37	Apple	38
Bread, heavy mixed grain*	30–45	Vermicelli	35	Mangoes	51
Apple juice	40	Ravioli	39	Popcorn (natural)	54
Orange juice	46	Rice, basmati	58	Fruit loaf	47
Pineapple juice	46	Tortellini	50	Milk, skimmed	32
Milk, full cream (for young children)	27	Sushi	48–55	Yoghurt, low-fat flavoured	33
Milk, skimmed	32	Tomato soup, canned	38	Soy drink, So-good™	31
Soy drink, So-good™	31	Corn (on cob)	54	Orange	44
Grapefruit	25	Bread, heavy mixed grain	30–45	Peach	42
Banana	52	Yoghurt, low-fat flavoured	33	Plum	39
Apple	38	Ice-cream, low-fat	50	Cherries	22
Mangoes	51	Butter beans, boiled	31		
Kiwifruit	53	Chickpeas, boiled	28		
Apricots, dried	31	Baked beans	48		
Peaches, canned in unsweetened juice	30	Kidney beans, boiled	27		
		Haricot beans, boiled	38		
		Lentils, boiled	28		

* Other breads such as white and wholemeal breads have a relatively high GI (about 70). Choosing low-GI breads is a very important factor in achieving low glycaemic load diet.

** Low-fat muffins often have a high energy content, so those with a weight problem need to be careful.

Sources: Brand-Miller, J. and Forster-Powell, K., *The New Glucose Revolution*, Hodder Headline, 1999. The GI website: www.glycemicindex.com

BMI weight chart

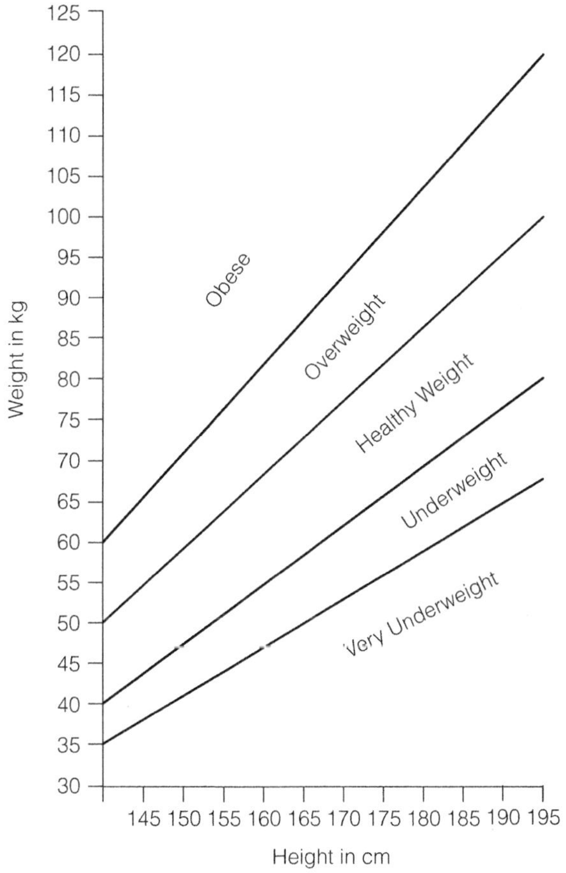

$$BMI = \frac{\text{weight (in kg)}}{\text{height in metres}^2}$$

Appendix 8 The evolution of vascular disease

Initial injury to the inner artery wall
(Numerous causes including ingested chemicals, forces from high blood preasure, high levels of body compounds such as homocysteine and oxidised LDL, infections.) Good vascular disease risk factor management helps reduce injury

LDL becomes oxidised inside the vessel wall by free radicals (oxidants) such as cigarette chemicals, environmental polutants etc. They are also increased in diabetes and perhaps even stress.

Increased permeability of vessel lining allows more LDL from the blood to enter the vessel wall.

Inflammatory reaction starts up as a response to injury. (Similar to the redness and swelling that occurs with a mild skin burn)

Oxidised LDL causes more injury. A self-perpetuating inflammation cycle is set up (shown by thick arrows).

Antioxidants help reverse/prevent LDL oxidation and slow the inflammation cycle.

Oxidised LDL is taken up by macrophages and cholesterol-filled foam cells are formed.

Substances produced by inflammation attract macrophage cells from the blood which enter the vessel wall

Foam cells die leaving a free deposit of cholesterol in the vessel wall which gradually builds up to form an early vascular lesion called a fatty streak.

This fatty streak gradually increases in size and starts to obstruct the lumen of the artery. As the lesion matures, it also accumulates calcium and fibrous tissue and becomes harder. This is termed an advanced lesion. This advanced lesion can have three different outcomes, depending on how well the person manages their vascular disease risk factors.

Risk factor management
Good ◄——► **Poor**

Minimal progression or regression (improvement)
Symptoms are unlikely or occur late in life.

Continued slow lesion enlargement—stable lesion
The inner artery wall that overlies the lesion is relatively thick, making the lesion unlikely to break open, i.e. they are stable.

More rapid enlargement—unstable lesion
The inner artery wall that overlies the lesion becomes relatively thin, making the lesion more likely to rupture, i.e. they are unstable.

Later onset of symptoms
Stable lesions tend to enlarge slowly and the body counteracts these blockages by creating new co-lateral vessels to bypass the blockage. This usually delays the onset of symptoms till later in life.
However, the blockage will eventually get large enough to cause symptoms.
The other option is that the lesion may change and become unstable.

Rupture—Heart attack
An increase in the pressure in the lesion or additional weakness in the wall due to inflammation causes the wall to rupture. Once a rupture occurs, a clot forms over the rupture site to help seal off the site, just like a clot forms over a cut on your skin. As this situation usually develops over a period of minutes, there is no time for co-lateral vessels to be established so that the blockage can be bypassed. Thus, the rupture and associated clot formation act to cause a sudden large blockage of the vessel and the tissue the artery supplies dies. (In the heart, this is called a heart attack or myocardial infarct.)

Dietary and other factors that influence vascular lesion formation

Appendix 9

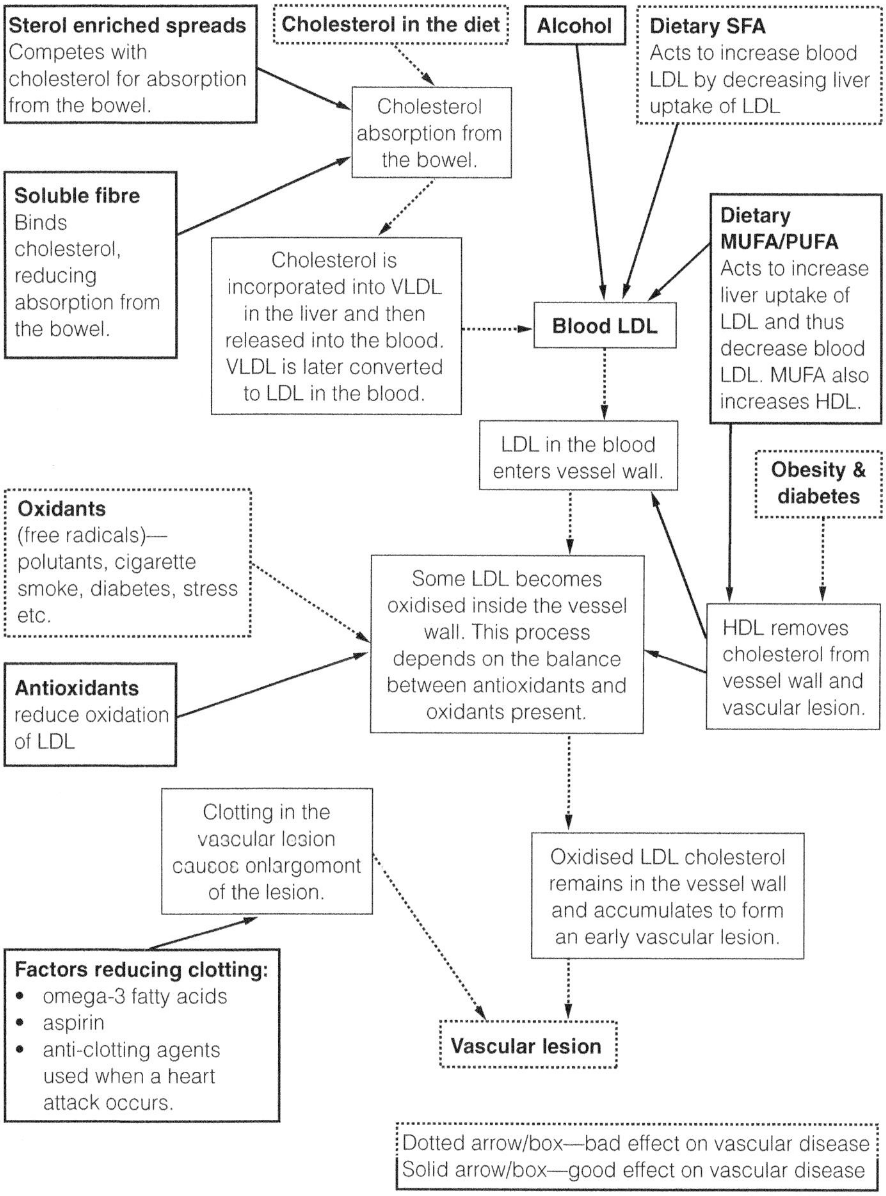

MUFA: monounsaturated fatty acids
PUFA: polyunsaturated fatty acids
SFA: saturated fatty acids
LDL: Low-density lipoproteins
HDL: High-density lipoproteins
Omega-3 FA: omega-3 fatty acids

Appendix 10

Diagnosing diabetes by testing blood sugars

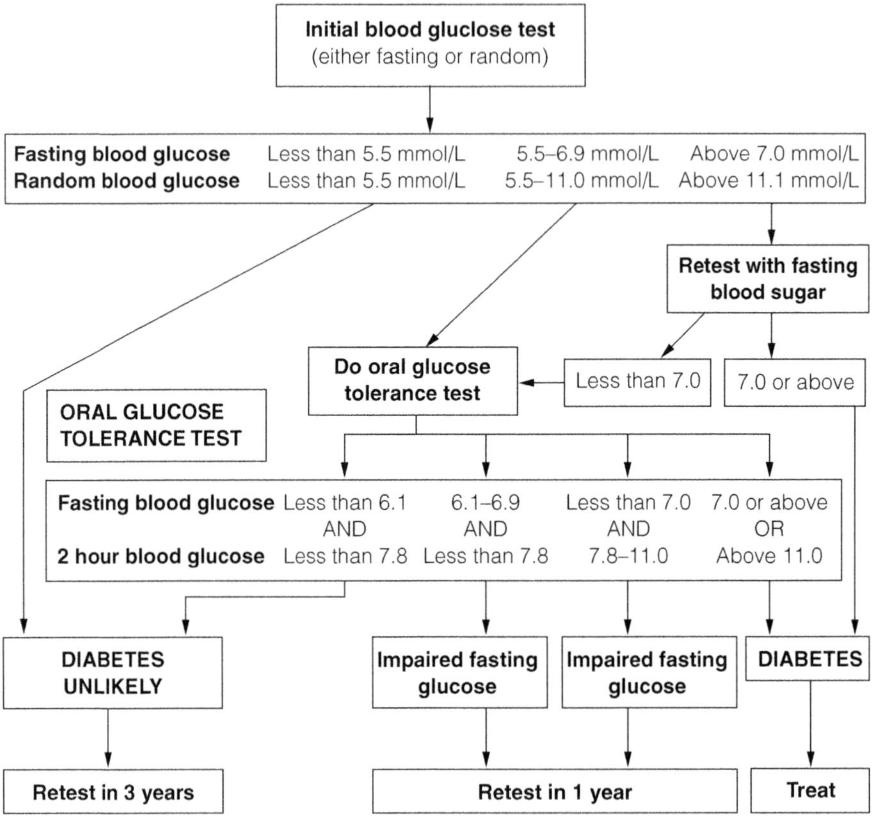

New Zealand cardiovascular disease risk calculator

Appendix 11

How to use these charts

Prognosis: To estimate a person's absolute five-year risk of a cardiovascular event (new angina, myocardial infarct [heart attack], death from coronary heart disease, stroke or transient ischaemic attack [TIA]), find the grey scale block which best describes your:

- gender
- age
- smoking habit
- diabetes status (on insulin, oral hypoglycaemics, or fasting blood glucose > 8.0 mmol/L Reflotron or laboratory measurement)
- BP (mean of two readings on each of two occasions sufficient for assessing risk but not for establishing pre-treatment baseline)
- total cholesterol/HDL ratio (mean of two non-fasting Reflotron measurements or one laboratory measurement sufficient for assessing risk but not for establishing pre-treatment baseline).

All people with symptomatic cardiovascular disease (CVD) (including angina, MI, chronic heart failure, stroke, TIA and peripheral vascular disease [PVD] or ECG diagnosed left ventricular failure), are assumed to have a CVD risk greater than 20 per cent in five years. Patients with a strong family history of CVD (first degree of relatives: male with CVD before 55 years, female before 65 years) or obesity (BMI of about 30 or more) are likely to be at greater risk than the tables indicate. These people should consider increasing one number category. Read off five-year risk from number code in key to table.

These tables have been produced with the kind permission of the New Zealand Guidelines Group. The charts normally appear in colour and are available at www.nzgg.org.nz/library/glcomplete/table1.cmf

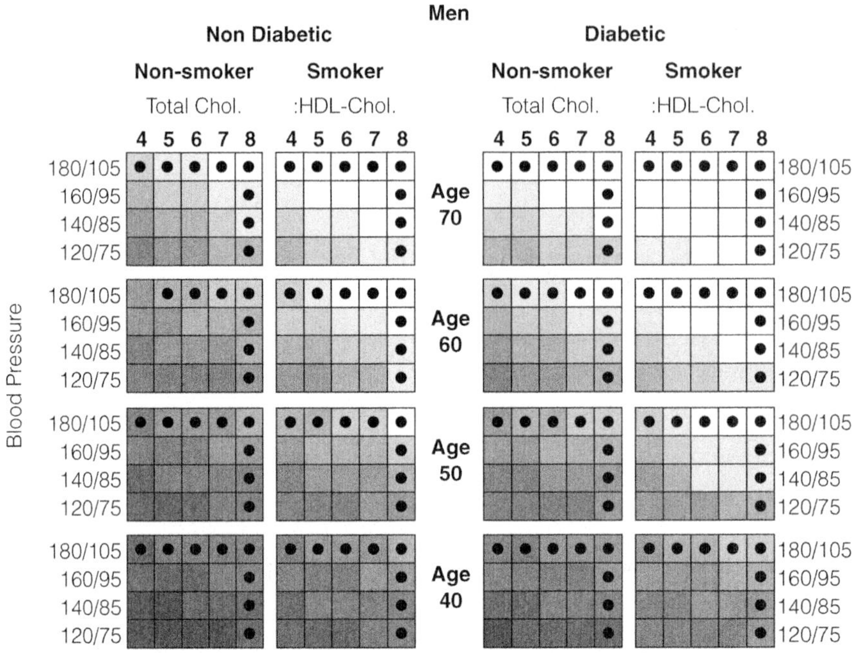
Men
Non Diabetic
Diabetic
Non-smoker
Smoker
Non-smoker
Smoker
Total Chol.
:HDL-Chol.
Total Chol.
:HDL-Chol.
4 5 6 7 8
Blood Pressure
180/105
160/95
140/85
120/75
Age 70
Age 60
Age 50
Age 40

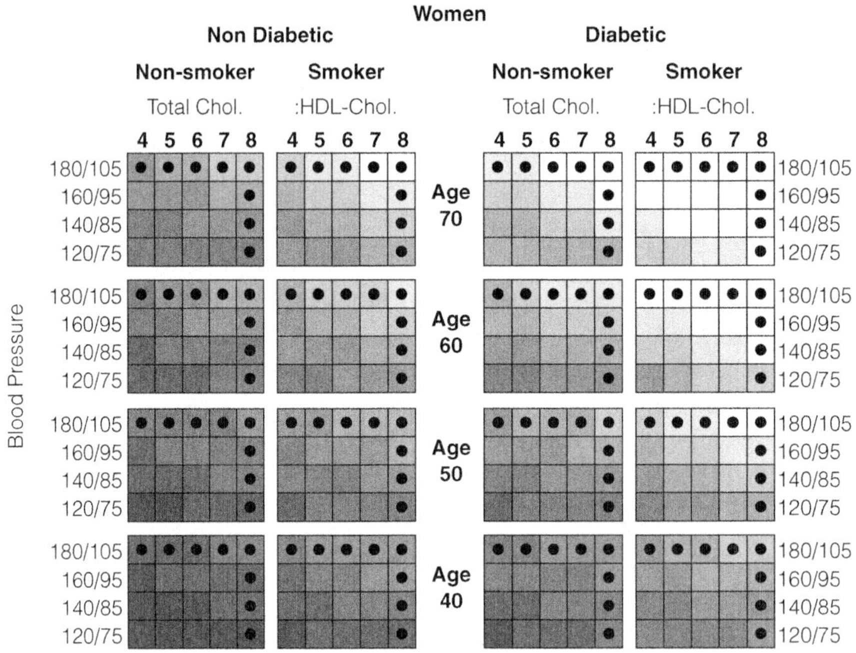
Women
Non Diabetic
Diabetic
Non-smoker
Smoker
Non-smoker
Smoker
Total Chol.
:HDL-Chol.
Total Chol.
:HDL-Chol.
4 5 6 7 8
Blood Pressure
180/105
160/95
140/85
120/75
Age 70
Age 60
Age 50
Age 40

Key to Risk Tables

Prognosis: 5 year CVD risk (non-fatal & fatal)	Benefit 1: CVD events prevented per 100 treated for 5 years*	Benefit 2: NNT for 5 years*
> 30%	> 10 per 100	< 10
25–30%	9 per 100	11
20–25%	7.5 per 100	13
15–20%	6 per 100	16
10–15%	4 per 100	25
5–10%	2.5 per 100	40
2.5–5%	1.25 per 100	80
< 2.5%	< 0.8 per 100	>120

Suggested starting point for discussion with patient about drug treatment. (15–20% and 10–15% rows: 6 per 100 / 16; 4 per 100 / 25)

- Cells with this marker indicate that in patients with very high levels of cholesterol (> about 8.5–9 mmol/L) or blood pressure (> about 170/100 mmHg), the risk equations may underestimate the true risk. **Therefore it is recommended that treatment be considered at lower absolute CVD risks than in other patients.**

* Assumes BP reduction of about 12/6 mmHg in patients with BP > 140–150/90, or cholesterol reduction of about 20% in patients with total cholesterol > 5.0–5.5 mmol/L, produces an approximate 30% reduction in CVD risk, whatever the pre-treatment absolute risk.

Benefit 1: This gives the number of CVD events (new angina, MI, death from coronary heart disease, stroke or TIA) that would be prevented by treating 100 people in this group with cholesterol-lowering medication for five years.

Benefit 2: This gives the number of people in this group that would need to be treated for five years with cholesterol-lowering medication to prevent one CVD event (new angina, MI, death from coronary heart disease, stroke or TIA).

Appendix 12 Cholesterol in the body

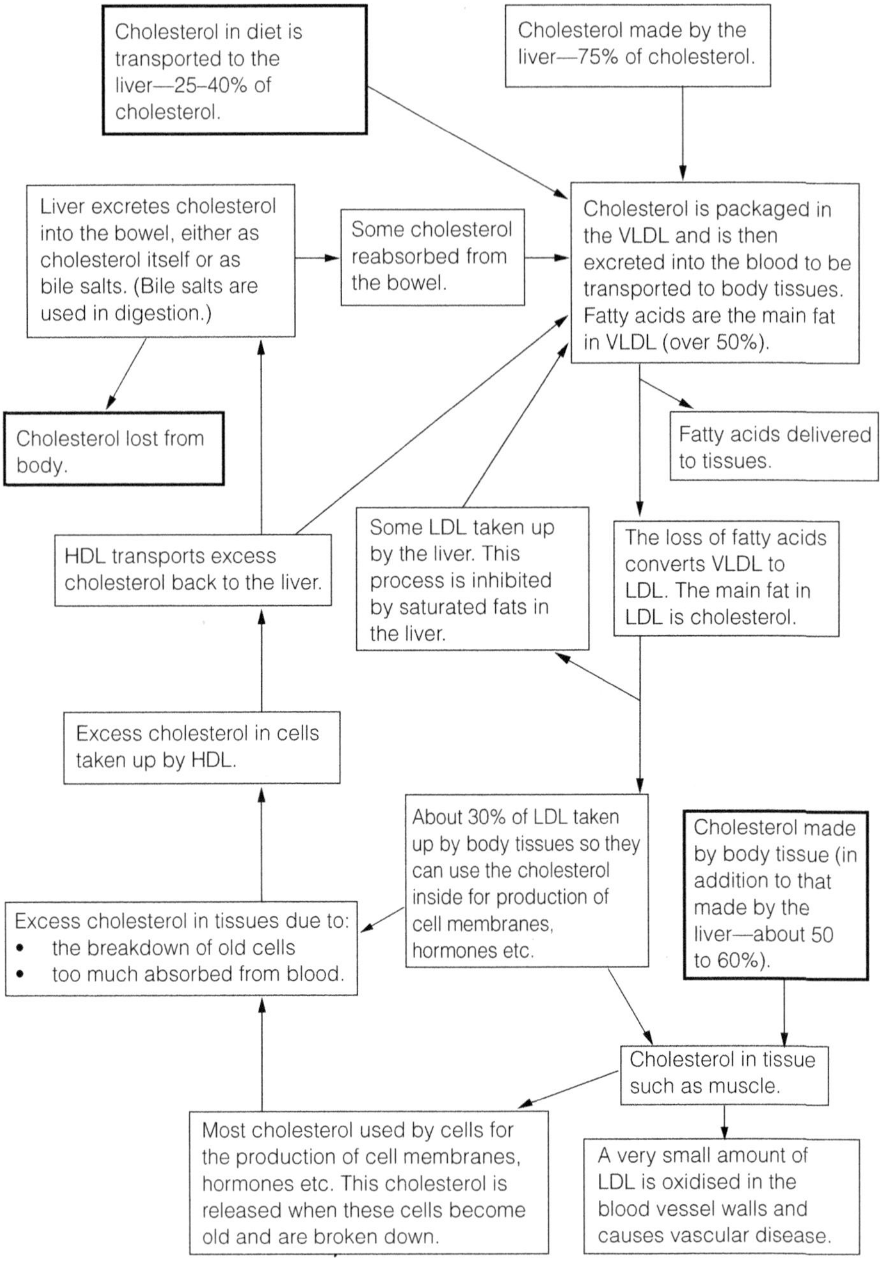

VLDL: Very low density lipoprotein
LDL: Low density lipoprotein
HDL: High density lipoprotein
Dark box: sources and losses of body cholesterol

Antioxidants in foods

Appendix 13

The table below includes a sample of the multitude of antioxidants found in many types of food.

Food	*Antioxidants present*
Apples	Bioflavonoids
Basil	O-cimene, cineol, esdragol
Broad beans	Flavonoids (especially quercetin)
Broccoli and other brassica family foods	Carotenoids, plant sterols, dithiolthiones, glucosinolates (indoles)
Capers	Biflavones, resins, glycosides
Capsicum	Capsaicin, carotenoids
Carrots	Carotenoids, flavonoids, coumarins
Citrus fruit	Carotenoids, flavonoids, limonoids, coumarins, monoterpenes, triterpenoids
Eggplant	Phenols, plant sterols, saponins
Fennel	Phenols, esdragol, anethole
Garlic	Glucosides, allyl, methyl trisulphide, allylic sulphides, allicin, allylic cysteines
Ginger	Curcumins, gingerols, diarylhptanoids
Horseradish	Isothiocyanates
Linseeds (flaxseeds)	Alpha linolenic acid, ligans
Marjoram	Terpineol, borneal
Mint	Menthol, cineol, menthoruran, terpenes
Olives and olive oil	Phenols
Onions	Flavonoids, many sulphur compounds
Oregano	Thymol, terpenes, carnarole, ursolic acid
Parsley	Coumarins, carotenoids, flavonoids, monoterpenes, phenols, phthalides, polacetalenes, aplin, pinene
Rosemary	Pinene, borneol, carnosol, ursolic acid
Sage	Borneol, camphor, cineol, tuyone, tannins, carnarole
Soy beans	Phytoestrogens, flavonoids, thymol
Tea, green or black	Tannins, catechins
Thyme	Thymol, terpenes, tannins, carnaroe
Tomatoes (red, ripe)	Carotenoids (especially lycopene), coumarins, plant sterols
Vegetables	Carotenoids, numerous antioxidants
Wine, red	Polyphenols

Source: Rosemary Stanton, 1997.

Appendix 14

Control of LDL levels by dietary fatty acids

The mechanisms by which saturated fatty acids cause an increase in LDL are still uncertain. However, the most likely explanation lies in the relative amounts of saturated and unsaturated fatty acids incorporated into cell membranes.

The shape of a fatty acid is determined by the presence or absence of double bonds in its carbon chain. Saturated fatty acids, with no double bonds, have the overall shape of a straight rod. The presence of one or more double bonds causes a kink in this rod-like shape and unsaturated fatty acids are thus the shape of bent rods. ('Trans' fatty acids are the exception to this rule. See the section on unsaturated fatty acids.) Their bent shape means that unsaturated fatty acids cannot pack as tightly together as saturated fatty acids and the bonds between them are therefore not as strong (see the figure on page 399). This explains why foods with a higher saturated fat content, such as butter, are solid at room temperature and those with more unsaturated fats, such as olive oil, are liquids.

Each cell in the body is surrounded by a thin continuous cell membrane which regulates what is allowed into and out of the cell. The main components used in their construction are phopholipids, which are compounds made from two fatty acids joined to a phosphorylated alcohol. When these phospholipids line up together, they form a sheet-like structure capable of surrounding the cell. How tightly these phospholipids can line up determines the rigidity of the membrane they form. A high concentration of straighter saturated fats allows a tighter fit and makes the membrane around the cell more rigid. Unsaturated fatty acids do the opposite—making the membrane more fluid or floppier. It is thought that these differences in cell membrane fluidity can alter the amount of LDL taken up by cells (especially liver cells), probably by altering the effectiveness of LDL receptors which are embedded in the cell membrane. These receptors are responsible for LDL uptake by the cell and an excessively rigid membrane is thought to reduce LDL uptake and thus increase blood LDL levels.

The cell membrane also contains cholesterol, so changes in the cholesterol content can also influence membrane fluidity and thus LDL levels.

Finally, it has also been postulated that unsaturated fats may act to increase cholesterol excretion by the liver. This would reduce the liver content of cholesterol and thus reduce the amount of cholesterol available for transport in VLDL. (VLDL is eventually transformed into LDL.)

As stated above, these explanations of how fatty acids alter LDL are not proven and more work needs to be done before the role of fatty acids in altering blood cholesterol is fully understood.

Unsaturated fatty acids—cis and trans types

The presence of a double bond in a fatty acid can cause the fatty acid to bend at the double bond site. Whether this occurs depends on the anatomical structure of the double bond and there are two possible configurations; the *cis* configuration and the *trans* configuration.

The cis configuration, which is the one that occurs in almost all naturally-occurring unsaturated fatty acids, causes a kink in their rod-like structure where the double bonds occur. The bent shape means that these unsaturated fatty acids cannot pack as tightly together as straight saturated fatty acids and the bonds between adjacent fatty acids are therefore not as strong.

The trans configuration does not cause a kink at the double bond site and this means trans fatty acids have a straighter overall shape and thus they more closely resemble the straight shape of a saturated fatty acid than their cis counterparts. If the trans fatty acid is monounsaturated, then it will have a straight rod shape that mimics the shape of a saturated fatty acid. A good example is the harmful trans fatty acid called elaidic acid, which, like almost all trans fatty acids, is produced in the making of processed foods such as margarines and cooking oils. As well as creating harmful trans fatty acids, such processing usually increases the number of saturated fatty acids in the fat. These fats taste better and are easier to use in processed foods but they are not good for you. Such trans fatty acids have similar harmful effects as saturated fatty acids.

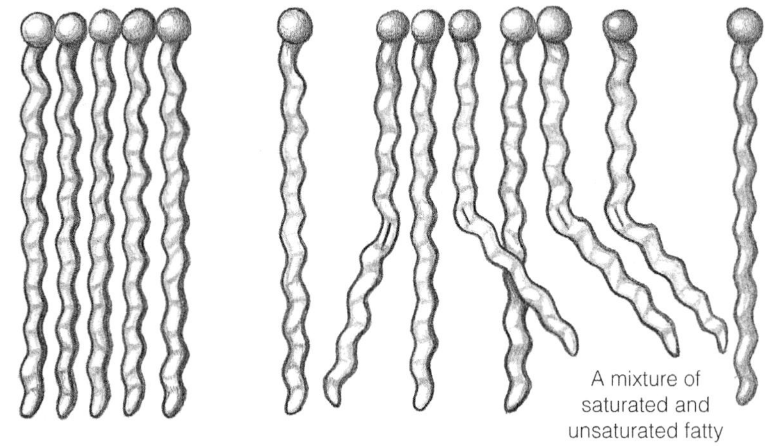

Packing of fatty acids

Saturated fatty acids are able to pack closer together due to their overall straight shape. This enables them to form stronger bonds between each other and means that fatty foods containing a high proportion of saturated fatty acids, such as butter, are solid at room temperature. Conversely, fatty foods that have a high proportion of unsaturated fatty acids, such as olive oil, are generally fluids at room temperature. Fatty acids also combine in a somewhat similar manner when creating cell membranes. Membranes containing a high proportion of saturated fatty acids tend to be more rigid in shape. This can alter the functions of membranes, such as how much of certain substances like cholesterol are allowed into the cell.

Glossary

Adipose tissue—Another term for body fat tissue.

Aneurysm—A blood vessel that has expanded due to a weakening in the vessel wall. This weakening can be congenital, as is often the case in strokes due to haemorrhages from aneurysms in the brain, or caused by vascular disease.

Angina—Heart pain caused by inadequate oxygen supply to the heart muscle. This is usually due to reduced blood supply to that muscle.

Anthocyanin—A type of antioxidant. (It is one of the main antioxidants in red wine.)

Antioxidant—A compound that prevents or reverses the oxidation of another compound. They do this by providing a spare electron either to a free radical or to a compound that has been oxidised by a free radical. Antioxidants are important in reducing vessel disease. They do this by preventing LDL (bad cholesterol) from being oxidised and it is only oxidised LDL that causes vessel disease. They can also reduce the incidence of other diseases such as cancers. There are many antioxidant compounds in our diet.

Aorta—The main artery taking blood away from the heart.

Artery—A blood vessel that transports blood flowing away from the heart.

Atheroma lesion—A fatty/fibrous lesion in the wall of a blood vessel that often leads to vessel blockage.

Atherosclerosis—The process by which fatty lesions cause blockages in arteries.

Australian Institute of Health and Welfare—An Australian government organisation that researches health issues in the Australian community.

Barium enema—An X-ray of the large bowel using radio-opaque dye.

BCC (Basal cell carcinoma)—This is a type of skin cancer. It does spread locally but usually does not spread through the body. It is related to sun exposure with initiation of the cancer appearing to occur relatively early in life.

BMI (body mass index)—This is a method of determining the level of a person's obesity using their height and weight.

BMR (Basal metabolic rate)—This is a measure of the minimum amount of energy the body uses. It is usually measured early in the morning after about eight hours of rest. It is usually very close to the resting metabolic rate, which is measured while resting during the day.

Burden of disease—A measure of the total amount of disease in the community. The contribution of each disease category is calculated using the severity and duration of the disease. It is measured in 'Disability adjusted life years' (DALYs). (See DALYs.) (See also Appendix 1.)

Calories—A unit of measurement for energy. It is often used to give the energy content of foods or to indicate the energy expended during exercise.

Carbohydrate—This is a compound made of carbon and hydrogen and oxygen. The main groups are sugars (e.g. glucose and glycogen) and starches (e.g. rice, flour, pasta, bread). It is an important source of energy in our food and the sugar glucose is the main energy source used by the body's cells. This glucose is stored in the body (mostly in the liver) as glycogen.

Carcinogen—A substance that can initiate cancer.

Cardiovascular disease—Vascular disease affecting arteries in the body, especially the aorta and those arteries supplying the heart muscle, the brain, the kidneys and the legs.

Cerebrovascular disease—A disease of the main arteries supplying the brain where the deposits of fats and other compounds in the artery wall leads to blockage of the artery. If severe enough, this can cause death of brain tissue (i.e. a stroke).

Cervix—The lower part of the uterus (womb) that projects into the vagina. Cancer can develop in this area of the uterus. It can be detected early before becoming life threatening by having a Pap smear.

Cholesterol—This is a type of fat. In our bodies it is an important component of the outside envelope surrounding all cells and it is also used in the production of steroid hormones. Cholesterol can be made by our bodies and is consumed in our diets. It is the fat that causes vascular disease.

Cholesterol ester—A cholesterol molecule that has been joined to a fatty acid. Cholesterol is usually stored in an ester form when being transported inside lipoproteins.

Chronic obstructive lung disease—This is caused by damage to the lining of the airways, mostly by smoking but can also be due to dusts such as coal dust. It causes the airways to produce extra mucous, makes this mucous more difficult to cough up and also narrows the airways which causes progressively increasing shortness of breath and eventually often death. It includes chronic bronchitis and emphysema.

Chylomicron—A type of lipoprotein that transports dietary fats absorbed from the bowel.

Colonoscopy—A procedure where the large bowel and rectum can be viewed through a fibre optic instrument.

Common carotid artery—The main vessel supplying blood to the head.

Coronary artery—A blood vessel that provides the heart muscle with its blood supply.

Coronary artery disease (coronary heart disease, coronary vascular disease, or ischaemic heart disease)—A disease of the coronary arteries where the deposits of fats and other compounds in the artery wall leads to blockage of the artery.

Coronary heart disease—see **coronary artery disease.**

Coronary vascular disease—see **coronary artery disease.**

C-reactive protein—A compound that, when measured in a blood sample, can indicate the degree of inflammation occurring in vascular lesions.

Decibel (dB)—A unit of measurement for the volume of sound.

Disability adjusted life year (DALY)—By adding the YLL and the YDL together, the total illness burden for a particular disease can be assessed (i.e. the total burden of disease). It is expressed in terms of DALYs. One DALY is one lost year of 'healthy life'. (See also Appendix 1.)

Embolus—A clot that breaks away from a lesion on the inner surface of a vessel wall. This clot travels further down the vessel, eventually causing a blockage further down.

Essential fatty acids—Fatty acids that need to be consumed in the diet as they can either not be produced in the body or not produced in sufficient quantity.

Faecal occult blood test (FOBT)—A test for determining the presence of blood in the bowel motions. As bowel cancers tend to bleed, it is a method used to screen people with no symptoms for bowel cancer.

Fatty acid—A fat that is basically a long chained hydrocarbon (usually 12 to 18 carbon atoms) used for providing energy. Most can be made in the body or can be ingested in the diet. It is converted to triglycerides for transport and storage.

Fibre—Fibre is defined as any food component that passes through the small intestine without being digested at all. Soluble fibre is that which can be dissolved in water. Insoluble fibre cannot be dissolved in water.

Foam cell—A cell containing cholesterol formed in an early atheroma lesion.

Free radical—An unstable compound that is short of an electron in its structure. Free radicals are able to oxidise other compounds in the body. They do this by taking an electron from them. The compound that has lost the electron is often not able to function properly in the body.

Gene—Each gene is made up of a varying length of double stranded chromosome material found in the cell's nucleus. The cell's 23 pairs of chromosomes are made up of thousands of genes and they control all functions of the cell by controlling the production proteins etc. by the cell.

Gestational diabetes—Diabetes that occurs when a woman is pregnant. This condition often resolves after the pregnancy although the woman is at greater risk of diabetes in later life.

Glomerular filtration rate—A measurement of the rate which the kidneys can filter blood. This gives an accurate indication of how well the kidneys are functioning.

Glycaemic index—A measurement of how quickly and to what degree a carbohydrate-containing food will raise a person's blood sugar after its consumption.

Glycogen—A series of glucose molecules joined together. It is a compound for storing molecules of the sugar glucose.

Haemorrhage—The inappropriate leakage of blood out of a blood vessel.

HbA1C—A type of haemoglobin (measured by taking a blood sample) that indicates how well blood sugars have been controlled in a diabetic patient over the last few months.

HDL—A lipoprotein that removes excess cholesterol from the tissues and returns it to the liver.

Heart attack (myocardial infarct)—The death of heart muscle tissue due to lack of blood supply (and thus oxygen) to that tissue.

High density lipoprotein (HDL)—A lipoprotein that removes excess cholesterol from the tissues and returns it to the liver. (Also called good cholesterol.)

Homocysteine—Homocysteine is an essential amino acid. (Amino acids are the compounds that we make proteins from.) When in excess, homocysteine can increase the risk of coronary artery disease.

Hypertension—High blood pressure.

HMG Co reductase—This is an enzyme that plays an important part in cholesterol production in the body. Drugs that inhibit this enzyme (statin drugs) are very beneficial in reducing cholesterol levels in the body.

Insoluble fibre—Insoluble fibre is fibre that cannot be dissolved in water.

Insomnia—Difficulty sleeping.

Insulin—The primary hormone responsible for regulating blood sugar levels in the body.

Insulin resistance—This occurs when the hormone insulin does not lower the blood sugar levels in the body by as much as would normally be expected. If severe enough, this problem can lead to type 2 diabetes.

Internal carotid artery—The main vessel supplying blood to the brain. (A branch of the common carotid artery.)

Intima—The inner portion of the wall of a blood vessel.

Ischaemic heart disease—See coronary artery disease.

Ischaemic stroke—The death of brain tissue due to a reduction in blood supply (and thus oxygen) to the affected brain tissue.

Kilojoules—A unit of measurement for energy. It is often used to give the energy content of foods or to indicate the energy expended during exercise.

LDL (low density lipoprotein)—A lipoprotein that basically transports cholesterol in the blood. (Also called bad cholesterol.)

Lipid—A term for any fat compound.

Lipoprotein—A large membrane bound compound used for transporting lipids in the blood.

Lipoprotein (a)—This is a lipoprotein that can increase the risk of vascular disease when blood levels in the body are elevated.

Low density lipoprotein (LDL)—A lipoprotein that basically transports cholesterol in the blood. (Also called bad cholesterol.)

Lumen—The 'inside' of the blood vessel through which the blood flows.

Macrovascular disease—Vascular disease that occurs in the large blood vessels, such as those supplying the heart muscle, the brain and the lower legs. It is mainly caused by fatty deposits in the artery walls (atheroma).

Mammogram—An X-ray of the breasts. There are two types of mammogram, that used for screening asymptomatic women for breast cancers and that used to investigate a woman who has an abnormality in her breast.

Melanoma—A serious pigmented (dark) skin cancer that spreads readily throughout the body (metastasises) and thus is very dangerous.

Mesothelioma—This is a type of cancer that occurs on the outside surface of the lung. It is caused by exposure to asbestos. (This exposure often only needs to be quite small and it is therefore important to stop all exposure to asbestos.) The cancer is often very aggressive and responds poorly to available treatments. The prognosis is usually poor.

Metabolic syndrome (Syndrome X)—This syndrome occurs in obese people (usually men) and is associated with a significant risk of heart attacks. It consists of all or some of the following features: a marked increase in atherosclerosis, an increase in blood pressure (hypertension), raised blood lipids, type 2 diabetes and protein in the urine.

Microvascular disease—Vascular disease that occurs in the small blood vessels, such as in the kidneys and the retina (eyes). It is usually caused by diabetes.

Monounsaturated fatty acid—A fatty acid which has a structure that includes one double bond between its carbon atoms.

Myocardial infarct (heart attack)—The death of heart muscle tissue due to lack of blood supply (and thus oxygen) to that tissue.

Mutation—A change in the structure in a gene in the nucleus of a cell. Such changes can cause the gene to malfunction and lead to diseases such as cancer.

National Health and Medical Research Council (NHMRC)—An Australian government body that researches medical topics and makes recommendations to the government about optimum treatments and health policy.

Nicotine—This is the addictive chemical in tobacco (cigarettes). It also causes narrowing of arteries in the body and therefore worsens vessel disease.

Occult blood—A small amount of blood that is not easily seen. The term is used in association with screening for bowel cancer. The faecal occult blood test (FOBT) looks for blood in bowel motions, which can signify the presence of bowel cancer.

Oestrogen—The princpal female hormone. It is made by the body and is also one of the two hormones in oral contraceptives and hormone replacement therapy (HRT) (along with progesterone). There are several types of oestrogen used in the pill and HRT.

Omega-3 fatty acids—A type of polyunsaturated fatty acid found in fish (especially oily ones) and vegetables. Increased consumption helps reduce vessel disease and also may help reduce inflammatory conditions such as asthma and rheumatoid arthritis.

Omega-6 fatty acids—A type of polyunsaturated fatty acid found mostly in 'vegetable sources' such as sunflowers. Increased consumption reduces vessel disease by lowering both total cholesterol and LDL. If consumption is too high, it can become out of balance with omega-3 fatty acids and this can cause an increase in inflammatory conditions such as asthma.

Oxidant—A compound that causes the oxidation of another compound. An antioxidant can reverse or prevent this oxidation effect. Free radicals are oxidants.

Peripheral vascular disease—A blockage in the large arteries supplying the legs with blood. It is mainly caused by fatty deposits in the artery walls (atheroma) and can lead to gangrene.

Polycystic ovary disease—In this disease cysts form on the ovaries. It is associated with several abnormalities including an increased risk of vascular disease due to increased blood lipids and hormonal problems including reduced fertility.

Phytochemicals—Chemicals found in plants.

Phytoestrogens—A group of chemicals found in plants that have properties similar to those of the human oestrogen hormone (17 beta-oestradiol). The most common ones occurring in food are isoflavones that come from soy beans and linseed (flaxseed).

Polygenic hypercholesterolaemia—This is the name given to the common problem of unexplained raised blood cholesterol. There are thought to be many contributing genetic factors. These may act independently or express themselves through interaction with external factors such as diet.

Poly-unsaturated fatty acid—A fatty acid which has a structure that includes more than one double bond between its carbon atoms.

Postural hypotension—This condition occurs when a person's blood pressure reduces when getting up from a lying position. (Normally the opposite occurs.) This often results in dizziness and can cause the person to fall. It is common in older people and is often caused by medications.

Primary (first-degree) relative—Your parents or siblings (i.e. brothers and sisters).

Progestins (Progesterones)—A group of female steroid hormones. Progesterone is produced in the body from cholesterol and is responsible, with oestrogen, for regulating the menstrual cycle. Progesterones are used in combination with an oestrogen hormone in the oral contraceptive pill and in hormone replacement therapy.

Psychosis—A major mental disturbance where people lose touch with external reality. It often includes delusions, such as thinking that you are some one you're not; feeling that you are being persecuted or continually watched; or seeing, hearing or smelling things that are not there. Schizophrenia is a mental illness characterised by such experiences. It is the most common psychotic illness. Such disturbances are also associated with some drug use.

Resistant starch—A type of starch that is slowly digested.

Resting metabolic rate (RMR)—This is a measure of the amount of energy the body uses while resting, say in a chair. (It is usually very close to the BMR, which is the minimum energy used by the body and is measured in the morning after about eight hours of rest.)

Saturated fatty acid—A fatty acid which has a structure that includes no double bonds between its carbon atoms.

SCC **(squamous cell carcinoma)**—This is a type of skin cancer. It spreads locally and can spread through the body. It needs to be excised. It is related to sun exposure with initiation of the cancer appearing to occur relatively later in life.

Screening—This is the process by which a selected group of the population (or all the population) are tested for the presence of a particular disease.

Second-degree relatives—Grandparents and aunts and uncles.

Sleep apnoea—A condition where relaxation of throat/tongue muscles causes an obstruction in the throat above the voice box, resulting in regular episodes where the person stops breathing for short periods. Each time this happens, the brain wakes the person just enough so that the person takes a breath (often as a snort or a gasp).

Soluble fibre—Fibre which can be dissolved in water.

Standard variation—A statistical method for measuring the extent to which a particular measurement varies from the average of a group of measurements. Positive levels indicate the reading is greater than the average and vice versa.

Starches—Starches are a group of carbohydrates. They are an important source of energy in our diets and include pasta, breads, potatoes, rice, cereals etc.

Statin drugs—These are the most common group of drugs used to reduce cholesterol. They act by inhibiting an enzyme called HMG Co reductase. This is an enzyme that plays an important part in cholesterol production in the body.

Stent—An expanding metal mesh tube used to open up blocked arteries. When placed in the artery it expands, acting to increase the size of the vessel lumen.

Stroke—The death of brain tissue. This can be due to reduction in blood supply (and thus oxygen) to the affected brain tissue (an ischaemic stroke) or due to damage caused to the brain tissue by a bleed into that tissue from a break in a blood vessel (a haemorrhagic stroke).

Sugars—A group of carbohydrates that are an important source of energy both in our bodies and in the food we eat. There are many different types of sugars. The main sugar in our diet is sucrose. The sugar glucose is the main energy source used by the body's cells and is transported in the blood.

Teratogenic substance—A substance, such as a drug or chemical, that causes foetal abnormalities when the mother is exposed to it.

Trans fatty acid—A type of polyunsaturated fatty acid that can act more like saturated fatty acids in causing vascular disease.

Transient ischaemic attack—A temporary interruption in the blood supply to a part of the brain, usually caused by a small embolus (clot) temporarily blocking an artery. Symptoms last for minutes to a few hours.

Triglyceride—A fat composed of 3 fatty acid molecules joined together by a glycerol molecule. It is the principal energy storage compound in the body and is also used as the 'transporting form' of fatty acids.

Unsaturated fatty acid—A fatty acid that has a structure which includes one or more double bonds between its carbon atoms.

Vascular disease—A narrowing or blockage of a blood vessel due usually to atheroma lesions in the blood vessel wall. This leads to blockage of blood flow through the blood vessel.

Vein—A blood vessel that transports blood towards the heart.

Very low density lipoprotein (VLDL)—A compound that transports cholesterol from the liver. It is the precursor of LDL (low density lipoprotein).

Years of life lost due to death (YLL)—This indicator is used to express death in terms of premature mortality (i.e. the burden of premature mortality). It indicates the years of normal life expectancy that is lost by a person due to their death. (See also Appendix 1.)

Years of life lost due to disability (YLD)—This indicates the years of healthy life lost due to poor health or disability (i.e. the burden of disability). (See also Appendix 1.)

References

Anderson, A., 'Maternal age and foetal loss: population based register linkage study', *British Medical Journal,* 320:1708–12, 2000.

Aronow, H.D., 'Effect of Lipid-lowering Therapy on Early Mortality after Acute Coronary Syndromes; an Observational Study', *Lancet,* 357:1063–68, 2001.

Australian Hearing, www.hearing.com.au

Australian Institute of Health and Welfare, *Australia's Health 2000; the seventh biennial health report of the Australian Institute of Health and Welfare,* Canberra: AIHW, 2000.

Australian Institute of Health and Welfare: Mathers et al., *The burden of disease and injury in Australia,* Australian Institute of Health and Welfare, Canberra, 1999.

Australia New Zealand Food Authority, *Food for Health,* Commonwealth of Australia, Canberra, 1991.

Australian Bureau of Statistics, *Australian Social Trends 1999 Family—Family Formation: Remarriage trends of divorced people,* ABS, 2000.

Barter, P. et al., 'Lipid Management Guidelines—National Heart Foundation of Australia/The Cardiac Society of Australia and New Zealand', *The Medical Journal of Australia,* 175:Supplement, 2001.

Bellamy, M., 'Herbal cocktail a risky mix', *Australian Doctor,* August 31, 45, 2001.

Blair, S.N., 'Physical Fitness and All-Cause Mortality. A prospective Study of Healthy Men and Women', *Journal of the American Medical Association,* 262 (17):2395–2401, 1989.

Brand-Miller, J. and Foster-Powell, K., *The New Glucose Revolution*, Hodder, 1998.

Brown, M.A, et al., 'Is resistant hypertension really resistant', *American Journal of Hypertension,* 14:1263–69, 2001.

Colagiuri, S., 'Screening for Type 2 Diabetes', *Current Therapeutics Diabetes Supplement,* May 13, 28–31, 2001.

Cole, T.J. et al., 'Establishing a standard definition for child overweight and obesity worldwide: International survey', *British Medical Journal,* 320:1240–3, 2000.

Conlin, P., 'The Effect of Dietary Pattern on Blood Pressure Control in Hypertensive Patients; Results from the Dietary Approaches to Stop Hypertension (DASH) Trial', *American Journal of Hypertension,* 13(9):949–955, 2000.

Continence Foundation of Australia, *Pelvic Floor Exercises for Women*, Continence Foundation of Australia (Ph (02) 9840 4165).

Crespo, C.J., 'Television Watching, Energy Intake and Obesity in US Children; Results from the 3rd National Health and Nutrition Examination Survey, 1988–1994', *Archives of Paediatrics and Adolescent Medicine,* 155:360–65, 2001.

Egger, G., and Binns, A., *The experts' WEIGHT LOSS guide,* Allen & Unwin, Sydney, 2001.

Field, A.E., 'Impact of Overweight on the Risk of Developing Common Chronic Diseases During a 10-year Period', *Archives of Internal Medicine,* 161:1581–86, 2001.

FRIENDS, www.friendsinfo.net

Gerstein, H.C., 'Albuminaemia and risk of cardiovascular events, death and heart failure in diabetic and non-diabetic individuals', *Journal of the American Medical Association,* 286:421–26, 2001.

Gilbert, L., 'Infectious diseases in pregnancy', *Australian Doctor,* 'How to treat' section, March 2, 2001.

Gillman, M.W., 'Family Dinner and Diet Quality among Older Children and Adolescents,' *Archives of Family Medicine,* 9:235–40, 2000.

Glazier, M.G., 'A review of the evidence for the use of phytoestrogens as a replacement for traditional estrogen replacement therapy', *Archives of Internal Medicine*, 161:1161–72, 2001.

Grundy, S.M., 'Early Detection of High Cholesterol Levels in Young Adults', *Journal of the American Medical Association,* 284:365–67, 2000.

Heley, Stella, 'Is a pap smear enough?', *Australian Family Physcian,* 30(6):535–538, 2001.

Henschke, C.I., 'Early lung cancer action project: Initial findings on repeat screening', *Cancer,* 92;1:53–59, 2001.

Hernandez–Diaz, S., 'Folic acid antagonists during pregnancy and the risk of birth defects', *New England Journal of Medicine,* 343:1608–14, 2001.

Jorgensen, O.O., 'A randomized study of screening for colorectal cancer using faecal occult blood testing results after 13 years and seven biennial screening rounds', *Gut,* 50:29–32, 2002.

Joshi, P., 'Preventing childhood allergies', *Australian Doctor,* 'How to treat' section, June 21, 2002.

Kang, M. 'Substance abuse in teenagers', *Australian Family Physician,* 2002; 31:18–11.

Kausman, R.A., 'New Perspective to Long Term Weight Management', *Australian Family Physician,* 29(4):303–306, 2000.

Keks, N.A. and Burrows, G.D., *MJA Practice Essentials—Mental Health Australasian,* Medical Publishing Company, 1998.

Kimmel, S.E., 'Risk of acute first myocardial infarction and use of nicotine patches in a general population', *Journal of the American College of Cardiology,* 37:1297–302, 2001.

Kramer, K., 'Lifestyle change key in type 2 diabetes', *Australian Doctor,* October 19, 37, 2001.

Kron, J., 'Incontinence in the active', *Australian Doctor,* June 30, 67–69, 2000.

Kron, J., 'No pain plenty to gain', *Australian Doctor,* September 24, 64–65, 1999.

Lily, A.A., Myers, D.L., and Jackson, N.D., 'Dietary caffeine intake and the risk of detrusor instability: a case-controlled study', *Obstetrics and Gynaecology,* 96:85–89, 2000.

Loane, Mark, 'Primary open angle glaucoma', *Australian Doctor,* 'How to treat' section, August 18: 2000.

McGill, H.C., 'Association of Coronary Heart Disease Risk Factor with Microscopic Qualities of Coronary Atherosclerosis', *Circulation,* 102:374–79, 2000.

McKay, R., 'Diabetic Retinopathy in Victoria, Australia; the Visual Impairment Project', *British Journal of Opthalmology,* 84:865–70, 2000.

Manson, J.E. et al., 'A prospective study of walking as compared with vigorous exercise in the prevention of coronary artery disease in women', *New England Journal of Medicine,* 341:650–58, 1999.

Marks, Sharon, 'The role of orlistat in weight management', *Australian Family Physcian,* 30(4), 2001.

Morgan, J.F., Reid, F., and Lacey, C.F., 'The SCOFF questionnaire: assessment of a new screening tool for eating disorders', *British Medical Journal,* 319:1467–68, 1999.

Myers, J. et al., 'Exercise Capacity and Mortality among Men Referred for Exercise Testing', *New England Journal of Medicine,* 346(11):793–801, 2002.

Myrtek, M., 'Meta-analysis of prospective studies on coronary artery disease in type A personality and hostility', *International Journal of Cardiology,* 79:245–51, 2001.

National Ageing Research Group, *Falls can be a problem for healthy, active older people,* NARG (PO Box 31, Parkville, Vic. 3052), www.nari.unimelb.edu.au

National Ageing Research Group, *Tips to avoid falls,* NARG.

National Breast Cancer Centre (NBCC), *Advice about the familial aspects of breast cancer and ovarian cancer,* National Breast Cancer Centre, 2002.

National Heart Foundation, *1999 Guide to Management of Hypertension for Doctors,* NHF, 1999.

National Heart Foundation, *Salt and hypertension: a paper for health professionals,* NHF, n.d.

NHMRC, *Australian Alcohol Guidelines—Health Risks and Benefits,* National Health and Medical Research Council, Canberra, 2001, www.nhmrc.gov.au

Nicodemus, K.K., and Folsom, A.R., 'Type 1 and Type 2 Diabetes and Incident Hip Fractures in Postmenopausal Women', *Diabetes Care,* 24:1192–1203, 2001.

NSW Health, *Quit because you can.*

NSW Cancer Council, www.nswcc.org.au

Obarzanek, E. et al., 'Long term safety and efficacy of a lipid-lowering diet in children with elevated low density lipoprotein cholesterol: Seven year results of dietary intervention study in children (DISC)', *Paediatrics,* 107:256–264, 2001.

Osteoporosis Australia, www.osteoporosis.org.au

Parker, R., 'Making marriages last', *Family Matters—The Australian Institute of Family Studies,* 60:80–89, 2001.

Pasco, J.A., 'Calcium intake among Australian women: Geelong Osteoporosis Study', *Australian and New Zealand Journal of Medicine,* 30:21–27, 2000.

Pepys, M.B., and Berger, A., '"Normal" blood glucose and coronary risk', *British Medical Journal,* 322:5–6, 2001.

Potter, J.D. et al., 'Food, Nutrition and the Prevention of Cancer: A Global Perspective', a report produced jointly by the American Institute For Cancer Research and the World Cancer Research Fund, 1997, www.aicr.org/report2.htm

Quayle, S., 'Escaping the sun trap', *Australian Doctor*, 'How to treat' section, February 9, 2001.

Robertson, M., 'Interpersonal counselling', *Australian Doctor*, 'How to treat' section, April 26, 2002.

Rouse, R., 'Folate: For or against', *Medical Observer*, January 24, 29–30.

Royal Australian College of General Practitioners; National Preventive and Community Medicine Committee, 'Guidelines for preventative activities in general practice', *Australian Fam Physician*, 2002; 31(5).

Royal Australian College of General Practitioners, CHECK PROGRAM—HRT, September 1998.

Royal Australian College of General Practitioners, CHECK PROGRAM—Genetics, March 2001.

Relationships Australia, www.relationships.com.au/advice/how_improve.asp

Relationships Australia Incorporated, *State of Australian Relationships Survey—2001 Survey Summary*, Relationships Australia, 2001.

Renner, P., 'A Stitch in Time Prevention—Preventing Anxiety Disorders in Children and Adolescents', *The Clinician*, Department of Psychological Medicine at The New Children's Hospital at Westmead, Sydney, 1(1):37–44, 2001.

Rey, J.M., 'Depression amongst Australian adolescents', *Medical Journal of Australia*, 175:19–23, 2001.

Roberts, R. et al., 'Are the Obese at Greater Risk for Depression?', *American Journal of Epidemiology*, 152:163–70, 2000.

Saunders, C., 'Incontinence linked with hysterectomy', *Australian Doctor*, September 15, 21, 2000.

Saxalby, C., *Nutrition for life*, Hardie Grant Books, 1999.

Seed, M. et al., 'Lipoprotein (a) as a predictor of myocardial infarction in middle-aged men', *American Journal of Medicine*, 110:22–27, 2001.

Sharp, T.J., *The Good Sleep Guide*, Penguin Books Australia Ltd, 2001.

Stampfer, M., 'Primary Prevention of Coronary Heart Disease in Women Through Diet and Lifestyle', *New England Journal of Medicine*, 343:16–22, 2000.

Stanton, R., *Good fats, bad fats*, Allen & Unwin, Sydney, 1997.

Stanton, R., 'Bean there drank that', *Australian Doctor*, March 9, 57-58, 2001.

Stanton, R., *Healthy vegetarian eating*, Allen & Unwin, 1998.

Stanton, R., 'Encouragement to eat well should start young', *Australian Doctor*, August 9, 55–56, 2002.

Stevinson, C. et al., 'Garlic for hypercholestereolaemia: A meta-analysis of randomised clinical trials', *Annals of Internal Medicine*, 133:420–29, 2000.

Stricker, P., 'Prostate cancer. Part 1. Issues in screening and diagnosis', *Medicine Today*, 2(7):20–31, 2001.

Terry, P. et al., 'Fatty fish consumption and risk of prostate cancer', *Lancet*, 357:1764–66, 2001.

Thompson, J.R. et al., 'Maternal folate supplementation in pregnancy and protection against acute lymphoblastic leukaemia in children: a case control study', *Lancet*, 358:1935–40, 2001.

Tice, J.A. et al., 'Cost-effectiveness of Vitamin Therapy to Lower Plasma Homocysteine Levels for the Prevention of Coronary Heart Disease: Effect of Grain Modification and Beyond', *Journal of the American Medical Association*, 286:936–43, 2001.

Vaillant, George, *Ageing well*, Scribe Publications Pty Ltd, Melbourne, 2002.

Wahlqvist, M.L, *Food and Nutrition*, Allen & Unwin, 2002.

Wakefield, M. et al., 'Effects of restrictions on smoking at home, at school and in public places on teenage smoking: cross sectional study', *British Medical Journal*, 321:333–337, 2000.

Woodhead, M., 'Early rubella vax does not harm foetus', *Australian Doctor*, April 13, 2, 2001.

Woodhead, M., 'Antioxidants fail to reduce rate of heart disease', *Australian Doctor*, Nov 23, 1–2, 2001.

Zobias, Helen, 'Breast change: Early recognition is vital', *Australian Doctor*, April 14, 64–65, 2000.

Index

(continues)